THE TASK

AN IDEOLOGY OF CARE

THE TASKS
OF MEDICINE

AN IDEOLOGY OF CARE

Edited by

PETER BAUME

Professor, School of Community Medicine
The University of New South Wales
Sydney

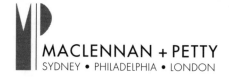

MACLENNAN + PETTY
SYDNEY • PHILADELPHIA • LONDON

First published 1998

MacLennan & Petty Pty Limited
ACN 003 458 973
809 Botany Road, Rosebery, Sydney NSW 2018, Australia

National Library of Australia
Cataloguing-in-Publication data:
The tasks of medicine: an ideology of care
Bibliography
Includes index
ISBN 0 86433 130 4

1. Social medicine. 2. Medical ethics. 3. Medical care.
1. Baume, Peter, 1935–
362.1

Printed and bound in Australia

CONTENTS

PART TWO: SOME UNDERPINNINGS

CONTRIBUTORS

Dorothy Angell, Professor and Head of the Caroline Chisholm School of Nursing, Monash University 1989–96, Dean of the School of Nursing, Chisholm Institute of Technology 1986–88, a trained nurse and registered midwife. She has 21 years experience in tertiary level nurse education.

Peter Baume, Professor of Community Medicine at the University of New South Wales, Chancellor of the Australian National University, Commissioner of the Australian Law Reform Commission 1993–97, Chair of the Australian Sports Drug Agency, Senator for New South Wales 1974–91, Government Whip, Minister for Aboriginal Affairs, Minister for Health, Minister for Education, Officer of the Order of Australia.

Peter Brooks, Professor of Medicine, St. Vincent's Hospital, Sydney, and Head of the Department of Medicine since 1991, Foundation Florance and Cope Professor of Rheumatology, University of Sydney 1983–91, Honorary Secretary of the Royal Australasian College of Physicians 1990–95, the author of a number of medical textbooks and many articles.

Eric Cassell is a practising internist in New York City and an attending physician at the New York Hospital. He is a Fellow of the Hastings Center, a member of the Institute of Medicine of the National Academy of Sciences and a Master of the American College of Physicians. He has written a number of medical books, most recently *The Nature of Suffering* (1991) and *Doctoring: The Nature of Primary Care Medicine* (1997).

Max Charlesworth, Emeritus Professor, formerly Professor of Philosophy and Dean of the School of Humanities, Deakin University, a member of the Monash Centre for Human Bioethics and co-founder of the Australian Bioethics Association, former member of the Victorian Standing Review and Advisory Committee on Infertility, the National Health and Medical Research Council, the National Bioethics Consultative Committee and the Australian Health Ethics Committee. He is an Officer of the Order of Australia. He has published extensively, for example, *Life, Death, Genes and Ethics* (the Boyer Lectures for 1989) and *Bioethics in a Liberal Society*.

John Ellard, Chairman of the Ellard Practice in Sydney and Editor of *Modern Medicine (Aust)* is the author of several books—*Psychiatry for the Non Psychiatrist* (1977), *Some Rules for Killing People* (1989), *The Anatomy of Mirages* (1994)—and has also published more than 100 papers in learned journals. He is a Member of the Order of Australia and holds the Reserve Forces Decoration.

Malcolm Fisher is Head of the Intensive Therapy Unit of the Royal North Shore Hospital of Sydney and a Clinical Professor in the Departments of Medicine and Anaesthesia, University of Sydney. He is currently President of the World Federation of Societies of Intensive and Critical Care Medicine and has received a number of international awards for his work in this area. He is the author of three books and 130 scientific articles and writes a weekly medical column that appears in three countries.

Richard Larkins, James Stewart Professor of Medicine and Head of the Department of Medicine at the Royal Melbourne Hospital, Dean of the Faculty of Medicine, Dentistry and Health Sciences, University of Melbourne, Chair of the National Health and Medical Research Council in Australia, Vice-President of the Royal Australasian College of Physicians, past President of the Endocrine Society of Australia and past Chairman of the Board of Censors of the Royal Australasian College of Physicians. He has written four textbooks and many scientific papers.

Stephen Leeder, Professor of Public Health and Community Medicine at the University of Sydney based at Westmead Hospital since 1986, Foundation Professor of Community Medicine, University of Newcastle 1976–85, Better Health Commissioner 1985–88, Dean of the Faculty of Medicine, University of Sydney and National President of the Public Health Association of Australia 1995–7.

David Leon is Senior Lecturer in Epidemiology at the London School of Hygiene and Tropical Medicine. He is co-director of the European Centre on the Health of Societies in Transition.

(John) Miles Little is Emeritus Professor of Surgery, University of Sydney. He was Foundation Professor of Surgery, University of Sydney, at Westmead Hospital 1977–96, co-founder of the World Association of Hepatic, Pancreatic and Biliary Surgeons 1987 and first President 1987–89, Founding Director, Centre for Values, Ethics and the Law in Medicine, Department of Surgery, University of Sydney 1995–. He has published several text books, including *Humane Medicine* (1995) on the philosophy of medicine and *Round Trip* (1977) which is a volume of poetry. He is a Member of the Order of Australia.

Robert Maxwell, Secretary and Chief Executive of the Kings Fund London since 1980, PhD, McKinsey and Company 1966–75, Administrator St Thomas' Hospital Special Trustees 1975–80. He has published several books and many papers and has several honorary Fellowships and honorary degrees.

Anthony (Tony) McMichael is Professor of Epidemiology at the London School of Hygiene and Tropical Medicine. Previously he was Professor of Occupational and Environmental Health at the University of Adelaide. He chaired the Scientific Council of the International Agency for Research on Cancer (WHO) from 1990 to 1992. During 1994–96 he chaired the scientific review of the potential effects of climate change for the UN's Intergovernmental Panel on Climate Change.

Paul McNeill is an Associate Professor in the School of Community Medicine, University of New South Wales, where he teaches law and ethics to medical students. He has degrees in law, psychology and the history and philosophy of science. He serves on the Professional Standards Committee and on the Medical Tribunal of New South Wales. He is author of a book *The Ethics and Politics of Human Experimentation.*

Jeff (Jeffrey Ralph James) Richardson is Professor in the Deparment of Economics, Monash University and Director of the National Centre for Health Program Evaluation since 1994 (co-Director 1990–93). He has held posts in several universities and has authored many articles and several books.

Deborah Saltman is Professor and Head of the General Practice Professorial Unit at Manly Hospital, Sydney. She has held academic positions at the University of New South Wales, the Australian National University and the University of Queensland. She is a Fellow, a former Councillor and former Treasurer of the Royal Australian College of General Practitioners. She is the author of several books and of many articles. She was Chairperson of the Board of the New South Wales Cancer Council 1996–97.

Chris Silagy is Professor and Head of the Department of Evidence-Based Care and General Practice, Flinders University, South Australia. He is the Director of the Australasian Cochrane Centre and holds positions with the Royal Australian College of General Practitioners and the National Health and Medical Research Council.

Ian Webster, Professor of Public Health of the University of New South Wales and Director of the Division of Population Health of the South Western Sydney Area Health Service, Chairman of the Faculty of Medicine of the University of New South Wales 1984–96, Clinical Dean of the South Western Sydney Clinical School and a member of the Board of the South Western Sydney Area Health Service, President of the Alcohol and other Drugs Council of Australia, President of the NSW Association for Mental Health and Honorary Visiting Physician to the Matthew Talbot Hostel for the homeless in inner Sydney. He was the Foundation Professor of Community Medicine at the University of New South Wales. He is an Officer of the Order of Australia. He has published extensively.

Judith Whitworth is Professor of Medicine and Head of the Department of Medicine at St. George Hospital in Sydney in the University of New South Wales. She is a nephrologist and has been an NHMRC Scholar and President of the Australian Society for Medical Research. In 1997 she was appointed Chief Medical Officer of the Commonwealth of Australia. She has published three textbooks and many papers. She was Chair of the Medical Research Committee of the National Health and Medical Research Council 1994–97.

John Yu has been Chief Executive of the Royal Alexandra Hospital for Children since 1978; before that he was Head of that hospital's Department of Medicine. He has served on the Council of the Royal Australasian College of Physicians, the Paediatric Research Society and the Australian College of Paediatrics. From 1990–95 he was President of the Australian Association of Paediatric Teaching Centres. He sits on the National Australia Day Council and the National Starlight Foundation Board. He was on the Board of Trustees for the Powerhouse Museum from 1993–96 and is an Honorary Associate of the museum. He is a Trustee of the Art Gallery of NSW and has published extensively on paediatrics, management issues and the decorative arts. On Australia Day 1996, he was named Australian of the Year and is a Member of the Order of Australia.

INTRODUCTION

Recently, in a class for advanced students, an experienced counsellor was making her obligatory oral presentation. She chose to recount how her medically qualified father had suffered a stroke which left him aphasic but able to hear and understand. The specialists attending him had come to the room and spoken to her—not to him. They had set out clearly the diagnosis and the poor prognosis to her in front of her father. At this point the student wept and continued to weep during the rest of her presentation. At the end I asked her how much she recalled about the diagnosis, taxonomy and outlook of stroke. 'Very little,' she replied. 'I am not medically qualified.' Then I asked her what she remembered about the conversation with the specialists. 'Every word,' she replied.

This story encapsulates many problems of modern medicine discussed in this book. The action by the specialists, while well intentioned, was cruel, inappropriate and improper. While it was necessary to have a scientific understanding of her father's condition and while the specialists' knowledge was probably excellent, it was not sufficient on its own to serve the needs of that patient or his daughter at that time. That scientific understanding has progressed during this century but seems not to have been matched by any advance in human capacities or sensitivity.

Medical science *has* made great strides in the twentieth century. No attempt is made to minimise or ignore those advances in this book. Indeed, experts have set out how clinical medicine and its associated sciences have advanced our knowledge and have been of benefit to us.

More is known today about human structure and function than ever before. New useful information emerges with each issue of every peer-reviewed journal.

People with disease today have more chance of finding relief and cure than ever before. And this tide of advance continues, with more and more understanding of more and more diseases, and with more and more treatments available for more and more conditions. There is no reason to suppose that the development of new and helpful knowledge will slow or halt. The Internet offers new possibilities for rapid transfer of information to providers and users of medicine and there is upon us a revolutionary 'information age' in medicine based on the Internet and on information technology. In this book one chapter (Chapter Ten) is devoted to the case for interest-driven research which has given us so much in the twentieth century and which forms the basis of the national research effort.

Yet all is not well in medicine today. Many practitioners have lost their idealism. Patients, once grateful, are unhappy with us and with what we offer.[1] Hospitals, once places in which it was good to work, generally have lost their purpose and their way, concentrating more and more on disease and less and less on people. They are dirty and run down, dispirited and uncertain about the future. The medical profession is demoralised and confused and many practitioners are looking wistfully at the mid-twentieth century, rather than forward to the twenty-first century. The associated helping professions seem to be interested as much in power accretion as they are in the welfare of patients. Alternative medical modalities continue to multiply in type and increase in popularity. Governments continue to pursue public cost reductions (including in hospital and medical services) without presenting clearly to the public the negative and inevitable collateral detriment of achieving money savings.

We have not achieved a sensible, transparent or acceptable way of rationing services—a phenomenon whereby some people miss out on care that is available somewhere for their condition (or receive care only after a delay) and, sooner or later, there are shifts in power[2] associated with all rationing. The public is still fed a diet of 'breakthroughs', and of the wonders of a science that is probably not cost-effective, by the media (aided and abetted by a naive or cynical research establishment) which seems to have a poor appreciation of its responsibility to advise and inform the public accurately of costs as well as of benefits.[3] The polity is shielded from knowledge of the constraints with which hospitals and practitioners work each day and has a romantic and unrealistic view of medical practice and of the capacities of medicine. Many participants in the sector continue to fight for their own narrow interests irrespective of the effects any action has on the whole.

A majority of practitioners is advising its own children not to undertake a career in medicine, and many young people, seeing these parents and authority figures unhappy, are devoting their lives to other professions.

It is a time of despair. Yet it is also a time of challenge and of hope. We are entering an information century which most practitioners still do not understand. Medical research continues apace. We may yet emerge into a new balance between the parts of medicine, into a new comprehension of the needs of society, and into new cooperative organisations of the parts of the healing professions.

To do this we need to identify those tasks which have as their focus the people we serve. We need to be sure of what the challenges are that we seek to meet, to know our own goals, to know our limitations and to know what the outcomes are that we wish to achieve. We are aware that Kerr White produced a book entitled *The Task of Medicine*[4] but both the messages and the derivation of contributions to this book are different from that earlier work. We are aware also that the Hastings Center has produced a recent report on the goals of medicine[5]—but again our insights are sufficiently different to warrant a separate report.

It is timely to look at the tasks facing medicine now. This book has been written to examine that question—what are our challenges today? Some outstanding colleagues have contributed their disparate thoughts on various aspects of a whole that presents both the triumphs and the shortcomings of modern bioscience and sets a context for medicine in the twenty-first century. No contributor has seen the writings of any other. So, if there are repetitions, this is a result of the way the collection has been constructed by the editor. Similarly, some authors disagree with one another in areas where there are several legitimate world views or where values differ—but this reflects the real world of the caring professions from which the authors come.

Each author has written on a single topic. Left to themselves, many would have chosen different subjects, and it would be wrong to attribute to any one author a narrowness of vision or view on the basis of what each has contributed. Good doctoring has always required an appreciation of the needs of people as well as an appreciation of the diseases they have. The group of authors that has written this book is aware of the needs in both areas; if some have written about the triumphs of modern biomedicine it is because those triumphs are real and because they have been asked to set them out. It is not correct to assume that those people have any of the narrowness of view which is criticised throughout the book. The achievements of modern medicine deserve proper contextual placement and proper recognition such as has been provided by our distinguished contributors.

The eminence of the group that has produced this work is testament to its belief that the work is timely and worth the involvement of each author. The writing is appropriate, balanced and relevant. To each author goes thanks and good wishes.

Thanks also from the editor to Jenny Curtis of MacLennan and Petty for continuing support and help throughout the project, to my wife Jenny who has read and criticised drafts, and to Peter Sinclair for help with many tasks. Valuable information was provided to Professor Judith Whitworth by Associate Professor David de Carle, Professor John Cade, Dr John Donovan and the National Health and Medical Research Council Secretariat, while Mrs. Marjorie McGrath provided valuable secretarial assistance to her. Associate-Professor Paul McNeill is grateful to Dr Peter Saul of the John Hunter Hospital and the University of Newcastle for his generous and helpful comments on early drafts of his chapter. Professor Jeff Richardson would like to thank Professor Dick Scotton, Leonie Segal and Richard Smith for comments on an earlier draft of his chapter.

PETER BAUME

Sydney 1997

REFERENCES

1. Stewart M, Weston WW. *Patient centered medicine.* Thousand Oaks, California: Sage Publications, 1995, pxv.
2. E.g., see Editorial. Multiple sclerosis drug prompts rationing fears. *Brit Med J* 1995; 311: 969.
3. Brody H. *The healer's power.* New Haven: Yale University Press, 1992, p6.
4. White KL. *The task of medicine: dialogue at Wickenburg.* Menlo Park, California: Kaiser Family Foundation, 1988.
5. The Hastings Center. *The goals of medicine: setting new priorities.* Hastings Center Report, 1996, 26 (6).

NOTE

PEOPLE, HEALING AND MEDICINE

CHAPTER ONE

Caring for the Sick

PETER BROOKS

C aring for someone who is sick is one of the greatest responsibilities that can be given to an individual. The tasks involved
are extraordinarily complex and, in Western society, are given
primarily to a doctor. Despite the continuing devaluation of the medical profession and the move across the world to embrace alternative
forms of therapy, it is likely that this medical approach will continue
well into the next century. Society's attitude towards each of the professions and towards the medical profession in particular has changed
enormously over the years and will continue to change. The medical
profession must be able to move with the times and if it is to survive
it must provide society with what it needs, or what it perceives it
needs, in terms of health.

In 1984 the Association of American Medical Colleges presented a
report *Physicians for the 21st Century*[6] which addressed the educational
requirements necessary to provide properly trained physicians for the
new millenium. This report provides an excellent review of the directions for medical education as we move towards the end of this millenium and, although it is over 10 years old, it still forms an excellent basis
on which to plan educational training for doctors in the next century.
Steven Muller points out in the introduction:

> Each patient expects the physician to respond to the patient's personal
> concerns and problems on the basis of professional knowledge.[7]

Patients expect that doctors will have a basic knowledge of diseases and
their treatments, but the doctor needs to know much more than that.
Doctors increasingly need to demonstrate that they have developed a
level of skill in a variety of practical tasks and to have an appropriate
set of values and attitudes.

What is being ill?

Illness is defined as an unhealthy condition of the body. The symptoms
that a patient experiences are a consequence of that disease which

may have a pathological and/or psychological basis. We all know that patients react very differently to a similar disease process and in fact the reasons why a person with symptoms (e.g., pain) becomes a patient (with pain) are complex. Presentation to the doctor, which converts the person with a symptom to a patient, is determined by many factors including the severity of the symptoms, the person's inherent beliefs, their educational and social status and previous experiences.

This must be particularly so with the so-called diseases of modern times—stress-related diseases which may present with pain, generalised fatigue, and a host of symptoms which have little, if any, physical basis. These conditions which are increasing rapidly in the community will pose a particular challenge to the physicians of the twenty-first century. To this has to be added the issue of compensation, either through workers' compensation insurance or through other legal channels.

Being ill has an enormous number of consequences. Apart from the physical symptoms of pain, loss of function of a body part or mental deterioration, there is frustration at loss of independence and autonomy. To this needs to be added loss of control of finances, inability to perform in one's job or even normal tasks of daily living, together with enormous emotional stresses which reflect both on the physical symptoms themselves and on a person's reactions to those symptoms.

Many of the diseases of modern times are chronic diseases, particularly in elderly persons. These chronic diseases have their added problems of fatigue due sometimes to a true physical weakness or having to deal with chronic symptoms such as pain. The frustration of never knowing what sort of day (in terms of symptoms) a person is going to have adds to an individual's problems. This is exemplified extremely well by the disease rheumatoid arthritis—a chronic rheumatic disease with recurrent exacerbations and remissions, where a patient's major frustration can be the uncertainty of waking each day and not knowing whether he/she is going to have a flare of his/her disease or be in relative remission.[8]

Those who care for the sick need to understand the close interactions between the mind and the body which have not changed since the observations of Plato (427–347BC):

> This is the great error of our day in the treatment of the human body, that the physicians separate the soul from the body.[9]

The inter-relationships between emotions and illness are very powerful and must be considered by all doctors once acute resuscitation and stabilisation of a patient has been attained. Interaction of emotions and disease is very well covered by Hislop[10] in an excellent monograph drawing on a series of patients over a long period of time and demonstrating

Figure 1.1 Influence of emotions on illness

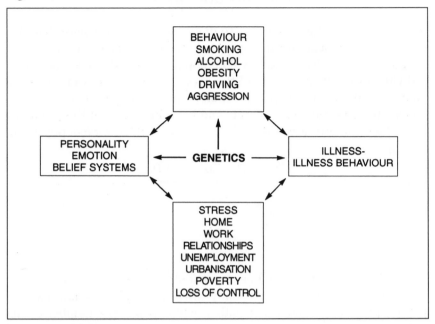

Adapted from Hislop[10]

how underlying attitudes, education, personality and emotions can influence the development and maintenance of ill-health. Doctors need to have a close appreciation of a person's underlying attitudes and personality so that an appropriate evaluation of the role of these factors on the illness can be made. Interactions of these factors are shown in Figure 1.1. These four major areas can all interact with each other. Behavioural issues such as smoking and alcohol may be a product of, and also play a role in determining, personality and emotions which are linked closely to stress at home or at work and to that underlying feeling of loss of control of one's destiny. The major smoking-related diseases, such as lung cancer, chronic lung disease, peripheral vascular disease and heart disease, are also associated with stress, as are peptic ulceration and many other diseases. Interestingly, the influence of genetics on behaviour, on illness and on personality, may be stronger than we think and it is certainly a fruitful area for research.

The issue of illness behaviour is a particularly relevant one in chronic disease where particular coping strategies are developed to a greater or lesser degree. In some situations the response to symptoms is unusual and the term 'abnormal illness behaviour' is adopted to define a specific group of individuals where response to usually mild situations is exaggerated.[11]

What do doctors do?

The task of a doctor is not only to diagnose and treat disease but also to act as an advocate for the patient. A doctor needs to have a foundation of basic knowledge, skills, values and attitudes, which will vary from individual to individual. One of the problems for doctors in a modern society with increasing specialisation is the perception that many specialists have become technocrats and have lost some of those important values and attitudes that are necessary for the *compleat* physician.

Table 1.1 The Tasks of a Doctor

• Diagnosis
• Investigation
• Treatment
• Education
• Support.

The diagnostic challenge in any particular patient should still be the theme driving doctors in their daily work. The ability to diagnose the problem affecting a particular patient will depend on a number of factors, but most importantly will depend on taking a careful history and performing a full physical examination. Doctors and patients seem to have forgotten that the most important investigation that needs to be performed is the history and examination. The history should not just focus on the symptoms of which the patient is complaining but also on a family and social history, past events and a number of other factors which might have either caused the disease or at least influenced its manifestation. Illness behaviour is becoming an increasing issue in medicine and, in many situations, chronic pain or chronic fatigue may be a manifestation of abnormal reactions to what in essence may be a simple and reversible symptom.[12]

The art of good history taking is being able to develop a rapport with the patient such that they will trust the health professional with information that is sometimes of a very personal nature. The development of this personal relationship and trust between doctor and patient is at the very basis of a good doctor-patient relationship and requires a degree of trust on both sides. The good doctor will also be able to pick up a lot of non-verbal cues which may help significantly in diagnosis and management. These include facial expressions, eye contact, voice tone, posture and gestures made by the patient.

Having taken the history and completed a physical examination, a differential diagnosis usually has been made. This comprises a list of the most likely conditions the patient may have. The doctor may then order a series of investigations to confirm or refute the diagnosis. These may include blood tests, imaging procedures such as radiology, ultrasound or a range of nuclear medicine procedures. Many of these are relatively expensive and some are invasive and the doctor should now take into account the cost/benefit of these procedures. Investigations in clinical practice have been driven to a certain extent (at least in the developed world) by a medico-legal imperative. This is particularly so in the United States of America but other parts of the world are now catching up rapidly. Decisions as to the appropriateness of investigations should be driven by clinical parameters based on a cost/benefit and risk assessment and should be discussed with the patient. Doctors should always ask themselves whether a particular investigation is going to alter diagnosis or alter management. If it is not, then perhaps it is better not to do the test and therefore to save the patient a risk, be it physical or financial. To this end the doctor needs to understand issues such as relative risk and positive and negative predictive value, as well as some economic issues involved.

It has been said that the most expensive piece of equipment a doctor has is a pen because it is with this that untold dollars are spent on investigations and medication. Appreciating the benefit of a particular test is very important to the optimal practice of medicine.

At this stage the diagnostic options can be discussed with the patient. This has to be done in a dispassionate fashion, but with integrity and openness, and again will depend on developing that trusting relationship with the patient. Other members of the family may also be involved at this stage.

Patient communication is a science in itself which has only recently had the time in the medical curriculum that it really deserves. Patients will not remember more than three or four concepts from an interview (and in this they are not different from any other group when they are being appraised of a new situation) and repeated interviews may need to be carried out. Provision of written material on a particular condition may be very useful in reinforcing certain concepts about a disease and its treatment. This is particularly so with the more chronic diseases. Doctors should be very careful in the terms that they use to describe disease. For example the term: 'you have a ruptured disc' to explain the cause of a person's back pain is probably not terribly helpful. Firstly, acute back pain is less commonly caused by a ruptured disc than by other things, but secondly, the patient imagines the discal material splattered over the inside of their spinal column and is, not surprisingly, very concerned about the issue.

In many situations an exact diagnosis may not be possible to make, at least on the initial consultation. This should be discussed with the patient and the concept that diseases sometimes have to evolve over a period of time accepted by both parties. This may require repeat clinical review and investigations of the patient. Many patients feel frustrated if an exact diagnosis cannot be made immediately, but this is usually because the uncertainty of the clinical situation has not been communicated to the patient in an appropriate manner. Denial may also be used by patients at this time, particularly when faced with diagnoses such as cancer which bring with them a whole range of fears about the future.

Educational role

Even at this early stage in the doctor-patient relationship, the doctor is assuming the role of an educator. Doctors must be able to inform the patient and the patient's family about the disease, about its prognosis and about the various management issues that will need to be embarked upon. At this stage the doctor also needs to appreciate the effect that the disease might have on the individual and the family in terms of the disruption of their lives. Patients are usually not frightened about facing the future but they do want some idea of what it holds. The doctor may provide the patient with educational material or put them in touch with one of the increasing number of patient organisations that deal particularly with the chronic diseases such as arthritis, diabetes, cancer, heart disease, blindness and deafness. Again, at an early stage in these chronic diseases, patients often go through a phase of denial and want to try to handle things on their own. They should probably be encouraged to participate in these patient organisations as they do provide an extraordinarily powerful network of individuals with these diseases and provide information which is related very much to maintaining the *locus of control* within the patient.

Management issues are also an important area where education needs to be carried out by the physician. Gone are the days when patients will blindly accept a physician's prescription for a drug or for an operation. Patients have a right to know the various treatment options available and their relative risks. Increasingly we are seeing that patient preferences need to be incorporated into medical decision making.[13] There are many situations described where patient perceptions are different from those of the doctor but those patient perceptions and views must be respected. This is referred to by Kassirer in commenting on a study by O'Meara et al[14] discussing a decision analysis of choice between heparin alone and streptokinase plus heparin in the treatment of deep venous thrombosis. Despite the results of a consensus panel suggesting that combination therapy with streptokinase and heparin was the treatment of choice for this condition, patient preference was clearly for heparin alone with patients being unwilling to accept the small risk of intracranial haemorrhage and death (associated with streptokinase plus heparin) to avoid the consequences of a chronically swollen and painful leg (associated with heparin alone).

The development of guidelines for good clinical practice and the move around the world to use evidence-based decisions where available will certainly help to provide doctors and patients with better information on which to base their choices. However, patient preferences will still need to be taken into account, particularly in the areas outlined by Kassirer:[13]

- Where there are major differences in the kinds of possible outcomes (death versus disability).
- When there are major differences between treatment in the likelihood and impact of complications.
- When choices involve trade-offs between near-term and long-term outcomes.
- When one of the choices can result in a very small chance of a serious outcome.
- When apparent differences between options are marginal.
- When a patient is particularly averse to taking risks.
- When a patient attaches unusual importance to certain possible outcomes.

These issues are sometimes made more difficult and frustrating for a doctor, who may be able to appreciate more clearly than the patient a relatively long-term positive effect on a disease outcome versus short-term risk of a side-effect. This is particularly so, for example, in treating rheumatoid arthritis with disease modifying drugs where there is good evidence of long-term benefit but also a risk (albeit minor) of an immediate adverse reaction to the drug.

How do doctors care?

Health care by doctors is delivered in a number of different ways. The majority of health care is usually delivered by one to one interaction in a consulting room where a patient shares his/her problems with a practitioner. Within hospitals care is provided by a team of individuals comprising nurses, junior medical staff, specialists and allied health professionals. Increasingly, medical students are considered part of the 'caring team'. Different groups of doctors will develop different types of relationships with their patients depending on the chronicity of the disease and often the type of disease. Psychiatrists, for example, may develop a very close relationship with the patient with a certain amount of dependency emerging from the relationship. Surgeons, on the other hand, will often have a relatively short-lived relationship with a patient before and during their operation until the patient has recovered. Physicians dealing with chronic disease will again develop longstanding relationships with patients, guiding them through exacerbations and remissions of their disease over many years. Increasingly, doctors are becoming involved in providing services for patients in the form of investigations—this is particularly so with endoscopy of the gastrointestinal tract. General practitioners may refer patients for a procedure to be carried out by a specialist physician rather than having the specialist actually take the history and provide an overall picture of the problem.

One of the big challenges for the profession is the care of the dying patient. This debate has been invigorated recently around the world by the issue of voluntary euthanasia. Appropriate care of the dying depends very much on symptom control and on guiding the patient and the patient's family through those last few weeks of life. More and more emphasis is being placed on keeping dying patients at home and offering support to them and their families so the death can take place in an environment that is familiar.

In the Australian context the big difference in the delivery of care rests between those general practitioners working in primary care and those doctors who work as specialists in a hospital or consulting rooms. In Australia, patients have to be seen initially by a general practitioner who then determines if a specialist consultation is required and who might be most helpful. Many consultations with specialists are generated by the patient and this must make things rather frustrating for the general practitioner. Patients should not necessarily feel bad about asking for a consultation with a specialist or for requesting a second opinion. This is certainly a right that the patient has and should be exercised by them if they wish. One might say that the good doctor is one who suggests a referral for a second opinion just before the patient asks for one. In this way the doctor often maintains the patient's confidence and helps to dampen any conflict that the patient has in requesting a second opinion. Referral to a specialist may be for diagnosis or treatment or perhaps to perform a particular investigation. There is a responsibility for the specialist to communicate with the referring doctor, providing his/her opinion on the patient and to return the patient to the general practitioner for follow-up. Ongoing review by the specialist may be justified in chronic disease where monitoring of the disease and treatment is important, but again the development of a shared care model is the most appropriate.[15]

How can we do better?

Doctors of the future will need to continue to hold the trust of their patients and will probably have to work harder to do it. Competition between doctors at all levels is increasingly driven by things such as 24-hour medical clinics which provide so-called one stop 'services'. The so-called advantages of the 24-hour medical service are that it is open at any time and in particular at weekends—useful for patients who work during the week. Other facilities are also provided such as pathology, radiology and often a range of specialists. Problems with this type of service are significant however. Firstly, the staff are on roster and continuity of patient care is less likely to occur. This will be particularly important if psychosocial factors are relevant to the disease process where building up a relationship with the patient and learning about the issues of stress within the home and the workplace are very important to appropriate diagnosis and management. There may also be a tendency to over-investigate because of the ready availability of pathology and imaging services.

Doctors of the future may also need to re-look at simple things such as appearance. Hippocrates for example stated that the physician should be 'clean in person, well dressed and anointed with sweet smelling unguents'.[16] There is little doubt that the standard of dress for young physicians in hospitals has changed dramatically over the years. Interestingly, a number of studies[17,18] have shown clearly that physician appearance is very important in provoking positive responses. The physician of the future should perhaps return to wearing a white coat and a tie.

Economic imperatives are likely to encourage third party payers to use primary care physicians in preference to specialists. This not only has economic advantages but may, in the long term, provide better care for patients. A number of principles of good outpatient shared care have been enunciated—these include:[13]

- Geographical and practice needs for a local clinic.
- A service sensitive to local needs.
- Referral criteria.
- Financial payment to secondary care providers.
- Clinical responsibility with the general practitioner.
- The patient remains in the community.
- Adequate resources.

- Specialist-GP equality.
- Consultations by the consultant.
- Good organisation with planning, definition of roles, protocols, and audit.

This model has been implemented in a number of specialties including psychiatry, obstetrics, cardiology, orthopaedics, ophthalmology and a number of others. Geriatrics is also an area where patient care has shifted away from hospitals. The shared care model depends on the development of agreed protocols and clinical guidelines between the general practitioner and the specialist. In the future it may be important to include the third major player in health care (the patient) in developing these protocols and clinical guidelines. Shared care models will also see the development of the nurse practitioner who will have a designated area of expertise and be able to assist and form a liaison between general practitioners, specialists and patients, particularly in rural areas. This model needs to be expanded and is probably more logical than trying to put a general practitioner in every small town in Australia.

Patients need to be encouraged to seek second opinions, particularly when there is going to be a radical change in therapy or perhaps an operation. Patients need to be encouraged to ask their treating doctors about the doctor's experience and his or her outcome data so that an informed decision regarding treatment can be made.

The push towards evidence-based medicine with the development of good data bases needs to be encouraged. Doctors should be aware of the outcome data of various treatments and need to be able to discuss these with patients. An increasing amount of this data is finding its way into the public domain through such means as the Internet, and doctors should be aware of this in an effort to remain at least one step ahead of their patients on the information super highway.

REFERENCES

6. Association of American Medical Colleges. Physicians for the twenty-first century—report of the project panel on the general professional education of the physician and college preparation for medicine. *J Medical Education* 1984; 59 (part 2): 1–208.
7. Muller S. Introduction. *J Medical Education* 1984; 59 (part 2): 1–3.
8. Anonymous. On living with rheumatoid arthritis. *Med J Aust* 1991; 155: 268–9.
9. Daintith J, Isaacs A. *Medical quotations.* London: Collins, 1989, p90.
10. Hislop I. *Stress, Distress and illness.* New York: McGraw Hill, 1991.
11. Pilowsky I. Abnormal illness behaviour (dysnosognosia). *Psychother Psychosom* 1986; 46: 131–7.
12. Block SR. Fibromyalgia and rheumatisms: common sense and sensibility. *Rheum Dis Clinics of North America* 1993; 19: 61–78.

13. Kassirer JP. Incorporating patients' preferences into medical decisions. *New Engl J Med* 1994; 330: 1895–6.
14. O'Meara JJ, McNutt RA, Evans AT, Moore SW, Downs SM. A decision analysis of streptokinase plus heparin as compared with heparin alone for deep vein thrombosis. *New Engl J Med* 1994; 330: 1804–9.
15. Orton P. Shared care. *Lancet* 1994; 344: 1413–15.
16. Strauss MB (ed). *Familiar medical quotations*. Boston: Little Brown and Company, 1968, p399; also Jones WHS (trans). *Hippocrates*. Cambridge, Mass: Harvard University Press, 1923, vol 2, pp311–12.
17. Gjerdingen DK, Simpson DE, Titus SL. Patients and physicians attitudes regarding the physician's professional appearance. *Arch Int Med* 1987; 147: 1209–12.
18. Taylor PC. Does the way the house staff physicians dress influence the way parents initially perceive their competence? Paediatric notes, 1985, 9: 1.

CHAPTER TWO

Caring for the Well

CHRIS SILAGY

Introduction—the need for strategies to care for the well

In many respects the task of promoting health and preventing disease is a more complex challenge than caring for the ill. The Ottawa Charter for Health Promotion emphasises that effective health promotion requires the following: development of personal skills; the creation of environments which support health; the refocussing of health and related services; the engagement of the community; and the development of healthy public policy[19] (see Fig 2.2). In order to fulfil the Charter, a broad based multi-sectoral approach is usually required. This can encompass strategies which are targeted community-wide (such as use of the media or legislation), as well as strategies targeted at subsets of the community (through specific health promotion programs and campaigns) and/or strategies targeted at individuals (particularly those at high risk of disease).[20] Despite the commitment and effort of many individual members of the medical profession, there has been substantial controversy and debate about how the medical profession can best make its contribution to caring for the well.

There is a strong argument in favour of the medical profession actively contributing to public debate about a range of social and welfare issues which impact directly or indirectly on the protection and promotion of health within the community. Within the last few years the profession, through its various representative and professional bodies, has been active in areas such as tobacco control, gun control, anti-violence, drug use, mental health initiatives, improved social and welfare conditions for indigenous people, and environmental protection issues. At a global level, groups such as the Physicians against Nuclear War have had a major impact on promoting appropriate international agreements and legislation safeguards against one of the world's major health threats.[21]

Furthermore, as a result of the high standing which the medical profession continues to enjoy within much of the community, there is an added social responsibility for its members to act as living role models in many of the areas referred to above. For example, smoking rates amongst physicians are generally well below that of the general population, and have been continuing to decline over the past few decades.[22] It is through personal example such as this that powerful role models can be provided to the community, and few would doubt its importance or value. What has been questioned, is the role that medical practitioners should play, if any, in terms of promoting health in their dealings with individual patients, their families and their local communities.[21]

If one considers a theoretical population of 1000 individuals, it has been estimated that 30 per cent will be acutely 'ill' at some stage during the year and will require the support of acute health care services. A further 10 per cent are chronically 'ill' and have multiple on-going requirements for health care services. This leaves 60 per cent of the population who remain healthy and have limited need for health care services.[23] Set against this, approximately 80 per cent of the adult population consult their general practitioner at least once each year.[24]

It is clear that much of the workload for general practitioners involves caring for the well.

Accurately quantifying the amount of caring for the well that is provided by medical practitioners is methodologically difficult. Survey estimates of physicians' self-reported involvement in preventive activities indicate a large amount of variability in rates of preventive activity.[25] For example, between 66 per cent and 98 per cent of physicians report asking all their patients about smoking compared with between 51 per cent and 94 per cent who report asking all their patients about alcohol consumption.[26] Similar analyses of patient surveys and chart audits suggest that the physicians' self-reports are a gross overestimate of what is recalled by the patient or recorded in the notes. In many key areas, such as smoking, alcohol consumption, immunisation, and cervical screening, the rate of providing preventive activity is well below the national authorities' recommendations.

In this chapter a framework of the medical profession's approach to caring for the well is described. Barriers and difficulties in implementing such an approach are discussed, as well as some of the potential strategies for overcoming these. Finally, the case will be argued for stronger and more effective partnerships between the medical profession and a range of professional groups across the health and welfare sectors to ensure the task of caring for the well is to become a community responsibility integrated within a broader public health strategy.

Figure 2.1 What does the health system do?

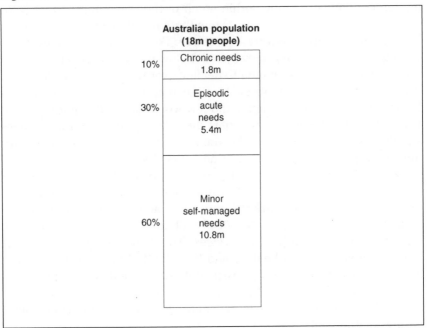

Adapted from Paterson J, National Health Care Reform. The Last Pictureshow, Department of Human Services, Government of Victoria, April 1996.

Distinguishing between wellness and illness

In many instances there is not a clear distinction between wellness and illness. It is best to consider health, and any of the potential problems which may arise, as a process rather than as a discrete event in the life of an individual.

Frequently this process begins years before the development of clinical illness. Along this spectrum, definitions of 'normal' versus 'abnormal' are often arbitrary and tend to reflect significant statistical deviation from the population norm rather than the presence or absence of a particular pathophysiological phenomenon. An example is hypertension. Blood pressure is a physiological measurement on a continuous scale. The level at which blood pressure changes from 'normal' to 'abnormal' is largely arbitrary and is based upon epidemiological information drawn from large populations suggesting that people with particular levels of high blood pressure have a greater risk of developing significant disease sequelae than people with lower levels of blood pressure.[26] Clearly it does not make sense to suggest that caring for someone aged 35 with

Figure 2.2 Natural history of disease and potential interventions

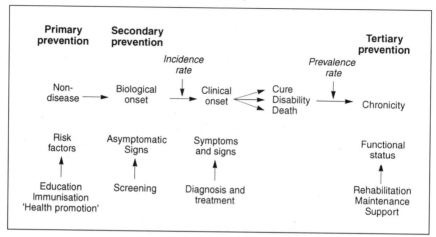

From Silagy CA. *Prevention in General Practice in a Textbook of Preventative Medicine* (McNeil JJ, King RWF, Jennings GL, Powles JW eds) Edward Arnold (Australia) Pty Ltd, Victoria, 1990, pp269–272.

a blood pressure of 140/90 mmHg is 'caring for the well', whereas caring for someone with a blood pressure of 140/91 mmHg is 'caring for the ill'. The situation is made more complex by the constant fluctuation that occurs in blood pressure, so that someone who is 'well' now may be 'ill' tomorrow and vice versa.

In other disease processes, there may be evidence of abnormal pathophysiology without any evidence of clinical illness. For example, atherosclerosis is commonly seen years before the degree of arterial blockage is sufficient to result in a reduced blood supply to the heart causing angina or a myocardial infarction. This situation has led to the concept of risk markers which reflect intermediate stages in the likely evolution of a disease. In other instances, identifiable disease may be present and yet not cause any symptoms of illness. Prostate cancer in males is a good example. Amongst older males the incidence of macroscopic cancer in the prostate gland rises, so that by age 80 approximately 43 per cent have macroscopic evidence of prostate cancer at autopsy.[27] However, the vast majority of these cancers are asymptomatic and never result in clinical 'illness'.

Superimposed on the pathophysiological basis of disease are complex psychological and social phenomena which influence the way individuals respond to illness. Adhering strictly to biological definitions of disease can be dangerous in assessing care needs of individuals. For example, two people may have identical degenerative changes in their knees (osteoarthritis), but their experience of pain and discomfort, and its impact on their daily lives, may vary considerably. One person may regard themselves as being 'well' and the other as being 'ill', despite no biological difference in disease severity.

The last two decades have seen considerable growth in consumer-driven definitions of 'wellness' and 'illness'. Concepts such as quality of life and functional capacity have emerged together with multi-dimensional constructs which allow them to be measured.[28]

Given the high degree of complexity in defining wellness, a fairly liberal definition, based on the perspective of the medical profession is utilised: 'caring for the well' encompasses providing holistic care to individuals, their families, and communities in order to promote health and well-being, in the absence of clinically symptomatic 'illness'. Furthermore, the acceptance of the notion that 'wellness' and 'illness' are part of a spectrum in which boundaries are blurred and frequently mobile, begins to highlight why the medical profession can not, and does not, ignore the task of caring for the well.

A framework for caring for the well

Ideally, one of the first steps in trying to care for the well is to predict those who are likely to become ill in order that preventive strategies can be appropriately targeted.[27] However, therein lies a major dilemma and challenge. With the exception of some congenital genetically determined conditions, it is almost never possible to determine with complete certainty whether a particular individual will, or will not, become ill. All one can assess is the *risk* (or probability) that an individual has of becoming ill based on previous patterns of disease within the community. In some cases the population 'at risk' of developing a disease may be very small (such as the increased risk of bladder cancer amongst workers in the rubber industry), however, in other situations almost the entire population can be 'at risk'. In the former scenario, preventive interventions can be specifically targeted to high-risk individuals. In the latter scenario, caring for the well may involve trying to target the entire population. Universal immunisation for some of the infectious diseases (tetanus, diphtheria, measles, polio, rubella, etc) is a good example of how such an approach is applied in practice.

Usually the level of risk varies throughout the population, from those who have a relatively low risk of developing disease to others at much higher risk.

In this case, the dilemma is deciding how to minimise the likely burden of illness within the community by appropriately targeting preventive interventions. Geoffrey Rose, a renowned epidemiologist, identified two different approaches to dealing with this problem.[26] The first

Figure 2.3 Distribution of risk

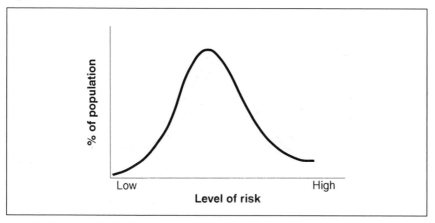

Figure 2.4 High risk approach to risk reduction

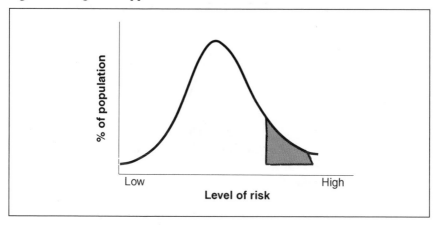

is known as the 'high-risk' approach, where efforts are targeted towards reducing risk amongst those most likely to become ill.

This approach gained popularity amongst many medical practitioners because of its application to the medical model. Doctors have a responsibility to identify and treat the sick, therefore extending that to identify those at highest risk of becoming sick seems logical and appropriate. However, from a population perspective most illness occurs amongst people with moderate risk rather than those at highest risk.

This presents a paradox for the medical profession because if the total burden of disease in the community is to be reduced, strategies are required which also target those in the low to moderate risk categories

Figure 2.5 Burden of illness in the community

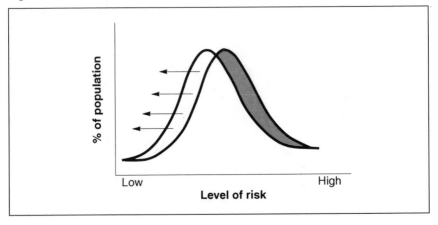

Figure 2.6 Population approach to risk education

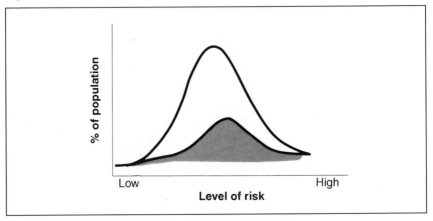

and shift their overall risk profile such that the whole community is at lowered risk of developing disease, as shown in Figure 2.6.

This second approach is known as the 'population approach' and requires the medical profession to use different strategies in order to be successful.

A practical illustration of this dilemma is deciding how to reduce the number of people who die from myocardial infarction. One perspective would be to seek to identify those at highest risk of developing myocardial infarction, for example, people with markedly elevated blood pressure or lipids, and then treating these aggressively. The problem with such an approach is that even though it targets those at highest *risk* of developing myocardial infarction, the majority of people who *actually* suffer a myocardial infarction do not have particularly elevated blood pressure or lipids. There is a trade-off between the effort and cost involved in identifying and treating a small number of high risk individuals in order to prevent one person dying from a myocardial infarction versus the effort and cost required to achieve a smaller change in the risk factor status of a large number of low to moderate risk individuals. Although both of these approaches potentially result in a similar outcome the caring strategies are quite different.

Whilst traditionally medical practice is much more suited towards utilising the 'high risk' approach to tackling prevention, the modern medical practitioner needs to be capable of adopting both approaches in order to maximise the public health benefits of caring for the well. Julian Tudor Hart highlighted this challenge two decades ago when he wrote of the need for a new type of doctor.

> GPs must translate the hard language of experimental medicine and epidemiology in the warm idiom of daily life, sufficiently sure of the value of their work to measure their work and consider its short-comings honestly. The world needs a new kind of doctor, one who combines clinical skill with the skills of population medicine.[29]

The first step towards responding to the Tudor Hart challenge requires medical practitioners to embrace the concept that they are responsible for caring for a practice population which comprises individuals and their families, rather than caring for individuals alone. Medical practitioners need to learn that it is not only the individual patient with whom they are consulting who is affected by any decisions that are made. This recognition is reinforced in settings where medical practitioners are responsible for resource allocation on behalf of their patients.

Maximising opportunities

The practical implementation of a strategy to care for the well that combines both a population and high risk individual perspective, requires use of both opportunistic and systematic prevention strategies. The former involves maximising the opportunity which arises when a patient happens to visit a doctor for 'illness care' by also targeting particular preventive measures. This targeting may either be 'cued' or 'non-cued'.[19] Cued strategies target the preventive measures to the presenting medical condition, for example, addressing smoking habits in a patient with bronchitis, or discussing dietary modification and increased exercise in a patient with angina.

Non-cued strategies are used in situations where the routine consultation does not generate any obvious areas for health promotion. In these cases, usually after relatively minor problems, random age/sex appropriate topics are selected. For example, discussion of contraception and pap smears with young women who present with a viral illness, or assessing cardiovascular risk factors in an apparently healthy adult who has presented following a minor sporting injury.

Systematic approaches for caring for the well involve targeting selected groups of individuals within the practice population at particular times in order to identify and/or treat those at particular risk. Recalling women for routine pap smears or assessing cardiovascular risk in middle-aged males are two examples of systematically caring for the well.

Usually, preventive efforts are targeted at particular behaviours or risk factors. However, in the last decade there has also been a trend towards encouraging 'periodic health checks'.[19] These involve measuring a battery of behaviours and risk factors on a regular (often annual or biannual) basis.[30] A few countries have gone as far as actively encouraging and financially supporting their medical practitioners to provide periodic health checks on a population-wide basis. Concerns about the effectiveness of such an approach led to several large-scale trials during the late 1980s and early 1990s, which almost universally found that these ambitious comprehensive screening and assessment programs produced extremely small benefits despite the large resource investment required.[30,31] Furthermore, there is risk of producing unnecessary anxiety as a result of generating false positive findings which require further investigation often with little or no clinical consequence.

With increasing computerisation of medical practices, it is likely that practice-based registers will greatly facilitate identification of 'at-risk' individuals on the basis of factors such as age and sex. Computerisation will allow patients to be recalled on a selected basis, as well as prompting doctors to undertake preventive activities that are due for patients presenting opportunistically.

Barriers to caring for the well

Bonevski, Sanson-Fisher and Campbell, in a recent review of current practices in health promotion amongst primary care practitioners, identified four levels of barriers: structural, office, patient, and practitioner.[25] The structural barriers included lack of education and training, both at undergraduate and postgraduate levels, lack of standardised guidelines for how to care for the well, and the lack of financial incentive to undertake preventive activities. As a result many physicians enter medical practice without the necessary skills or knowledge on how to care for the well. The quality of their continuing medical education is often poor and this is not aided by the mixed messages that are conveyed in guidelines from different reputable organisations. For example, recommendations about the frequency of cervical screening vary from annually to three-yearly depending on the country and professional organisation responsible for developing the guidelines.

At the office level, three barriers were identified: time restrictions, inadequate support staff, and forgetfulness. The first of these reflects the busy nature of medical practice, much of which is devoted to accomplishing the illness-oriented agenda. The time available for preventive procedures is relatively limited, and this is compounded by the fact that many preventive activities require dedicated and extended periods of time, such as lifestyle counselling and cervical screening. It is not surprising that under these circumstances a busy practitioner often forgets to undertake preventive activities. In a recent Australian study of general practitioners 43 per cent cited 'forgetting' as the main reason that women did not receive cervical screening. In some countries, such as the UK, this problem has been partly overcome by greater use of practice support staff (such as nurses and allied health professionals) and financial incentives for higher screening levels.

At the patient level, reluctance and competing priorities are cited as barriers to prevention. At the practitioner level, lack of feedback and confidence are the common barriers. Lack of positive feedback for the practitioner arises because, unlike the benefits that arise from treating individuals who are ill, the immediate individual health gains that arise from caring for the well are often small and take many years to emerge. As a result, many medical practitioners become despondent about the effectiveness of investing effort in caring for the well. The situation is compounded by the increasing proportion of preventive activity which involves achieving behaviour change.

This is a complex area that requires special skills and training in order to be effective. Traditionally, medical practitioners have not received any formal training in behaviour change and, as a result, have been unable to maximise their potential effectiveness in this area. A recent systematic review of general practitioners' ability to change four key behaviours (smoking, alcohol consumption, exercise, and diet) found that whilst many of the general practice-based lifestyle interventions show promise in effecting small changes in behaviour, none appears to produce substantial changes.[32]

One of the major advances in the application of behaviour change techniques in medicine has been the development of simple models which help explain the process and provide a framework for practitioners to more appropriately target their intervention. One of the most widely used frameworks is the 'stages of change' model developed by Prohaska and DiClemente.[33] This distinguishes five separate stages in achieving behaviour change: pre-contemplation, contemplation, preparedness for action, action, and relapse. An example of the practical application of this in medical practice is in facilitating smoking cessation. There would be little point in a medical practitioner discussing aids to smoking cessation with someone who is not even contemplating quitting. It would be far more appropriate to try to move such a person from the pre-contemplation stage to the contemplation stage by discussing the potential adverse effects of smoking.

How successful have health care professionals been?

Despite the barriers referred to above, the medical profession has made significant achievements as a result of caring for the well. Immunisation and hypertension are two such examples. Balanced against this has been the much more limited success in achieving behaviour change in areas such as diet and smoking cessation. In these areas, the real advances have come largely from community-wide initiatives often using mass media and/or legislative strategies.

Setting goals and targets

Over the last decade almost every Western country has developed goals and targets, in one form or another, directed towards reducing the amount of premature death and disability. Specific outcomes have been set in areas such as cardiovascular disease, cancers, immunisation, accidents and injuries, and mental health which provide a framework against which to measure performance both in caring for the ill and the well in the future.[34]

Many of the goals and targets emphasise achieving population-wide lifestyle changes, in areas such as smoking cessation, physical activity, diet, alcohol consumption, sun exposure, oral hygiene, appropriate use of medicines, and safe sex practices. Developing and refining strategies to achieve these goals and targets will shape the way in which the medical profession embarks on the task of caring for the well into the next millennium.

Future challenges

There are very few, if any, medical practitioners who would disagree that caring for the well is very much a part of their professional responsibility. Increasingly, their daily routine involves reassuring patients that they are well and not suffering from any life-threatening or debilitating illness. As Mant argued in a recent *Lancet* article, medical practitioners are willing to embrace prevention in their practices, because they experience a feeling of personal responsibility for the stroke patient whose hypertension had been unmeasured and uncontrolled, and the woman with invasive cervical cancer who has never had a pap smear.[35] He goes on to argue that the real challenge for the future is not the identification of disease risk, but the subsequent provision of effective intervention and long-term care to deal with the risk identified.

The second challenge in caring for the well in the future will be to develop methods which incorporate the care process into the routine consultation in a way that does not discount the patient's presenting symptom. This means placing the emphasis on secondary prevention before primary prevention.

The third challenge in the future is to target behaviours and risk measures for which there is good evidence that the available interventions are effective. Such evidence needs to address not just the efficacy of interventions under controlled research settings, but their effectiveness in the 'real world'. Where there is evidence of effectiveness, it is important that meaningful goals are set both at the practice level, as well as at regional and national levels. This ought to encourage medical practitioners to see their caring function as part of a broader public health strategy.

The fourth challenge is to create a practice environment which maximises the likelihood of being able to care effectively for the well. With the rapid uptake in practice computerisation and exploration of alternative funding strategies and structures to reimburse preventive activities appropriately, many of the often cited barriers to caring for the well are being dismantled.

The fifth challenge in the future will be to remind the medical profession constantly that caring for the well is not solely its province. Given the evidence that other members of the primary care team can provide equally effective, and perhaps even more cost-effective, care[36] their role in this process needs to be further exploited.

The final challenge, and perhaps the most important, is for the medical profession to embark on the task of caring for the well in partnership with public health efforts designed to influence and engage community-wide change. The very real reductions in the rates of smoking in Western society are an example of how such a partnership has worked well in the past. For example, doctors can, and ought to, advise their smoking patients to quit, and counsel young patients not to take up the habit. At the same time, doctors can act as role models themselves by not smoking and being seen to actively support public health campaigns by placing posters in their surgeries which advertise positive health messages. Beyond that, there is still an important and indispensable role for public health action such as appropriate tobacco control legislation and pricing policies. The combination of the individual and population approach represents the most powerful partnership possible in caring for the well and is the strategy most likely to be effective in the future.

REFERENCES

19. World Health Organization. The Ottawa Charter for health promotion. *Health Promotion International* 1986; 1 (4): iii–v.
20. Oldenburg B. Health promotion and disease prevention in the primary health care setting: setting the scheme. *Behavioural Change* 1994; 11 (3): 129–31.
21. Smith R. What now for IPPNW? Comment in: *Brit Med J* 1991; 303: 145–6.
22. Winstanley M, Woodward S, Walker N. *Tobacco in Australia: facts and issues 1995.* Victoria Smoking and Health Program, Australia (Quit Victoria), 1995, p415.
23. Paterson J. *National healthcare reform—the last picture show.* Department of Human Services, Government of Victoria, 1996, p41.
24. Commonwealth Department of Health and Family Services. *General practice in Australia: 1996.* Canberra: Australian Government Publishing Service, 1996, p346.
25. Bonevski B, Sanson-Fisher RW, Campbell EM. Primary care practitioners and health promotion: a review of current practices. *Health Prom J Aust* 1996; 6 (1): 22–31.
26. Rose G. *The strategy of preventive medicine.* Oxford: Oxford Medical Publications, 1992.
27. Commonwealth Department of Health and Family Services. *Prostate cancer screening.* Canberra: Australian Government Publishing Service, 1996, p111.
28. Fitzpatrick R, Fletcher A, Gore S, Jones D, Spiegelhalter D, Cox D. Quality of life measures in health care. I: Applications and issues in assessment. *Brit Med J* 1992; 305: 1074–7.
29. Hart JT. *A new kind of doctor.* London: Merlin Press, 1988.
30. ICRF Oxcheck Study Group. Effectiveness of health checks conducted by nurses in primary care—results of Oxcheck study after one year. *Brit Med J* 1994; 308: 308–12.
31. Family Heart Study Group. Randomised controlled trial evaluating cardiovascular screening and intervention in general practice: principal results of British Family Heart Study. *Brit Med J* 1994; 308: 313–20.
32. Ashenden R, Silagy C, Weller D. A systematic review of the effectiveness of promoting lifestyle change in general practice. *Family Practice* 1997; 14; 2: 160–175.
33. Prohaska J, DiClemente C. Toward a comprehensive model of change. In: Miller WR, Heather N (eds). *Treating addictive behaviours: processes of change.* New York: Plenum, 1986.

34. Nutbeam D, Wise M, Bauman A, Harris E, Leeder S. *Goals and targets for Australia's health in the year 2000 and beyond.* Sydney: Department of Public Health, University of Sydney, 1993.
35. Mant D. Facilitating prevention in primary care. *Brit Med J* 1992; 304: 652–3.
36. Buntinx F, Knotterus JA, Crebolder HF, Essed GG. *In search of good quality cervical smears: a literature review.* Netherlands: Vlaams Huisarten Institut, 1992.

CHAPTER THREE

Non-medical Care

PETER BAUME

Introduction

W e rely on the medical care, and support, given in Western societies by non-medically trained people, whether or not conventional care exists, although in some countries care given by non-medically trained workers is the only care available.[37] In Eastern countries, and especially in China, there has been a long tradition of care, given within different paradigms, but accompanied by systematic observation and an emphasis on the preservation of health.[38] Indeed, some alternative practitioners sell 'wellness', a concept that is peripheral to the daily lives of many practitioners trained in orthodox medical schools to concentrate on the causes and treatment of loss of health.

Since most diseases (perhaps 80 per cent)[39] are self-limited, it may make little difference medically who cares for us while most illnesses resolve, although those of us who value communication, a concern for us as individual people, may have a distinct preference for non-medically trained carers where an attractive persona and personal interest may play a part in the choice. The portfolio of attributes mentioned above is sometimes subsumed under the phrase 'holistic care' —although Rosalind Coward has mounted a forthright and vigorous counter-attack against alternative care, including the concept of 'holistic care'[40]—and Chapter Two on 'Caring for the Well' makes clear that 'holistic care' is part of the remit of many orthodox practitioners. It is even possible that we will recover more rapidly where our carers, sometimes medical carers, sometimes other carers, share emotional rapport with us.

A majority of the population of the world does not have access to, nor does it use, Western trained medical practitioners. A respectable discussion could take place about what, in a global context, is 'orthodox' and what is 'alternative' medicine in view of the numbers of persons adhering to the concepts of each.

One difference between orthodox and alternative practitioners is the communication style they use. Orthodox practitioners (for the purpose of this chapter those trained in medical schools) are generally not as good as alternative practitioners at reflective and active listening, and often project their own paradigms.[41,41a] Indeed, they often ignore or misunderstand messages which the patient is trying to send. Another and different view is that alternative practitioners (for the purpose of this chapter those trained other than in medical schools), rather than possessing any communication advantage, may have a 'gentle spirituality' in their approach to people that is lacking in many orthodox practitioners.[42] A third view is that alternative practitioners reject 'scientism' and that adherents of alternative medicine are challenging medicine's strict adherence to science.[43] But communication within orthodox medicine is often sub-standard—certainly medical teachers complain about the communication capacity of many students. There is no *a priori* reason why orthodox practitioners cannot be just as good at listening and communication as alternative practitioners. What militates against this at present is a narrow paradigm and a restrictive tradition of orthodox medicine rooted in bioscience and in the treatment of disease, so that Little has declared that:

> Western medicine has evolved very strongly in the traditions of empiricism, realism, materialism, and positivism. For these reasons, the scientific or experimental method is highly valued by medical scientists.[44]

That these are not the only ways in which medicine can develop or in which healing can occur is lost on some colleagues.

Background

With many illnesses there is no prospect of cure, but there is still a great need of the application of effective treatment to intercurrent illness or to symptoms. Good examples are the very old with permanent disabilities, those with AIDS (the end stage of infection with the HIV), those with advanced cancer, those with chronic illness such as rheumatoid arthritis or diabetes mellitus, in each of which cure is not an option but care is important. It is vital that medical practitioners should detect and treat a few important diseases, but, having done that, should be broad-minded about what any of us chooses to do next in seeking amelioration of troublesome symptoms. There are many routes to relief of symptoms, only some of which are medical. Indeed the medical paradigm—sometimes called 'the medical model'—is only one among a number of ways of understanding illness.[45]

In any community in any one month, many people do not feel well.[46] Most of us look after ourselves when we feel unwell. Either we do not use any treatment at all, or we medicate ourselves to relieve symptoms[47] while the curative forces of natural healing (*vix mediatrix naturae* to an earlier generation) have time to take effect.

Only a minority of us seeks advice from anyone for our sicknesses. Many of us seek advice from non-medical people, either non-medical carers, relatives, pharmacists, or friends. Usually the advice which we receive from these 'non-medical' sources is sufficient to relieve our symptoms and to sustain us while we return to normal functioning.

A smaller number seeks advice from a primary care practitioner. This advice might include treatment for the symptoms and/or might include reassurance. For only a minority of the people who see the primary care practitioner will more specialised advice be sought, and for only a tiny minority of these will hospital admission be recommended.[48] Professor Charles Bridges-Webb studied a community in rural Victoria and found that people had, on average, 10 illnesses each in a year, saw general practitioners for only 17 per cent of these and went to hospital with only 1 per cent of illnesses.[49] Kerr White and his colleagues asserted that only one in a thousand is admitted to a teaching hospital[50] in any one month.

For many years orthodox opinion was that diseases now recognised as infectious were due to miasmas, or to faults of 'nature' within the sufferer. Then bacteria were discovered and the germ theory of infectious disease emerged. So 'facts' within medicine represent too often just the majority orthodoxy of the moment—they change over time. In the same vein, the Catholic Church insisted, for theological reasons, on the 'correctness' of the geocentric theory of cosmology even after Copernicus and Galileo had published their works* and then took about 350 years to recognise officially that Galileo was probably correct.

The contribution of science to medical outcomes may be less important than generally thought,[51] although its major contribution to the understanding of human function and disease in individuals is not questioned and is set out in other chapters. Another important part of medical practice is reassurance—the explanation of phenomena in terms which people can understand and accept—for which medically trained people do not have a monopoly.

If we look at health outcomes the available measures are few and relatively crude. We use life expectancy at birth,[52] age adjusted mortality,[53] infant mortality,[54] variants of the preceding, potential years of life lost (PYLLs),[55] disability adjusted life years (DALYS),[56] quality adjusted life years (QALYS),[57] and a few more. The latter two measures involve

---

* Galileo is reputed to have said: 'E pur si muove' ('Yet it does move') when forced to recant his heliocentric doctrine.

some value judgments and depend on some assumptions being made by the observer.

At present there are many non-classifiable diseases and symptom complexes without a label. Thomas[58] has indicated that about half of the patients coming to a general practice have no identifiable pathology and he has coined the name 'temporarily dependent patients' for such persons, to give them a label which allows the 'openness' of the diagnosis to be kept in mind. Labels, diagnostic tests and treatment will be provided over time for some conditions at present not understood. But we practitioners should seldom assert that 'there is nothing wrong' with those for whom we cannot give a diagnosis and we might need to accept, more than we have, that people generally (there are some exceptions) do not see a healer without cause and that relief or reassurance, rather than diagnosis, is what many patients want.[59,60]

Cassell asserted[61] that about half of the problems of medicine relate to caring and 'art' rather than to diagnosis or cure or 'science.' Indeed, some of the benefits of the 'art' of medicine depend upon expectancy and suggestion, each of which may produce lasting benefit.[62] Experienced community practitioners include both 'art'[63] and 'science' in what they do, drawing upon long-used and ancient healing skills[64] and building upon the long recognised effects of 'the doctor' as a therapeutic agent.[65]

Without science modern medical practitioners are dangerous. Without humanity they are monsters. Some alternative practitioners have no science; some orthodox practitioners have no humanity.[66] The best practitioners have always combined both sets of skills and have given recognition, along with science, to empathy,[67] authority, cultural affinity and sympathy.[68]

Much of what orthodox practitioners say may be good science, but is mumbo-jumbo to patients. Patients do not understand the technical jargon or the concepts with which some orthodox practitioners bombard them. Some wise practitioners give patients written material to take away and to read at leisure.

That patients do not understand, matters less than it might when one realises that perhaps more than two-thirds of all communication[69,70] is non-verbal, and that patients are well able to read non-verbal signals. Sometimes people become aware quickly that what is being said by the practitioner does not accord with the signals received from posture and gestures.[71] Such a discordance, when it occurs, probably inhibits the process of healing. Most people accept the non-verbal signals in preference to words if forced to choose between them.

If medical practitioners meet the needs of those who see them, the transaction will be valuable to the persons concerned. Should the practitioner not meet the needs of people, however irrational or unworthy the practitioner considers those needs to be, then he/she should not be surprised that people seek increasingly either a more empathic medical practitioner or those alternative practitioners who will respond to their needs.

Who are these alternative practitioners, and what do they offer which is often so valued by people? First, they differ from conventional practitioners in that they generally reject the paradigms of orthodox medicine.[72] They are generally (though not exclusively) people without formal medical training who work within paradigms that are at variance with orthodox medical belief and inconsistent with orthodox medical paradigms. In a Popperian sense, much of what they claim is not disprovable, and is therefore not scientific[73] whereas much of what is taught and practised in the basic sciences of medicine can be disproved and is, therefore, 'scientific'. It is interesting that much basic science (for example, the existence of sub-atomic particles) is disprovable (that is, 'scientific') only in a few laboratories in the world and then only with equipment which is expensive—which makes the acceptance by most people of the basic beliefs of science a matter of faith in fact, however disprovable and scientific those beliefs might be in theory. More clinical medicine is 'scientific' than used to be the case, but even today, part of clinical medicine rests more on faith, fashions, magic, orthodoxy and authority than its adherents care to acknowledge.

Much of what is offered by alternative practitioners is conventional advice about diet, rest and moderate regular exercise, combined with active listening and a capacity to respond to people as people. It is this last characteristic that many care-users find particularly attractive and effective; conventional practitioners are sometimes so busy detecting and treating disease that they have no time left for the needs of troubled people whose symptoms may seem trivial.

There is more use of so-called alternative healers than is often recognised. A survey of children attending an oncology service and receiving orthodox therapy revealed that 46 per cent had used at least one alternative therapy[74] and Begbie et al[75] reported extensive use of alternative therapy by cancer patients. McKnight and Scott[76] reported widespread use of alternative therapy by patients infected by the HIV and Leeder[42] gives an eloquent account of the secret use of multivitamin therapy by his own parents during times of serious illness.

Human history and the progress of medicine

In the early days of civilisation life was brutish and short. For most of recorded history disease was rife and maternal and child mortality were high. Nature has been called 'red in tooth and claw'[77] and it certainly

Figure 3.1 Survival curve

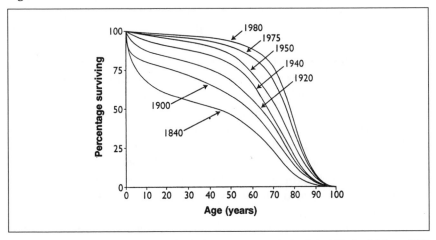

Adapted from Coni N, Davison W, Webster S, eds. *Lecture notes on geriatrics*. Oxford: Blackwell Science, 1988. Reproduced with permission.

was not, and is not, benign in its dealings with humans. There was little that could be done to prevent, detect, or treat diseases which today are within the capacity of medical science to address. Many people died and many others suffered greatly. In 1700 the average European could expect to live 25 years, a figure which had risen only to 35 years in 1800.[78] In the first third of the nineteenth century the average expectations of life were, in Derby in the United Kingdom, 49 years for the gentry, 28 years for tradesmen and 21 years for labourers,[79] and others have drawn attention to marked social inequalities in health, even then.[80] Increases in average longevity are shown in Figure 3.1.[81]

So people tried to come to terms with sickness, death, loss and grief—'seeking some understanding of the world in which our patients struggle to survive'.[82] They did this first by invoking magic (e.g., possession by evil spirits),[83] then by using religion, and then by using authority. Wizards, shamans, prophets, diviners and interpreters were the forerunners of priests and clergymen. Religion used, and still uses, authority as one means of 'making sense' of otherwise incomprehensible things. The teaching 500 years ago that this earthly existence is a vale of tears which prepares people for eternal bliss helped people to cope with a hard, brutal and unfair life. That medieval proposition is not disprovable. It serves to illustrate too just how much of what we do is determined by 'baggage'—social norms, cultural, political or philosophical assumptions, and by faith. Religion introduced both sin (which is a necessary element in an imperfect world) and punishment (which followed logically from the concept of sin).

The scientific revolution which began with the Renaissance has helped us to see things differently, but it does not explain everything. An early Cartesian view (see Chapter Six 'Cartesian Thinking') was that the body was a machine[84,85] which, if studied sufficiently, would yield up all its secrets and allow disease to be conquered. This view, although rejected now by philosophers, is still the paradigm within which some medical scientists operate. But neither science nor religion can explain yet why innocent children get fatal illnesses, or why many people who have harmed no-one suffer so much agony and die horrible premature deaths. Neither does such a restricted view see death as the natural end of life. Today, too often death is seen as 'alien', as 'the enemy', as 'failure', as something to be fought and rejected. Indeed, the activities of some medical scientists are death-denying in terms of the assumptions on which they take place.

The prevailing orthodox paradigm derives from allopathy—'the treatment by opposites'—in spite of contrary protestations from many well-trained, present-day practitioners. Allopathy arose from the view that disease was caused by noxious influences within people. In accordance with that view it made sense to purge and bleed people to reduce the amount of noxious substances. That paradigm continues to affect practice today—the pharmacopoeia contains antibiotics, anti-hypertensives, antipyretics, analgesics, anti-cancer drugs, anti-emetics, contraceptives, antihistamines, anti-viral drugs, and many more agents which are grouped by what they are against, and whose desired action is to oppose something.

But there remains a large group of patients (often those with 'unclassifiable' symptoms) for whom 'best practice' interventions depend on the 'art' of medicine, for whom diagnosis is not the most important purpose, for whom expectant treatment might be justified, and for whom specific 'cure' is not sought. Further it may not matter a lot what treatment is given for the 80 per cent of patients with self-limited disease— provided always that the treatment does them no harm. But, depending on the skills of the practitioner, there might be considerable differences between different encounters in their effect on reducing anxiety.

Many conventional medical practitioners assert that alternative medicine is a form of pseudo-science although in practical skills (e.g., manipulation and massage) some alternative practitioners may be better operators than many practitioners trained in conventional medical schools. Nevertheless, listening, relief of symptoms and a 'whole person' approach is what some 'healers' do provide in amounts, and with skill, not matched by many conventionally trained practitioners. Many of those who practise alternative medicine (sometimes called 'complementary medicine')[86] produce at least part of their benefit through use of the 'art' of healing. Some scientific practitioners who sneer at alternative medicine do not understand the particular skills that many alternative practitioners have, the elements of good non-specific care, the 'active listening', the use of the 'art' of medicine, or of the desire of people for an approach which is holistic, personal, and spiritually satisfying.

If a complementary practitioner misses an important condition the consequences can be catastrophic. But equally, the failure of any medical practitioner to respond to the human needs of patients represents a catastrophe of a different kind.

Some of the more prominent kinds of alternative healers are described in the paragraphs which follow.

Traditional healers

Traditional healers do not use Western medical paradigms but operate organically within their own societies, of which they are a valued and important element. Their systems of belief are logical if their assumptions are accepted and those beliefs and assumptions are generally part of their culture.[87] Indeed, this cultural affinity with the society is, and has always been, one substantial source of their strength and much of the source of their influence.[88] They are sometimes experienced healers in whom there may be a family tradition or in which healing is seen as part of a 'priestly' occupation. Indeed, both in their use of power and their association with faith, traditional healing has been more like orthodox medicine than many will admit. Throughout history, traditional healers represent a more consistent thread of healing than does orthodox medicine which is limited in its areas of geographical influence and is recent in its history, its achievements and its paradigms.

Because many conditions require simple interventions only, because there is much good general advice (rest, diet, exercise) given by healers of many kinds, and because many communities believe in the efficacy of traditional healers, they have real value in the management of many community problems. Germany's reliance on 'taking the waters' at spa towns is a form of therapy which depends on sensible, but non-specific, interventions. The placebo effect (which requires belief on the part of the patient) may operate in those who 'take the waters' and may lead to release of endogenous opioids with powerful, important and effective assistance to many troubled people.

Traditional healers in many countries often assert that much disease is due to possession by evil spirits, to spells cast on the sufferer,[89] to the 'evil eye', or to malice from enemies. Activities directed towards propitiation and exorcism become important in freeing sufferers from illness and often whole families or communities are involved in common cause (which has its own value) in these prescribed activities.

But people continue to suffer and die. Sensibly, traditional healers have a capacity to do nothing active on some occasions and to 'explain' events such as death or progression of disease that occur in spite of their interventions. Their explanations are often related to sorcery and may have dire consequences for third parties.

Homeopathy

Homeopathy (or homoeopathy) was introduced by Samuel Christian Friedrich Hahnemann in the nineteenth century. He expounded a main principle of homeopathy 'Let like be treated by like', sometimes referred to as 'the law of similars'. Paracelsus is said to have used a similar principle, 'the law of signatures', in his practice and writings.[90]

Homeopathy teaches that much illness responds to tiny doses of drugs—so it promotes use of dilute tinctures. At least homeopaths are observing the ancient medical dictum *'primum non nocere'*—'first do no harm' as their dilute tinctures may be pharmacologically inactive —and therefore harmless. Homeopaths postulate that there is a loss of poisonous elements with dilution, associated with retention and accentuation of pure creative energy.[91] There is no scientific evidence to support this assertion. Homeopathic approaches may be useful where one is filling in time waiting for the healing forces of nature to take effect—as for any rational basis for homeopathy we may have to await more developments and more evidence.

It is hard for those trained in orthodox paradigms to imagine that homeopathic remedies have any specific pharmacological benefit. The minority of people with more severe symptoms want some rapid benefit from treatment, and homeopathy is limited in what it can deliver to them. Further, part of the training of students of orthodox medicine, is to understand the significance of certain symptoms or signs as evidence of serious and treatable underlying disease. So, while symptoms may be treated, they are understood as evidence of more subtle disease elsewhere (but see Chapter Fifteen 'The Disease Model Challenged'). This is an area which is not addressed credibly by homeopathy.

Chiropractic

Under this heading we will, for convenience, consider chiropractors, osteopaths, manipulative therapists, and masseurs. That they are different is acknowledged and understood—but there is a common thread to the activities of all of them that allows them to be considered together here.

Chiropractic was introduced by an American practitioner named Daniel David Palmer in 1895. There is a limited number of schools of chiropractic around the world and many Australian chiropractors with no formal qualifications were admitted under a 'grandfather' clause when the School in Melbourne was established.[92]

Chiropractic is said to rest on the thesis that most, if not all, human ailments result from a slight misalignment or subluxation of contiguous vertebrae.[92] Most chiropractors use standard treatments except for drugs or surgery—and so include many standard commonsense health promoting activities in what they offer to patients.

The idea of the chiropractic subluxation is what sets the chiropractor apart from the osteopath or other manipulative therapists. It was the abandonment of simple manipulative skills by the orthodox medical profession in the nineteenth century that created the window of opportunity which allowed Andrew Still to introduce osteopathy and D.D. Palmer to introduce chiropractic.

It is likely that most soft tissue injuries are self-limited and most heal within 10 days or so. For such injuries, it may not matter whether chiropractic or some other technique is used—provided that serious treatable disease has been excluded first by an orthodox practitioner. If the practitioner (whether an orthodox practitioner or a chiropractor) has real manipulative skills he/she may give more rapid relief of symptoms and will be well regarded by grateful patients. If the skills include caring, good communication, a coherent general philosophy and kindness, then a need is being satisfied that some orthodox practitioners ignore too often.

Naturopathy

Naturopathy is closely allied to homeopathy and to herbalism. All three assert that nature will heal if allowed to do so (true in most illnesses—but not all) and that 'natural' substances are to be preferred over synthetics.

Naturopathy teaches that 'natural is best' and that artificial substances poison people. Much of the basis of naturopathy is that the adoption of a healthy lifestyle will promote health—and most orthodox practitioners would agree with this proposition.[93] Indeed, the adoption of a healthier lifestyle is one thing that is promoted within conventional medical schools—even if it is unequally acted on in society. But naturopaths then go on to say that most diseases can and should be treated with 'natural' substances. Some schools devoted to naturopathic teaching and training have emerged.[94]

An assertion that only natural substances should be used in treatment has serious flaws. Mortality remains at 100 per cent and those adherents who practise 'natural' therapeutic methods have no advantages in survival over their more conventional brothers and sisters. It is true that much disease is 'iatrogenic', resulting from medical interventions, from infection with resistant bacteria in hospitals, or from drugs used by medical practitioners, and so adherents of natural therapy would avoid at least some of these untoward effects. But until contraception was introduced (an 'unnatural' intervention) women had high mortality and morbidity associated with pregnancy and childbirth. Many natural products are poisonous—botulinus toxin, oleander leaves, snake venom, box jellyfish venom, blue-ring octopus venom, to name just a few. Many synthetic substances are single pure compounds. Some are made chemically under artificial conditions while some are made 'naturally' by bacilli that have been treated genetically so that they produce the substances in large volume in pure form. Doses of single pure chemicals can be standardised in ways that are impossible where plant extracts are used.

Naturopathy also uses (manufactured) 'tissue salts' which are mineral salts which should be present in any balanced diet. Additionally, use is made of vitamins, sometimes in megadoses, with some consequent ill effects from vitamin overdoses.[95] The use of either of these groups of substances is closer to conventional drug therapy than it is to a reliance on nature.

Not only that, but orthodox medicine has some strengths which naturopathy cannot match. Orthodox medicine is good at detecting some diseases, and patients in whom such detection is delayed unreasonably may suffer from the delay.

Some of the practitioners of naturopathy use concepts and terms that are foreign to medical science and which rest on concepts which cannot be disproved. Segal[96] lists a number of terms which would be poorly understood by orthodox practitioners, including 'life energy fields', 'orgone', 'bioplasma bions', 'shimmering blue vesicles in the blood', 'blue bions', 'vivaxis energy', 'auras of radiation'. Naturopaths sometimes discuss 'radiesthesia'[97] to describe and detect energy fields which are supposed to surround the body.

The training of natural therapists was considered in extenso by an expert committee, chaired by a noted biochemist Emeritus Professor Edwin Webb, which was set up in 1974 and which published its report in 1977.[98] That report was scathing about some of the training of naturopaths, as it was of 'zone therapy' which is one of the naturopathic techniques.

It is just as possible that everything said by naturopaths is correct as it is that it is all incorrect (or that some parts are correct or incorrect). Testing of the hypotheses of naturopathy has, so far, turned up little evidence to support the assertions of its adherents. And this is the problem for people of good will—how to keep an open mind on matters that await scientific testing and which remain, for the present, as speculations and the ideas of enthusiasts.

Herbalism

Herbalism[99] involves the use of plants and plant extracts and of 'natural' plants. It is, accordingly, closely allied to naturopathy. But the use of plants may have drawbacks (for example, poisons, unpredictable doses, mixing of active therapeutic agents with poisons), sufficient to have led to the almost complete abandonment of plant use by orthodox practitioners who used to champion it, and who studied it in the old subject Materia Medica. Today most drugs are produced as single, pure compounds, the doses of which are predictable and free from contaminants.

With plants the doses are variable and the extract used may be a combination of several substances, some of which may be toxic.

Iridology

Iridology was introduced by Ignatz von Peczely who was born in 1826. Constable[100] records a description of iridology as:

> a science (*sic*) whereby the doctor or operator can tell from the markings or signs of the iris of the eye the reflex conditions of the various organs of the body.

It is asserted that different regions of the iris equate to different internal organs and the right and left eyes are supposed to have different diagnostic significance.

Practitioners of iridology employ terms which are foreign to orthodox practitioners. Terms such as 'nerve wreath' and 'psoric spots', 'calcium-sodium ring', 'lymphatic rosary', 'scurf ring', 'vascular arc' have no correspondence to conventional medical language. The use of these terms does not of itself make them either correct or incorrect, but does indicate at least a need for some efforts to make language and concepts correspond more than they do between practitioners of different kinds.

Much advice given by iridologists is common sense and many iridologists have good communication skills.

Again, there is a need to submit many of the assertions, the theories, and the observations of iridology to critical test and examination. Until this is done there must remain healthy scepticism about some of the statements and conclusions of iridologists.

Meditation

This covers a variety of practices in which people enter a hypnoid state between waking and sleeping. There is a number of meditation techniques, ranging from commercial hypnotism, to auto-hypnosis (used effectively by some orthodox medical practitioners), to Zen Buddhism, and so on. Indeed, prayer is a distinguishing feature of the monotheistic religions today; many other religions have a preference for meditation and altered consciousness.

The advantages to individuals of these techniques are many. For some it may enable them to cope with pain from a malignant process (some medical practitioners teach the technique of auto-hypnosis as one tool in the armoury of controlling such pain)—perhaps by enhanced release of endogenous opioids; for others it may produce general relaxation and a sense of well-being, for others still it may produce beneficial alterations in various autonomic functions (fall in blood pressure, slowing of pulse, altered skin conductance) as a result of which they may feel better. In a later chapter the earlier use of hypnotherapy in surgery is discussed.

Most of the benefits of meditation remain to be tested critically but the adherents of meditation techniques feel often that their lives have been improved by what they regard as simple processes which they can control. Meditation techniques appear to be harmless, and there is no sensible reason why orthodox practitioners would wish to decry or sneer at patients who practise one of the meditation techniques.

Acupuncture

Acupuncture is derived from traditional Chinese practice and is combined often with moxibustion. In the former, treatment is directed towards redirecting or 'normalising' the Chi or supreme nourishing force within the body which flows along certain meridians[39] while the latter involves the application of heat from moxa sticks for the same purpose. Tai Chi is a martial art designed to stimulate the flow of

Chi through the normal meridians or channels. Acupuncture has been defined as:

> the most direct of the manipulative therapies in that the network of meridians which connect with deeper internal organs and other body parts are precisely outlined and accessible. . . . used to redirect and normalise the flow of Chi. Acupuncture is the insertion of fine needles into surface points[39]

of which 722 are known but less than 50 are commonly used.

Acupuncture is recommended for a wide variety of conditions and has been used to produce analgesia sufficient to allow performance of major surgery. Acupressure uses fingertip pressure to the same external points.

Acupuncture is safe in practice (although the use of invasive needles carries a potential risk of infection), and some of the analgesic effect may be due to release of endogenous encephalins.

Miscellaneous

New forms of non-conventional care are emerging continually, driven partly by a sense of resentment at the failure of orthodox medicine, in spite of its real achievements this century, to address (often even to respond to) many problems of individual troubled people, partly by an unwillingness of persons to face the realities of finite life and of human frailty, and partly by failures to understand (or to be told) that many illnesses (and at least one illness for every mortal being) remain beyond the capacity of orthodox practitioners to address effectively. Equally, there are fashions that make one unproven modality popular for a time, after which it disappears for decades.

So we need to be aware of phrenology, imagery, commercial weight loss programs, lifestyle diets, macrobiotics, self-help groups, biofeedback, megavitamin therapy, radionics, spiritual healing, aromatherapy, crystal healing, Shiatsu, to list just a few. They are not considered separately in this chapter because each represents the application of general principles already outlined and discussed.

Such emerging forms of non-medical care are a testament to the troubled nature of humanity, to our unwillingness to submit completely to the doctor-priests set over us with the approval of society, and to a feeling that answers to eternal questions can be discovered if only the key can be found. It can be predicted that more modalities of alternative medicine will appear and will become popular and that the popularity of existing modalities of care, orthodox and alternative, will wax and wane.

Conclusion

Alternative medicine is flourishing in the Western world. This is partly due to an inchoate desire for immortality and to a denial of death[101] by people, irrespective of the type of care they seek, but is due too partly to the failure of many orthodox practitioners to meet the needs of people for coherent explanations, for sensitive communication, for care, and for interest. Much of the advice from many alternative practitioners is sensible 'general' advice and, as such, does no harm to the many people without an underlying treatable serious disease.

The existence of alternative medicine, and its popularity,[102,103] should encourage orthodox practitioners to be more ready to challenge or to change the paradigms within which they work. Put bluntly, there is likely to be more progress from paradigm change (or at least paradigm widening) than there is from the continued application of existing paradigms to problems of medical care.

If we look back 150 years, to the paradigms and practices of that time,[104] we are likely to smile indulgently. Many of us can see clearly that the belief systems then operating were inadequate to explain events, and have been overtaken. But too many of us lack a capacity to learn from that observation about our current paradigms. If we go forward 150 years in our imagination and then look back it seems likely that practitioners of that day will smile again at *our* belief systems. There is nothing wrong with this—we are using the best paradigms we have. They are not perfect and they will be overtaken. We need to be relaxed and ready—and not to be prisoners of the paradigms of today.

Perhaps more people might attend an orthodox 'doctor' for initial assessment and advice, and might then, if they wish, attend a 'healer' (if that is their choice), and might return regularly to the 'doctor' for re-assessment and review. Such a practice would require an alteration to the 'proprietorial' view of patients and therapy possessed by many recognised healers today. But it gives to the patient the best of both worlds—it has few drawbacks and is something that we may wish to use more.

REFERENCES

37. Djukanovic V, Mach EP. *Alternative approaches to meeting basic health needs in developing countries.* Geneva: World Health Organization, 1977.
38. Chow EPY. Traditional Chinese medicine: a holistic system. In: Salmon, JW (ed). *Alternative medicines: popular and policy perspectives.* New York: Tavistock, 1984, ch 4, p114.
39. Segal W. Naturopathy, homeopathy and herbalism. In: Joske R, Segal W. *Ways of healing.* Melbourne: Penguin Books, 1987, p97.

40. Coward R. *The whole truth: the myth of alternative health.* London: Faber and Faber, 1989.
41. Little JM. *Humane medicine.* Cambridge: Cambridge University Press, 1995, see p5 for an explanation of this word.
41a. Goulston S. The humanities in medical education. The place of literature. Thesis submitted to University of Sydney for degree of Master of Philosophy, 1997.
42. Leeder SR. Alternative medicine: alternative to what? *Medical Observer*, 24 June 1994; 7.
43. Maddocks I. Alternative medicine. *Med J Aust* 1985; 142: 547–51.
44. Little JM. *Humane medicine*, ibid, p31.
45. Little JM. *Humane medicine*, ibid, pp30–49.
46. Wadsworth M, Butterfield W, Blaney R. *Health and sickness: the choice of treatment.* London: Tavistock, 1971.
47. Thomas DHV, Noyce PR. The interface between self-medication and the NHS. *Brit Med J* 1996; 312: 688.
48. Marmot MG, Zwi AB. Measuring the burden of illness in general populations. In: White KL, Connelly JE. *The medical school's mission and the population's health.* New York: Springer-Verlag, 1992, p83.
49. Bridges-Webb C, quoted in Hetzel BS. *Health and Australian society.* Ringwood, Vic: Penguin Books, 1974, p235.
50. White KL, Williams TF, Greenberg BC, quoted in: McWhinney IR. *An introduction to family medicine.* New York: Oxford University Press, 1981, p39.
51. Joske R, Segal W. *Ways of healing*, ibid, p4.
52. Australian Institute of Health. *Australia's health 1988.* Canberra: AGPS, 1988, p25.
53. Australian Institute of Health and Welfare. *Australia's health 1994.* Canberra: AGPS, 1994, p5.
54. Australian Institute of Health. *Australia's health 1988.* ibid, p41.
55. Australian Institute of Health and Welfare. Mathers C. *Health differentials among adult Australians aged 25–64 years.* Canberra: AGPS, 1994, p14.
56. World Bank. *World Development Report 1993: investing in health.* New York: Oxford University Press, for World Bank, Washington DC, 1993.
57. Loomes G, Mackenzie L. The use of QALYs in health care decision making. *Social Science and Medicine* 1989; 28: 299–308.
58. Thomas KB. The placebo in general practice. *Lancet* 1994; 344: 1066.
59. Lennard-Jones JE. Foreword to Wulff HR. *Rational diagnosis and treatment.* London: Blackwell, 1976, pviii.
60. McDonald IG, Daly J, Jelinek VM, Panetta F, Gutman JM. Opening Pandora's box: the unpredictability of reassurance by a normal test result. *Brit Med J* 1996; 313: 329–32.
61. Cassell EJ. *The nature of suffering and the goals of medicine.* Oxford: Oxford University Press, 1991, p21.
62. Rosenthal D, Frank JD. Psychotherapy and the placebo effect. *Psychological Bulletin* 1956; 55: 294–302.
63. Sartorius N. Foreword to White L, Tursky B, Schwartz GE (eds). *Placebo: theory, research and mechanisms.* New York: Guilford Press, 1985.
64. Shapiro AK, Morris LA. The placebo effect in medical and psychological therapies. In: Garfield SL, Bergin AE (eds). *Handbook of psychotherapy and behaviour change: an empirical analysis*, (2nd edition), 1978, New York: John Wiley.
65. Balint M. *The doctor, his patient and the illness.* London: Pitman Medical, 1957.
66. See for example German GA. The traditional and the modern in the practice of medicine. In: Joske R, Segal W. *Ways of healing*, ibid, p22.
67. Nisselle P. Empathy: another tool in the bag. *Australian Doctor*, 17 May 1966; 54.
68. Little JM. *Humane medicine*, ibid, p160.

69. Birdwhistell RL. Kinesics and context. University of Pennsylvania Press, 1970, quoted by Pease F. *Body Language.* Sydney: Camel Publishing Company, 1981, p6.
70. Mehrabian A. *Silent Messages.* Wadsworth, California: Wadsworth Publishing Co, quoted in: Northouse PG, Northouse LL. *Health Communication: strategies for health professionals.* Connecticut: Appleton and Lange, 1992, p117.
71. Windschuttle K, Windschuttle E. *Writing, researching, communicating.* Sydney: McGraw-Hill, 1988, p338.
72. Joske R, Segal W. *Ways of healing,* ibid, p3.
73. Popper KR. *Conjectures and refutations: the growth of scientific knowledge.* London: Routledge, 1989.
74. Sawyer MG, Gannoni AF, Toogood IR, Antoniou G, Rice M. The use of alternative therapies by children with cancer. *Med J Aust* 1994; 106: 320–2.
75. Begbie SD, Kerestes ZL, Bell DR. Patterns of alternative medicine use by cancer patients. *Med J Aust* 1996; 165: 545–8.
76. McKnight I, Scott M. HIV and complementary medicine. *Med J Aust* 1966; 165: 143.
77. Tennyson A. *In Memoriam,* quoted in Cohen JM, Cohen MJ. *The Penguin dictionary of quotations.* London: Penguin Books, 1960, p385.
78. McKay JP, Hill BD, Buckler J. *A History of Western society: volume II: from absolutism to the present,* 3rd edition. Boston: Houghton Mifflin, 1987, p647.
79. Flinn MW (ed), Chadwick E. *Report on the sanitary condition of the labouring population of Great Britain.* Edinburgh: Edinburgh University Press, 1965, pp219ff.
80. Snow J, quoted in Harper AC, Holman CD'A, Dawes VP. *The health of populations: an introduction.* Edinburgh: Churchill Livingstone, 1994, p49.
81. Asscher AW, Parr GD, Whitmarsh VB. Towards the safer use of medicines. *Brit Med J* 1995; 311: 1003–6.
82. O'Donnell M. The toxic effect of lanuage on medicine. *Journal of the Royal College of Physicians of London,* 29: 525–9. 1995.
83. Cawte J. Aboriginal medicine. In: Joske R, Segal W. *Ways of healing,* ibid, p55.
84. Russell B. *History of Western philosophy.* London: George Allen and Unwin, 1940, p383.
85. McKeown T. *The role of medicine: dream, mirage or nemesis?* Princeton, New Jersey: Princeton University Press, 1979, p4.
86. Joyce CRB. Placebo and complementary medicine. *Lancet* 1994; 344: 1279.
87. Lovell J. A visit to the witch-doctor. *Modern Medicine of Australia,* September 1966, 39: 51–5.
88. Buckman R, Sabbagh K. *Magic or medicine? An investigation of healing and healers.* London: Macmillan, 1993.
89. Cawte J. *Healers of Arnhem Land.* Sydney: University of New South Wales Press, 1996.
90. Quoted in Coulter HL. *Divided legacy: a history of the schism in medical thought. Volume 1: The patterns emerge; Hippocrates to Paracelsus.* Washington, DC: Wehawken, 1975, p432.
91. British Homeopathic Association. *A guide to homeopathy,* 8th edition. London: British Homeopathic Association, 1979, pp6, 14.
92. Hay MC. Chiropractic. In: Joske R, Segal W. *Ways of healing,* ibid, p139.
93. Segal W. Naturopathy, homeopathy and herbalism. In: Joske R, Segal W. *Ways of healing,* ibid, p95.
94. Steele FR. Washington State, Bastyr University lead natural medicine charge. *Nature Medicine* 1996; 2: 619.
95. Evans CDH, Lacey JH. Toxicity of vitamins:complications of a health movement. *Brit Med J* 1986, 292: 509.
96. Segal W. Naturopathy, homeopathy and herbalism. In: Joske R, Segal W. *Ways of healing,* ibid, p91.

97. Segal W. Naturopathy, homeopathy and herbalism. In: Joske R, Segal W. *Ways of healing*, ibid, p93.
98. Webb E (chair). *Report of the Committee of Inquiry into chiropractic, osteopathy, homeopathy and naturopathy*, (known as the Webb Report), Canberra: AGPS, 1977.
99. Discussed in extenso in Robbins C. *Herbalism: Thorson's introductory guide*. London: Thorsons, 1993.
100. Constable I. In: Joske R, Segal W. *Ways of healing*, ibid, p117.
101. Mendelsohn RS. *Confessions of a medical heretic*. Chicago: Contemporary Books, 1979.
102. Little JM. *Humane medicine*, ibid, p55.
103. Editorial. Complementary medicine is booming world wide. *Brit Med J* 1966; 313: 131–3.
104. Wulff HR. *Rational diagnosis and treatment*. Oxford: Blackwell Scientific Publications, 1976, p44ff.

CHAPTER FOUR

Healers and their Society

JOHN ELLARD

Human beings are not well designed and are poorly constructed. At best they fail structurally or functionally after a few decades; at worst they do not function at all. Manifestations of disintegration or of dysfunction appear long before the end. Worse, they damage themselves or attack each other, producing injuries or an untimely finish. They must be refuelled and emptied with great frequency; if these operations are not carried out correctly they malfunction and may die.

These are the disorders which confronted our ancestors and confront us now. Some attempts at repair may be instinctual; their limits are obvious. Thus dogs lick their wounds but there are no canine veterinarians. Here we are concerned with mankind's attempts to repair itself, and—where possible—defer death. We shall call that treatment. We shall not consider the further ambition—to live forever in one form or another. It preoccupies many still; the results of their endeavours are not easy to evaluate.

We are very complicated creatures and the probability is that the desire to heal arose before there was any understanding of how we are constructed and how we work. The universe at large presented exactly the same difficulty; it too needed management. There were storms to be tamed, droughts to be broken: how was it all to be done? This is a familiar situation with a customary solution: when confronted with a resistant mystery mankind turns to magic.

We have reason to believe that in that early world, spirits—good and bad—were thought to be everywhere and to control everything. There are some who believe this today. Therefore all disasters—earthquakes, droughts, accidents and diseases—were due to the malfeasances of evil spirits. The only hope of appeasing them lay in prayers, incantations and sacrifices, for these practices were thought to be pleasing to spirits. It would be even more advantageous to be able to communicate directly with the entities controlling the universe. Still to be found in some cultures are shamans—men and women who are believed to have this power. They are not merely medicine men, but pathways to the hidden secrets of the universe. Finding the way was made easier by anything which overturned the normal functioning of the brain; thus exhaustion, sensory deprivation, persistent strong rhythms and hallucinogenic drugs all had their uses and in some cultures still do.

Specialisation set in early and continues. Thus Sigerist[105] records that the Havasupai of Arizona had 'three types of medicine men—one who has power over the weather, one who cures diseases and one who treats wounds, fractures and snake bites'. In our community now we have clergymen who confine themselves to spiritual matters and others who conduct healing ceremonies.

Even in a world dominated by magic there were some observations of fact to be made. A broken leg has a bend in it which should not be there—reference to the other leg establishes that. Common sense would suggest that a good strong pull would straighten it out and that if it persisted in bending it would be rational to tie it to a straight stick until it mended itself. Skeletons last a long while; there is evidence to suggest that this was done.

It is difficult to know when observation and reason became firm partners of magic and faith. As we shall see they are neck and neck now.

Magic and science at the dawn of writing

We have an important insight into what happened. It is impossible to put a firm date to the beginning of writing for at first there were no sharp boundaries between pictures, tally marks and signs made to represent sounds. But we know from the reporting of a particular event that there were medical treatises some 5000 years ago. The Pharoah Neferirkere was congratulating his chief architect Weshptah on the construction of a new building and became alarmed when he could not respond. Priests and physicians were summoned and the Pharaoh had brought to him a 'case of writings' to assist them.[106] It may be that amongst the writings in that case was the surgical papyrus of which the Edwin Smith papyrus[107] is a later copy.

The Edwin Smith papyrus was put down by a Theban scribe some 3700 years ago. On the front the scribe copied a surgical text which was then probably more than 1000 years old; its language was archaic and difficult for him. The text began with disorders of the head and proceeded logically downwards through the body. For some long forgotten reason the scribe stopped in the middle of a case and turned the papyrus over to copy a series of incantations about pestilence, and other magical remedies as well. Miraculously it was preserved and we have it today.

The surgical cases are arranged logically. The clinical features of each are described, as is the examination. Then a diagnosis is made and treatment prescribed unless recovery cannot be expected. If that is so the surgeon states it. It reads like an educational text and is in no way alien to modern readers. The medical procedures on the back of the papyrus are incantations and petitions to the gods. There is no hint of science.

The importance of the Edwin Smith papyrus is that it demonstrates that thousands of years ago, at the beginning of written history, treatment rested upon both science and magic. We shall need to reflect upon how true this is today and upon why this is still the case.

Ancient Egypt also had its medical bureaucracies. There were specialists (e.g., 'guardian of the anus') and there were grades of physicians. They were Physicians, Chief of Physicians, Inspector of Physicians, Superintendent of Physicians, and Greatest Physician of Upper and Lower Egypt. There was also the 'Administrator of the House of Health and Chief of the Secret of Health in the House of Thoth.'[108] We still have these medical bureaucracies.

We have other relics of the past as well. Quite often some well meaning person in modern times is struck by the great insight that it would be better to prevent diseases than to treat them after they have arrived. Amulets, fetishes, taboos and dietary rituals have been used for this purpose since time immemorial; some of these practices are founded upon good observation. Variolation was practised in Africa and Asia in the seventeenth century; Western medicine got there later.[109]

Galen: a scientist made into an authority

The growth of what we might call scientific medicine continued into the second century AD. Galen (AD 130–200) is an important figure. On the one hand he used experiment to advance knowledge and on the other he (and Aristotle) were to be promoted by the forces of religious conservatism as authorities whose words must not be questioned.

One of Galen's experiments will suffice as an example. Until his day it was believed that since speech came from the chest, the chest must be the centre of thought. The heart was the likely source. Even today one 'speaks from the heart'. Galen, observing the results of cutting the recurrent laryngeal nerve—deliberately in pigs, by accident in man—demonstrated that respiration went on unimpeded but phonation was much damaged. The brain, not the heart, was the source of the mind.[110]

He wrote extensively on treatment, being primarily concerned with antidotes not only against poisons but against all diseases. He noted that even in his day prescriptions were badly written so that many errors were made in transcribing them.[111]

Galen referred to one form of investigation not uncommon in the ancient world. Two centuries previously Mithridates VI, King of Pontus in Asia Minor, devised many antidotes and tried them out on prisoners. Pompey, who defeated him in 66 BC, found in his palace a notebook written in Mithridates' hand with the recipes for many such prescriptions. Translated, they reached Galen.[112] They were still famous and used almost 2000 years later.

After Galen the light of enquiry slowly darkened in Western culture and the forces of conservatism reigned. For them scientific enquiry is anathema, for it may discover a fact which would disturb the status quo. Galileo was made to realise that.

During those dark years the physicians of Islam continued to experiment and to extend such knowledge as there was. In addition they preserved, translated and in many cases improved upon the classical writings which we might have lost without their efforts. They too were limited by religious scruples. Since both autopsy and dissection were forbidden they did not anticipate the great anatomical discoveries which began in the sixteenth century.

Their respect for treatment can be seen in that pharmacy first became a separate profession in the Arab world. Their pharmacopoeia was in two parts; the first comprising compound medicines, the second medicines directed towards the treatment of each part of the body.

The Renaissance, which began in the fourteenth century, was in medicine a curious mixture of the old and the new. On the one hand Galen was rediscovered and revered. On the other the antidotes which began with Mithridates and Galen—Mithridatium and Galene—were looked at critically. They had been supposed to be effective agents against every poison and disease but had not been of much use against the Black Death. Nevertheless they survived in the Pharmacopoeia of the Royal College of Physicians of Edinburgh until 1756 and of the Royal College of Physicians of London until 1788.[113] The extract of viper or lizard remained a component until the last.

After the Renaissance came the Enlightenment. In the eighteenth century evidence and enquiry began to challenge dogma and belief and medicine began to move slowly towards what we see now. Before science overwhelms us it is time to look more closely at magic and see what its powers are.

The power of the mind

Two hundred years ago when physiology was still understood in terms of the rising and falling of the humours of the body (as believed by

Galen) Franz Anton Mesmer—a scientist, not a physician—wondered how he might influence their movements and so produce benefits in the treatment of diseases. The movements of the humours were thought to be determined in part by the movement of the moon and the planets. He decided to try the effects of magnets and was gratified to discover that some patients seemed to benefit from his laying them in certain places.

Pursuing his experiments, he made the surprising discovery that non-ferrous objects produced exactly the same results as the magnets. Reflecting on this he saw that the common element was himself—he placed the objects where they were, therefore the curative force must lie within him and not within the objects.[114]

He had, he believed, discovered a new form of magnetism—animal magnetism. Remember that he was a scientist and not a doctor. Now turn your mind to an operating theatre in the eighteenth century. There were no effective anaesthetic agents; limbs were amputated, breasts removed and other major procedures performed as rapidly as possible while the patients were restrained forcibly. The agonies endured are almost beyond our comprehension. By 1840 animal magnetism had excited an enormous amount of interest in Britain, Europe and the United States. Cures of all kinds were reported and there had been several Royal Commissions and similar inquiries by learned bodies.[115]

One anecdote will illuminate what was happening. In 1842 James Wombell, a 42-year-old labourer in Britain, had his left leg amputated above the knee. He was put into a mesmeric sleep and the operation— an unusually protracted one—was performed.

> During the operation Wombell moaned a little as if in a troubled dream, but gave no other sign of pain. The moaning did not increase when Ward thrice touched the divided end of the sciatic nerve. After the operation Wombell blessed the Lord to find it was all over and stated that he had felt no pain. He made a good recovery and survived for more than thirty years.[116]

To put it shortly, some hundreds of painless operations were carried out thereafter using the same principle, with no rise in pulse and no experience of pain. There were expert observers on many occasions. There was no hard science in it but the benefits were enormous. This was treatment at its best.

Not only were the patients spared from agony but the method used was simple and without dangerous side-effects. Let us avoid a very complicated argument and attribute the results to suggestion. If suggestion can produce results of that magnitude it is difficult to know where its limits may be. More than that, it is important to discover where suggestion is operating, for it could be that the more difficult and spectacular the procedure the greater its psychological impact.

For example, some 30 years ago, before the development of the modern operations on the heart and its arteries, it was believed that if a surgeon opened the chest and tied off a particular artery which ran down inside the chest wall—the internal mammary artery—the blood supply to the heart was increased, with great benefit to the patient. In support of this, some 40 per cent of those who had received the operation reported that they were improved.

Then the surgeons operated on a series of patients, making the same incision on each of them, tying off the artery in some and leaving it intact in others. Those patients whose arteries were still intact (which fact they did not know) reported the same amount of improvement as those whose arteries had been tied off.[117] The operation was abandoned even though it had produced the significant belief in improvement. In these days of informed consent it would be impossible to conduct such an experiment so we do not know how much suggestion contributes to the results of some of the more recently devised operations. Objective tests will show blood flowing in arteries where it did not flow as well before the operation but this is not quite the same as the patients' evaluation of the benefits that they have received.

There are still arguments about the contribution that suggestion makes to medical and surgical treatment overall. In some cases—such as serious infections—scientifically based treatment will be of the greatest importance while in others suggestion may provide a large part of the benefit. Since there are many serious conditions it is important for treating doctors to have a firm and up-to-date grasp of what can be achieved by scientific medicine. This is not to say that they should ignore suggestion for, as we have seen, it can improve the patients' sense of well-being very greatly.

Although suggestion can produce remarkable results it has its limits. It has been remarked that though a shrine may exhibit crutches discarded by those who no longer need them, one does not find artificial limbs abandoned by those who have grown new ones.

Any system of medicine which disregards science or disregards suggestion is incomplete and will not meet the needs of some of those who come for help. This is a major issue right now.

The growth of scientific medicine

The growth of scientific medicine in the last century has been awesome. Living human brains can be seen in great detail and the mechanisms of the whole brain or its parts monitored as they occur. To put it shortly, the structure and function of the body can be examined now in life with little risk and modest discomfort to the patient. The details of the biochemistry, the arrangements and disorders of genes, and the microscopic structures of the organs are now accessible in a way unimaginable when I was a medical student. The exploratory operation is virtually a procedure of the past.

The benefits of these advances are obvious. Breast cancers can often be detected while they are still curable and cancer of the cervix would almost be eliminated if women were examined early enough and often enough. The principal arteries of the body can be seen more clearly in life than they are at autopsy, for their flow is both visible and audible. No system escapes the prying eye of the investigator.

The changing role of the doctor

When doctors had little scientifically based treatment to offer, their efforts were mainly limited to reassurance and the use of traditional remedies. Some of these remedies were very powerful. Withering learned of digitalis when investigating a cure for the dropsy, long kept secret by an old woman in Shropshire.[118] Some remedies were dangerous, such as bleeding and the deliberate production of an abscess to let the 'bad' out. Scepticism began late—if one reads Heberden published in 1802[119] one is struck by the number of treatments then in existence for all sorts of diseases and Heberden's often reiterated opinion that the treatment in question had little or no value in spite of its reputation to the contrary.

At an accelerating pace in the last century doctors have had more proven treatments available to them and therefore, at least in some diseases, a secure knowledge of what to do and what the results will be. Also accelerating is the amount of knowledge about those treatments, investigations necessary to establish which will be appropriate, and the possible undesirable consequences of using them.

There are now more than 100 000 medical journals. Granted that there is much repetition and that some of them are so specialised that few beside their authors can understand them, nevertheless the amount of knowledge required of the ordinary practitioner is daunting. More than this there are peer review committees, quality assurance mechanisms and complaints commissions to make sure that their knowledge and their use of it is up to the mark.

A natural consequence of this is that when doctors are confronted with a patient their minds turn towards establishing as precise a diagnosis as possible and instituting the logical therapy. Modern patients are better educated and much less inclined to accept authority than once they were and quite reasonably want to know what is wrong with them, what can be done about it and what the possible outcomes are.

Very often the patients are sent off for complicated investigations. Even the simple ones—such as a chest x-ray—can be associated with much anxiety. There is the fear of the outcome—what will it show? —and the unfamiliar environment. One must remove some of one's clothes and maintain what is often an uncomfortable position while one's body is firmly applied to a cold table. Meanwhile half-seen people move about and do mysterious things. Colonoscopy is both uncomfortable and undignified, and MRI can produce claustrophobia even in the stout-hearted.

Then one returns to the doctor who instigated these ordeals to be told the result, which will often threaten experiences which are even worse. This is a marked contrast to the procedures of a few decades ago when the diagnosis was reached by a detailed physical examination and a simple blood test. There is no doubt at all that diagnoses reached by today's methods are much more likely to be correct but one cannot be surprised if patients felt much more comforted by the slow hands-on personal approach than is the case now where doctors spend a few minutes setting up disagreeable experiences for you and later on a few more minutes telling you the bad news and what comes next.

Treatment would require a book in itself. True it is that modern surgical techniques have made many operations less painful and less formidable but they are still a far cry from having nothing done at all. Again the prognosis for some cancers is much better but the chemotherapy and radiotherapy can produce ordeals of their own. Even when nothing more than medication is offered many people are very anxious about their adverse effects—sometimes with good reason.

To generalise, doctors have no option but to make use of modern technology and therapeutics and as a result their image has changed. No longer are doctors kindly people who examine you and carefully reassure you and then prescribe some simple treatment. No longer do they have the time—nor in many cases, the inclination—to deal with the anxieties and emotional needs which could be dealt with before. Nowadays you are much more likely to remain alive; the price is often an unsatisfied need for magic.

The future

We have seen that in the past many forces have determined the nature of medical practice and that scientific knowledge is but one of them. If we can combine that realisation with what we can observe today then perhaps we can make some predictions about what will happen in the next few decades. The auguries are not good.

First there are some wild cards which may turn up at any time and change things greatly. It can be argued that the most successful form of life on earth are the bacteria. They have been here since the beginning and are still doing very well. It seems possible that they may exist in other worlds as well; perhaps they came here as space travellers. Viruses are no less successful. It is always possible that a mutation will produce another and much worse Black Death. We have seen what HIV can do: next year we may be attacked by a more virulent organism spread by the droplets we disseminate when we speak and sneeze. It should be noted also that bacteria and micro-organisms generally are getting the measures of our antibiotics. It is not as easy to treat pulmonary tuberculosis as it once was.

Enormous sums of money are spent on searching for a cure for cancer. So far the results have been patchy. Imagine that someone discovers a final common path in the genesis of all the cancers and the cure arrives. The impact on medical services would be enormous. Great enterprises devoted to researching the disease and others specialising in looking after the sufferers would become redundant. The sufferers would survive to die from other disorders. The facilities which exist for the care of the aged are inadequate now; it would be optimistic to believe that the money saved by the cancer cure would be directed towards their improvement.

The final outcomes of successful ventures in prevention are also difficult to predict. Prevention can certainly be effective, as we have seen in the case of smallpox and poliomyelitis. It can also be difficult to achieve when the knowledge is there, as in the case of malaria and cancer of the lung.

Outcomes can be more complicated than one might imagine. What would happen, for example, if not only the malignant effects of smoking tobacco became universally understood but that as a consequence everyone stopped smoking. It has been shown that since a substantial proportion of smokers die young, and die rapidly, there is a net saving of public money. They do not survive to die from prolonged and complicated diseases and they do not require old-age pensions. More than this, tobacco attracts a variety of taxes and is an important source of income for governments, as well as many large corporations. If everyone stopped smoking taxes would rise, bankruptcies would occur and medical facilities would be even more overloaded than they are now.

If all this seems fanciful, reflect upon the fact that every now and then Earth collides with an asteroid: remember the dinosaurs.

Social forces

Social disorder can also make prediction very difficult. At the end of the second millennium central Africa is in chaos; who knows what the world will be like at the end of the third? What will happen in those regions where it can be predicted water will begin to run out early in the next century? There can be no compromise about an insufficiency of water.

Some social changes are visible now. In a number of developed countries the middle class is contracting and one can see the emergence of two classes, the rich and the poor. In Britain, wages for the lowest paid hardly changed from 1978 to 1992 while those of better paid workers rose up to 50 per cent.[120]

> In 1993 the top 20 per cent of US households received 48.9 per cent of the total income, whereas those in the bottom 20 per cent shared only 3.6 per cent. Between 1991 and 1992, 1.2 million more Americans became poor for an estimated total of 36.9 million citizens living below the federal poverty level.[121]

Changes such as this are in part a product of the naive belief that if one removes all government controls then the economy will burgeon and everyone will benefit. The reality is that some will be much better off and some will be worse. If we project this tendency into the reasonably near future then we might predict that there will be the rich, who will be well looked after and the rest—an underclass—will be lucky to get their basic needs.

Alternative medicine

One might expect that as the benefits of scientific medicine become more widely known people would be more inclined to entrust their health and their future to medications and procedures which have been carefully tested under controlled conditions. The evidence suggests otherwise.

A large survey conducted in South Australia in 1993 involved 3004 interviews with persons aged 15 years or more.[122] The survey found that 48.5 per cent of the total population had used at least one non-medically prescribed alternative medicine. By far the most common medicines taken were non-prescribed vitamins. The significance of this figure is not as straightforward as one might think. For example, at present there is no certainty about the value of vitamin E in the prevention of cardiovascular disease. It is harmless and cheap; it is not irrational to take it. However something like one in ten took herbal medicines, mineral supplements and homoeopathic medicines where faith might seem to be more important than logic.

It was estimated that the Australian population was at that time spending a little under one billion dollars each year on alternative medicine and alternative practitioners.[123] Of this total it was estimated that $621 million was spent on alternative medicines: this contrasts with $310 million of patients' contributions for all pharmaceutical drugs purchased in 1992–1993. (It will be understood that much more than this was spent on pharmaceuticals; the $310 million is the amount that came directly and immediately out of people's pockets.)

The Australian experience is not unique. In the United States, where the general practitioner does not have such a central role as is the case in Australia, one study[124] found that more visits were made to alternative practitioners than to all the United States primary care physicians.

The reasons for the use of alternative medicines are not completely clear. It is certainly not that those using them lack education. There is anxiety about the dangers and side-effects of conventional medicine and a recognition that in certain disorders it is ineffective. There is a belief that alternative medicine involves the whole person, which belief is more likely to be based on the personality of the therapist and the time taken with the patient than the particular remedies used.

To put it shortly, we still have a dichotomy as marked as that revealed in the Edwin Smith papyrus and there is no reason to believe that there will be much change from this state of affairs.

Other professionals

As the techniques of medical care become more complicated other professionals become more involved. Nurses, psychologists, social workers, pharmacists and many others have a more prominent role in the system than used to be the case. The same blurring of boundaries is happening within the medical profession—procedures once carried out only by surgeons are now performed by physicians and radiologists.

The doctor's ability to act autonomously, or even to be the leader of the team, is more and more under challenge. Doctors are often surrounded by a horde of administrators, ethicists, lawyers and regulatory persons and bodies. In 1968 hospitals in the United States employed 435 000 administrators and clerks while handling an average daily patient load of 1.4 million. In 1990 the clerks and managers totalled 1.2 million and the patient load was 853 000.[125] I was reminded of this when, on a recent visit to the large public hospital in which I was trained, I was informed that as wards were closed and emptied of patients because of a shortage of funds they were turned into offices for more administrators. I do not believe that doctors should be able to act as they think fit but I fear that the day will come when it will be difficult for them to act at all.

Litigation

This is a difficult area. Medical judgments and procedures can be difficult and complex. The most skilled and conscientious practitioners do not get everything right every time. More than that, there are times when doctors cannot avoid making decisions even though there are not enough data available to make a properly based judgment. The risk of doing nothing may be greater than the risk of doing something; action cannot be avoided.

Later, after the die is cast, and the result is evident, a court which has the great advantage of knowing the final outcome may spend a leisurely week or two examining a decision which a doctor had to take in the middle of the night. It is not difficult to be both wise and critical under these circumstances. On the other hand there is no doubt that there are doctors who are incompetent, corrupt, unscrupulous or all of those things. There are others who because of impairments of one kind or another should not be practising or should be practising under strict conditions. There must be checks on medical practice and redress for those patients who suffer because of factors such as these.

The problem is to decide how this is to be done.

In Australia the courts have decided that they, and not the medical profession, shall determine what the proper standards of conduct and medical practice shall be. This has left us with some curious results, with the courts restoring to practice some doctors whom their peers thought should be excluded, and the courts embracing some clinical procedures in the teeth of professional opposition.

Even worse, juries have the power to make decisions on scientific questions—such as the complications of certain medications and surgical procedures both when the evidence does not exist to sustain a proper decision or when the evidence points in exactly the opposite direction. Worse still—particularly in the United States—they can award enormous damages which seem to have little relationship with anything in the real world.

There are many consequences. One is that fewer and fewer practitioners are prepared to practise obstetrics, for only too often it is believed that if a perfect baby is not produced then it must be the fault of the doctor. It may be apocryphal but I was told some time ago that a bumper sticker could be seen in the United States which read 'If

you want your baby delivered, see your attorney'. Not only does litigation drive doctors away from some essential procedures but it makes
medical practice much more expensive. Expensive tests are done to
exclude rare possibilities. It has been held that it is negligent not to
refer a patient with a particular disorder to someone more knowledgeable than oneself, even if that person is some hundreds of kilometres
distant. Since most of us concede that we are not at the absolute top
of the tree in anything one must wonder where it will all end.

Medical indemnity insurance becomes progressively more expensive. Doctors must recover this from the patients they see, for they
have no other source. How much patients have benefited from all this
activity is difficult to estimate. As we look into the future it seems that
it is more likely that things will get worse than that they will get better.

Avoiding trouble

If the trends that we can see now continue to operate we can guess
how medical treatment might be conducted in perhaps 50 years time.
First of all it will be necessary to avoid being in the underclass; how
to achieve that I must leave to the readers' imagination.

Then your disorder must fall within one of the defined diseases managed by your health care organisation. The final decision about that
will not be made by your doctor but some sort of generic health professional who may be in another city or even another country.[126]

Having achieved a diagnosis, you and the person caring for your
health—whoever and whatever he or she may be—will be controlled
by a program which states that for a particular disease certain specified services will be available for a limited number of days. If after
that number of days you have neither recovered nor died then obviously either you or your medical carer are not conducting yourselves
properly and there will be no more money for treatment.

Needless to say there will be penalties for both participants. What
they will be in the future is difficult to say but what they can be now is
quite clear. *The Wall Street Journal* of 31 May 1996 reported that under
the provisions of the Kennedy-Kassebaer Bill passed by the Congress
there can be a five-year prison sentence for the patient who neglects
to mention a pre-existing condition, no matter how trivial it might be.
For doctors, the fine for making an incorrect billing code is US$10 000
($A12 700).[127]

On the other hand the rewards can be great. The Chief Executive
Officer of US Health Care has a salary compensation package and stock-
holding totalling US$783 million;[128] there are others as well above the
$100 million mark per year.

A final word

What then of the future? The history of medicine reflects the history of mankind and we can conjecture that the same themes will be projected into the future as long as *homo sapiens* is about. The original author of the Edwin Smith papyrus, looking about him, could have surmised that the need for both magic and careful observation which existed then would persist for a long time. Five thousand years later there is no need to alter this prediction.

Again, in the days of the Pharaohs, there were masters and slaves, rich and poor, hierarchies and elites. We still have them and I cannot imagine them going away. Never has there been an equitable distribution of medical services. There is much talk about it now but I do not know where it is to be found. As the diagnosis and management of disease becomes more complicated and expensive I cannot imagine the future succeeding where the past has failed. Those who believe that the day will come when the poor and disadvantaged will receive exactly the same medical services as the rich and powerful can believe anything.

Certainly the means will exist for a proportion of the total world population to live longer and better than has ever been the case before. An inspection of the current state of affairs, country by country, suggests that those who receive those benefits should count themselves fortunate. It will be a great day when the human genome project is completed and the mysteries of our heredity are unravelled. Who knows which other diseases will join smallpox on the list of those defeated? For a large proportion of the world's population it will be a miracle when they have access to clean running water and efficient treatment of their common infections.

To be a doctor is to be immersed in the human condition and all its vicissitudes. It is a turbulent domain in which there is anguish and triumph, rescue and loss. Over the millennia, science and professionalism have served us best, with kindness and suggestion as admirable handmaidens. Paradoxically the successes of medicine are threatening its destruction. It remains to be seen whether the current invasion of those from other fields will provide its salvation or a cure worse than the disease.

REFERENCES

105. Sigerist HE. *A history of medicine. Volume I: Primitive and archaic medicine.* Oxford: Oxford University Press, 1951, p171.
106. Sigerist HE. *A history of medicine. Volume I: Primitive and archaic medicine,* ibid, p300.

107. Breasled James Henry (ed). *The Edwin Smith Papyrus:* published in facsimile and hieroglyphic transliteration with translation and commentary in two volumes. Chicago: University of Chicago Press, 1930.

108. Sigerist HE. *A history of medicine. Volume I: Primitive and archaic medicine,* ibid, p321.

109. Sigerist HE. *A history of medicine. Volume I: Primitive and archaic medicine,* ibid, p150.

110. Galen. *On the usefulness of the parts of the body.* Translated from the Greek by May MT. New York: Cornell University Press, 1968, p63.

111. Watson G. *Theriac and mithridatium. A study in therapeutics.* London: The Wellcome Historical Medical Library, 1966, p7.

112. Watson G. *Theriac and mithridatium. A study in therapeutics,* ibid, p35.

113. Watson G. *Theriac and mithridatium. A study in therapeutics,* ibid, pp145–50.

114. Gauld A. *A history of hypnotism.* Cambridge: Cambridge University Press, 1992, p3.

115. Gauld A. *A history of hypnotism,* ibid, pp25–38.

116. Gauld A. *A history of hypnotism,* ibid, p220.

117. Frank JD, Frank JB. *Persuasion and healing,* 3rd edition. Baltimore: The Johns Hopkins University Press, 1991, pp135–6.

118. Withering W. *An account of the foxglove and some of its medical uses.* Birmingham: Swinney M, 1785; p2.

119. Heberden W. *Commentaries on the history and cure of diseases.* London: Payne T, 1802.

120. Thomas P, Romme M, Hamelijnek J. Psychiatry and the politics of the underclass. *Bri J Psychiatry* 1996; 169: 401–4.

121. Bassuk EL, Browne A, Buckner JC. Single mothers and welfare. *Scientific American* 1996; 275: 36–40.

122. MacLennan AH, Wilson DH, Taylor AW. Prevalence and cost of alternative medicine in Australia. *Lancet* 1996; 347: 569–73.

123. Maclennan AH, Wilson DH, Taylor AW. Prevalence and cost of alternative medicine in Australia. *Lancet* 1996; 347: 569–73.

124. Eisenberg D, Kessler RC, Foster C. Unconventional medicine in the United States. *New Engl J Med* 1993; 328: 246–52.

125. Greenberg DS. Safe targets: fraud and paperwork. *Lancet* 1993; 342: 670.

126. Bodenheimer T. The HMO backlash—righteous or reactionary? *New Engl J Med* 1996; 335: 1601–3.

127. *Australian Doctor,* 26 July 1996, 104.

128. Nader R. *ABC Health Report,* 11 December 1995.

CHAPTER FIVE

Choices in Health

IAN WEBSTER

'Our purpose is to enlarge human freedom—to set people free,
so far as we can, from the disability and suffering that so easily
mar their lives and hamper their fulfilment'.[129]

In the 1970s community health and medicine were new ideas. The
new academics at that time had aspirations which are now the preoccupation of their successors. Social issues, poverty and illness,
population ageing, impairment and disability, prevention, the need for
support services, de-institutionalisation and the need for a social justification of the use of expensive resources were on their agenda.[130] The
boundary between technical decisions and social objectives in health
was a problem then, and is of greater magnitude and even more pressing now.

The welfare of people

No medical textbook has isolation or loneliness in the index, yet both
engender health problems and affect outcomes. Textbooks of psychiatry eschew the social conditions of patients, and the commonplace views
of mental illness,[131] as if the mind is not only separate from the body
but separate from the social world as well. Medical students are taught
to look for one disease to explain the patient's symptoms. But many
patients bring life predicaments, social and material circumstances and
not one but a set of diseases to the consultation. Can decisions about
a person's welfare[132] be made without cognisance of these factors? To
exclude contextual and non-medical factors, and to isolate the parameters for clinical decisions to those which are manageable medically,
diminishes the efficacy of treatment—at least in the eyes of the patient.

In health, choices are made at two levels—health policy and clinical
practice. Public decisions can affect patient care, and the sum of individual patient care decisions can influence public welfare. A decision
now is not an event isolated and disconnected from other choices. There
are antecedent events, preceding decisions and a context with inputs

and a set of potential impacts. It is a process that combines scientific data, values and evaluation. Any choice will involve appreciating the evidence, weighing options, adoption of a course of action and evaluation of outcomes. Appreciation involves fact and value, as do all health and medical decisions.[133] They are multi-valued choices and involve different ways of seeing (appreciating) the situation and a process that anticipates and balances the range of potential outcomes. That is the art and science of clinical practice.[134]

The medical and health professions are expected to act ethically, making decisions which are essentially other-centred in clinical and public health circumstances. In health care Alistair Campbell considers that medical ethics refers to whether health care actions are right or wrong, or whether relationships are good or bad in an objective sense.[135] In a democracy competing claims are reconciled and public choices are publicly accountable. Public health decisions involve multi-valued choice and are therefore political. Bernard Crick said:

> In politics, not economics, is found the creative dialectic of opposites: for politics is bold prudence, a diverse unity, an armed conciliation, a natural artifice, a creative compromise, and a serious game on which free civilisation depends.[136]

The implications of this reasoning is that partisanship can be set aside in an other-centred ethos. It is a naive idea as governments turn to the market for social and economic policy, through which competing needs and claims are to be rationed. The ethos of competition is being transported from business to health care as the instrument of efficiency. But it does not mean that this public good should be jettisoned in favour of banal competition simply because it is naive.

How then can clinical decisions be 'other-centred' and concerned with the person's welfare? With this objective, treatment will aim for an acceptable level of physical and social functioning, not only to overcome disease or to correct injury. That will be possible when consumers and professionals better understand the limits of medical treatment. As hospital admission rates rise, medical visits and costs increase, the dynamics of the demand for treatment sets an agenda for over-utilisation and a psychology of aggrievement for people whose demands are not met.

Welfare and the community

WHO promulgated a view of health in 1946 as:

> a state of complete physical, mental and social well-being, and not merely the absence of disease and infirmity.[137]

The word 'infirmity' has the quality of disability and in turn reflects function. Health is also about the response to change, expectation and adaptation. It is a life trajectory, in which 'disease' represents departures from the trajectory. Diseases are artefacts on the changes of development and ageing. Others see health as a relative concept,[138] akin to the idea that poverty is relative deprivation and not an absolute state.[139]

At another level, health may be understood as a means to achievement,[140] fulfilment and ultimately of survival. A person's health enables them to function physically and emotionally in a particular community. This is in line with the idea that health is a resource for everyday life. These concepts are appropriate to health promotion since to achieve health, people need food, a certain level of education, relationships with other human beings, and housing, in addition to determinants in the environment and heredity and access to health services.[141]

Lindstrom, a Norwegian sociologist, has outlined a framework for quality of life based on the spheres and dimensions of life and personal freedoms.[142] Since these constructs embrace subjective experience and personal perceptions it offers a framework for collective health that is more comprehensive than usual measures of public health. In addition it includes the community valuation that is needed in choices for public health.

Table 5.1 Quality of life[143]

Spheres	Dimensions (objective/subjective)	Examples
Global	1. Macro environment 2. Human rights 3. Politics	Clean environment Democratic rights Culture
External	1. Work 2. Economy 3. Housing	Employment Income Type of housing
Interpersonal	1. Family 2. Intimate 3. Extended	Structure and function of social relationships
Personal	1. Physical 2. Mental 3. Spiritual	Growth, development activity, self-esteem, meaning of existence

Thus material circumstances are not the only pillar on which community well-being is founded, but includes the other half of the Cartesian dichotomy—a collective sense of mental health. Indeed, the prerequisites for mental health are key conditions that will promote health as a whole. Jahoda has said:

> When individuals are assured good conditions for mental health, they will also be able to improve their quality of living.[144]

The public's health is not sufficiently described by the epidemiology of disease, it needs also to include a wider range of factors relevant to health.

Table 5.2 Three components of quality of life[143]

Objective conditions	Preferences	Subjective perceptions
Global, external, interpersonal, personal.	Freedom of choice, solidarity, to read, to exercise, to participate in politics, to play music, to contemplate, to relax.	Perceived satisfaction of objective conditions (happiness, general satisfaction).

In the democracies interest groups make claims on the community's resources. The political process encourages the expression of these interests and through politics they are reconciled. In the delivery of health services and promoting community health, choices occur at a number of levels. The important point is that citizens are able to provide input at a number of points and health service managers and professionals have defined opportunities to contribute, as illustrated in the table below.

Table 5.3 Points of input to decisions

Choices	Level of decision	Public input/access
Allocation of state resources, direction and priorities	Political/government	Democratic processes, parliamentary debates
Health priorities	Regional community, management professionals	Boards of health, health councils or advisory groups
Quality of outcome	Service directors, consumers, professionals	Management, consumer and professional advisory groups

The argument so far has been that health is served when open processes foster accountable policy decisions. This assumes that a consensus is possible or indeed exists on the quality of life and how it is to be maintained.

Causes of dislocation

Both in clinical and public health practice, health problems can be constructed from different frames of reference. In discovering causes, the perspective of the inquirer will define the variables and the relationships analysed. In public decision-making, different communities will have different priorities and see health problems in different ways.

The student in pathology soon learns that the disease found at autopsy differs from diagnosis in life. At the time I studied pathology, the discrepancies were most obvious in kidney disease. The pathophysiology of kidney disease was being unravelled with immunological techniques and electron microscopy. These were more accurate descriptions except that the physicians still diagnosed the syndromes of nephritis type I and type II which were poorly correlated with these findings. The correlation between the diagnosis of pneumonia and post-mortem findings was similarly poor.

These issues of construct, of how disease occurs and how to act in clinical situations are bound up with the way health and disease is described and analysed. Much of the thinking assumes there is one cause and one action, when in reality there are often multiple causes, and systems of causation, as well as proximate and distant causes.

The concepts of disease causation and nature, especially a unitary as distinct from multi-causal view, have a profound influence on the decisions in clinical medicine and public health.

Common sensibility

In spite of criticisms of the medical consultation, the relationship, or its variants, is the basis for personal health care. To the interaction between doctor and patient, the patient brings their previous experience, and the physician knowledge, 'medical rules' and experience of similar health problems. The matching of 'medical rules' to life circumstances involves a multi-valued choice which typifies much of clinical practice. The majority of medical interactions require that the doctor and patient understand what is happening and what will happen following a particular course of action.

Given that there are risks in the disclosures made in a medical consultation, it is remarkable that it is so accepted. Symptoms are recounted and detail explored. The person is physically examined: clothes are removed, the person is touched, stethoscopes and clinical instruments used. Differences in social class are accommodated. In this ordered relationship there is a level of personal trust and disclosure. At the same time the interaction aims to maintain emotional distance. The ritual is known and expected. From the patient's point of view the process offsets the risks in disclosure. However, in modern medical practice this trust may not survive.

Medical discourse drives towards certainty and reduction of ambiguity. The language is precise and focussed. The frameworks of technology, objective data and economics mean there is pressure on clinicians to exclude from their interactions with patients, their common sensibilities. The art of conversation, the use of eyes, hearing, touch and smell seem to be undervalued in this context. Ordinary people, too, put their faith too often in test data rather than their own senses.

The medical record becomes a catalogue of bare and efficient facts. The question is whether this is as efficient as it appears, or whether it effectively describes the evolution and nature of health problems.

The hospital grand round reifies these styles. Here we see the upcoming doctor performing before his/her seniors and peers. A performance is judged to be good if it involves a difficult case—one that has a plethora of data, conflicting evidence, an uncertain diagnosis and a rare condition. There is a staccato of fact, images and challenges. When the young doctor appears confident, precise and speedy the performance is praised. Yet it is the opposite characteristics, which are so lacking in modern health care, which should be encouraged and rewarded.

Medical decisions are often taken in situations where the diagnosis is uncertain. Time during which change can be observed is a key parameter to appreciate the evolving disease and its urgency. Time is at a premium and fragmentation of the elements of health care mean that continuity is easily broken.

In the time-urgent health service there is little room for stories (see Chapter Seven 'Reason and Emotion in Medical Ethics'). Wanderers waste time. Does it really matter where this person is from? Their roots? Their life trajectory? Their predicament? These questions are seen to be redundant in an environment of economic choice. The evolving sequence of 'disease', the patient's investment in their condition and their background takes a back seat to 'hard' data. To discover the patient's disease is more important than to discover who the patient is. Perhaps this exploration is the province of psychiatry, but here too, the social circumstances come second to psychic phenomena.

The 'story' in the medical history is the metaphor for 'other centredness'. In old age, in the dislocation of homelessness, in migration, these 'other person' attributes assist the doctor to appreciate the patient's predicament. Their actions and preferences are better understood then.

There is a recent trend for guidelines for clinical management to be promulgated but implementation is patchy. For effective implementation, local ownership of the process is needed in which the unique aspects of settings and communities can be taken into account.[145] The guidelines for clinical conditions are usually based on data obtained from large scale studies which do not incorporate the variation in settings and the personal characteristics of primary care and general physicians. Neither do these studies follow the natural history of disease and the interaction of patients with treatment plans.[146]

In old medical texts disease was compellingly described; the language full and evocative. Could it be that these pictures helped the clinician come to terms with uncertainty? The person's syndrome, albeit non-specific, could be matched with the textbook account and some certainty attained. To say the diagnosis was mucous colitis when in truth diarrhoeal disease was poorly understood and the cause unknown, allowed the doctor and patient to reach some common ground and comfort for dialogue (see Chapter Fifteen, 'The "Disease Model" Challenged').

In a paradoxical way our ability to characterise the minutiae of disease has decreased the capacity to cope with uncertainty and to communicate this to patients.

Subjective health/illness

Much of the work in health care is with symptoms unrelated to pathology. Such subjective experience is difficult to validate but the physician is expected to respond to the patient's distress. When symptoms recur or are unrelieved the physician is faced with a sense of failure, frustration and anger. This is common with chronic pain syndromes such as recurrent headaches, back and lower abdominal pain and in sleeplessness.

Table 5.4 Parsons' model of sickness roles in addiction

Usual sickness role	Sickness role in addiction
Exemption from social responsibilities.	Reinforces social withdrawal.
Illness a legitimate basis for exemption.	Addiction is defined as an illness.
Not held responsible for the outcome so long as he/she is a 'good' patient; relapse is accepted.	Addicts are unpredictable and revert to previous patterns of drug use.
No blame.	Highly blameworthy.
Desires to be well.	Addiction is less hurtful than the real world.
Medical treatment is sought and the patient is co-operative.	Medical treatment is sought to maintain addiction. Compliance is problematic.

The dissonance that can develop between doctor and patient is illustrated in addiction. Parsons' model of sickness helps to understand this type of interaction.[147]

Addiction

The behavioural and sociological aspects of addiction mean that conventional disease models fall short and more appropriate models are required. Some current alternatives are based on minimisation of harm, managing relative risks and containment of behaviour. These management strategies are especially important in dealing with the health problems of illegal drugs.

Drug addiction demonstrates starkly the range of value judgements in clinical management and in public policy. The diverse elements of the definition of alcoholism are illustrative:

> Alcoholism is a primary chronic disease with genetic, psychosocial, and environmental factors influencing its development and manifestations. The disease is often progressive and fatal. It is characterised by impaired control over drinking, preoccupation with the drug alcohol, use of alcohol despite adverse consequences, and distortions in thinking, mostly denial. Each of these symptoms may be continuous or periodic.[148]

Addiction disrupts the functioning of the person and the underlying disorder persists for a long time with ready relapse to active drug taking. The drugs activate neuronal circuits that reinforce behaviour and involve motivation as well as powerful emotions. Like other chronic diseases addiction requires lifelong treatment. It has a multi-factorial aetiology—heredity, childhood and development, exposure to risk factors and lifestyle—as do other chronic conditions.[149]

Compared with those who suffer from diabetes, hypertension and asthma, addicted persons are believed to have brought the condition upon themselves. But the spectrum of influences is not widely different. There are non-voluntary factors, such as peer pressure, availability and advertising to promote substance use. Vulnerability may in part be genetic. The initial psychological response of pleasure, at some point moves beyond misuse to addiction.

The conundrum of issues in the clinical management of addiction is mirrored in the confusion of values and ambivalence in the community about drug abuse.

The problem is seen in different ways. The moral/legal view defines drug abuse as a legal, ethical or religious matter. The health approach includes drug abuse as a disease suitable for treatment. It may be seen as a psycho-social phenomenon of dysfunctional individuals and in socio-cultural terms it may be defined as a problem of society.[150] The first two constructions imply the problem should be controlled or eradicated. In the other two, drug abuse is considered to arise from the needs of individuals or of society[151] in which underlying causes have to be corrected.

The dissonance in values is no more evident than in the illegal status of certain drugs such as the narcotic analgesics and the legal status of other addictive drugs such as alcohol and tobacco. When certain drug use is defined as a problem of law enforcement, police will act economically. Their efforts are to drive up the price which, it is conjectured, will reduce demand. In a suburb of Sydney, Australia, the Bureau of Crime Statistics and Research found 'the rate of arrest from heroin use and/or possession exerts no effect on street-level price of heroin or on the rate at which heroin users seek methadone treatment'.[152] That is, police action had no effect on price and availability. On the contrary, intravenous drug use becomes urgent and unhygienic with increased exposure to blood-borne viruses.[153] The street level police action has the social costs of increased health risks to users and the local community.

In developing drug policy the views, social values and human rights within the community have to be reconciled with the facts of epidemiology, known public health risks and potential benefits of interventions.

Homelessness

In a book on clinical ethics Jonsen et al. observe:

> The ethics of any case arises out of the facts and values embedded in the case itself. Ethics is not added to a clinical case by imposing on it some alien principles or values. Clinical ethics is a discipline that provides a structured approach to decision making that can help a doctor identify, analyse, and resolve ethical issues in clinical medicine.[154]

Patient care is a personal interaction located in an institutional setting within resource constraints and social circumstances. These characteristics are crucial in clinical decision-making. The health problems of disadvantaged people illustrate this particularly, for example, among the urban homeless.

Like disease, homelessness has many causes. There are societal causes—lack of affordable housing, high unemployment, mal-distribution of work opportunities, social inequality and poverty. There are individual causes—physical and developmental disability, physical injury and chronic disease; and a set of proximate factors—alcohol and drug use, injury, sickness, onset of mental illness, family break-up, death of a parent or loss of a job.

This is a transient state for some people, for others it is long-term. Young people cycle through the scene, and there are the less visible women and families. Males, rural people, itinerant workers, immigrants, illiterate people and people with disabilities are over-represented. Some live on the verge, in inner city boarding houses and single rooms. In 'skid row' areas violence, poverty and health risks are endemic. The doss houses and hostels are impersonal, overcrowded and alien places.

Life is short. In 1994 the age-adjusted mortality for 6308 homeless persons in Baltimore was four times that of Philadelphia's general population.[155] A study in New York City found:

> Diseases of the extremities were 14 times higher; neurological disorders were six times higher; liver diseases were five times higher; nutritional disorders were four times higher; acute respiratory conditions were four times higher; teeth and mouth disorders were four times higher; infectious and parasitic diseases were two to three times as common; venereal diseases were two to three times as common; blood diseases were two to three times as common; eye and ear diseases were two to three times as common; gastrointestinal conditions two to three times as common; skin conditions two to three times as common; and, trauma two to three times as common; than in a demographically matched sample of urban respondents in the National Ambulatory Medical Care Survey.[156]

Not only is the severity and incidence of disease in this group important but the multiplicity of problems, their interactions and context are predominant factors in any choices to be made. Multiple problems create special needs, since each social program defines the limits of its eligibility and excludes other needs. These additional needs compound as homeless people are rejected when they do not fit through the gate. The person may have both a mental illness and a large hernia, have problems with alcohol and at the same time be breathless, require a disability pension but need treatment which is unobtainable. A cycle of rejection is established.

Medical management in these people illustrates the ethics of choice. In terms of the patient's preference, the patient may not want to follow advice, such as to go to hospital. The patient may be confused by mental illness and have no real preferences. They may prefer to stay where they are—in their home as they see it. They may want to continue drinking. The assessment they make of their quality of life will differ from the physician's assessment. Life is harsh and a small change may represent a large gain for them.

There are few options in the environment of 'skid row', few options for treatment, and for accommodation and support. The essence of choice in these circumstances is a balance between what is possible and what people will accept. The medical 'rules' have to be reconciled with the hope of achieving an optimum quality of life, which for the homeless is very different from those who are well fed and housed.

Governments have a role to assist those who suffer misfortune. Public programs are based on social values which may conflict. For example, in the environment of a teaching hospital, the homeless person will be treated like anyone else for their medical condition. A king—for a day! Medical need is the primary goal. If you speak to the doctors and nurses they feel proud of what they do.

But outside the hospital different values prevail. Does this person qualify for income support, for a sickness or disability benefit, housing and primary medical care? Access to these programs is through eligibility criteria defined in Acts of Parliament or regulation. In social security, access is through economic need; in compensation through cause and damage (e.g., work injury); in rehabilitation, potential for work; and, education and training through merit.

Contrast these with the essential value underpinning health care—medical need. Medicine can respond to the needs of the most disadvantaged individuals when the goals are humanitarian and focus on medical need. When other values of a utilitarian nature are added, the needs of marginalised groups are compounded and less likely to be met. Choice is indeed multi-valued in this environment.

In sum, choices in health are multi-valued choices. They involve appreciating the evidence, decision, action and evaluation of outcomes. These choices are rarely unitary. The values which individuals and the community bring to a health problem or issue need to be reconciled with the scientific rationale for intervention through processes which are honest and open to scrutiny. That is the art of good medicine and politics for public health.

REFERENCES

129. Fox Theodore. The purposes of medicine. *Lancet* 1965; ii: 801–5.
130. Webster IW. Where healing starts. In: Walpole R (ed). *Community health in Australia*. Melbourne: Penguin Books, 1979, pp37–52.
131. Patel V. Recognition of common mental disorders in primary care in African countries: should mental be dropped? *Lancet* 1996, 347: 742–44.
132. Welfare is used to denote qualities of well-being.
133. Vickers G. *Value systems and social process*. England and Australia: Pelican Books (Penguin), 1970, p198.
134. Vickers G. *Value systems and social process*, ibid, p132.
135. Campbell AV, Higgs R. *In that case: medical ethics in everyday practice*. London: Darton, Longman & Todd, 1982, p2.
136. Crick B. *In defence of politics*. Harmondsworth, England: Penguin Books, 2nd Pelican edition, 1983, p161.
137. World Health Organization (WHO), preamble to the WHO Constitution, 7 April 1948. In: Hobson W (ed). *Theory and practice of public health*, 5th edition. Oxford: Oxford University Press, 1979, p763.

138. Downie RS, Fyte C, Tannahill A. *Health promotion models and values*. Oxford: Oxford University Press, 1990.
139. Townsend P. *Poverty in the United Kingdom: a survey of household resources and standards of living*. Harmondsworth, England: Penguin Books, 1979.
140. Seedhouse D. *Health and the foundations of achievement*. New York: John Wiley, 1986.
141. Davy J, Parker R., Patterson J. *Personal and community health*. Melbourne: Heinemann Educational, 1992.
142. Lindstrom B. Measuring and improving quality of life for children. In: Lindstrom B, Spencer N (eds). *Social paediatrics*. Oxford: Oxford University Press, 1995, ch 35, p575.
143. After Lindstrom. Measuring and improving quality of life for children, 1995, ibid, p575.
144. Jahoda quoted in Lindstrom B. Measuring and improving quality of life for children, 1995, ibid, p574.
145. Grimshaw JM, Russell IT. Effect of clinical guidelines on medical practice: a system review of rigorous evaluations. *Lancet* 1993, 342: 1317–22.
146. Noble J. Influence of physician perceptions on putting knowledge into practice. Commentary in *Lancet* 1996, 347: 1571.
147. Parsons T. *The Social System*. London: Routledge and Kegan Paul, 1951.
148. Meyer RE. The disease called addiction: emerging evidence in a 200-year debate. *Lancet* 1996, 347: 162–6.
149. O'Brien CP, McLellan AT. Myths about the treatment of addiction. *Lancet* 1996; 347: 237–40.
150. Brown VA, Manderson D, O'Callaghan M, Thompson R., *Our daily fix: drugs in Australia*. Canberra: Australian National University Press, 1986, p54.
151. Nowlis H. Prevention is not easy. In: Drew LRH, Stolz P, Barclay W (eds). *Man, drugs and society—current perspectives: proceedings of 1st Pan-Pacific conference on drugs and alcohol*. Canberra: Australian Foundation on Alcoholism and Drug Dependence, 1981, pp218–22.
152. Weatherburn D, Lind B. *Drug law enforcement policy and its impact on the heroin market*. Sydney: NSW Bureau of Crime Statistics and Research, 1995.
153. Maher L. personal communication.
154. Jonsen Albert R, Siegler Mark, Winslade William J. *Clinical ethics: a practical approach to ethical decisions in clinical medicine*. New York: McGraw-Hill, 3rd edition, 1992.
155. Hibbs JR, Benner L, Klugman L, Spencer R, Macchia I, Mellinger MD, Fife D. Mortality in a cohort of homeless adults in Philadelphia. *New Eng J Med* 1994, 331: 304–9.
156. Wright JD, Weber W. *Homelessness and health*. Washington, DC: McGraw-Hill Healthcare Information Centre, 1987, p103.

SOME UNDERPINNINGS

CHAPTER SIX

Cartesian Thinking in Health and Medicine

MILES LITTLE

'He regarded the bodies of men and animals as machines. . . .'
Bertrand Russell.[157]

Introduction

I t may seem curious, particularly to the general medical reader, to present an extended examination of the philosophical and scientific thinking of a man dead for nearly 350 years. Yet Descartes' name resonates with associations in a way which distinguishes him from almost any other philosopher.

While few non-philosophers can say what distinguishes the thinking of Socrates, Plato, Aristotle, Francis Bacon, Hobbes, Locke, Hume, J.S. Mill, Hegel or Nietzsche, most can repeat the Cartesian slogan *Cogito ergo sum*; most know that Descartes constructed an intellectual system on that slender foundation; some know that he was a founder of rationalism, a great mathematician and a less successful natural scientist. Many will also know that critiques of Descartes have dealt harshly with much that he proposed. Most non-philosophers will feel that what he did was a long time ago, and that it has been passed over in modernity because we know and understand more than he could, given the context of his time. This is not quite the case. The influence of Cartesian thinking has been immense, and continues to be so. Admittedly, we may now think that Descartes erred in his ontology, epistemology, logic, physiology and psychology—which only leaves his mathematics intact. And yet, a modern commentator could write:

> Descartes—like other philosophers whose works continue to repay study—altered the problem space of philosophy in such a way that his failures bequeath problems that take their peculiar shape only against the background of his enormous success.[158]

How can this be?

75

To understand the peculiar impact of Descartes and his work, we need to understand the intellectual climate of his times; what he did to change that climate; what intellectual processes and constructs he bequeathed to Western philosophy; how these have affected scientific thinking, particularly in medicine; what shortcomings these bequests may have; and what we, his successors, may have to do to rectify those shortcomings. In order to do these things, we will need to cover both familiar and unfamiliar intellectual ground.

A brief biography

René Descartes was born in 1596 at La Haye, near Tours in France. The details of his early life are imperfectly known, but he certainly attended the Jesuit school of La Flèche in Anjou, regarded by Descartes himself as one of the best schools in Europe. There he studied classical literature, rhetoric and history, and later mathematics, moral philosophy, theology and 'natural philosophy' or physical science. Jesuit scholastic pedagogy was dominated by Thomist theology and Aristotelian logic, ethics, metaphysics and natural philosophy, and Descartes absorbed what he was taught, though he was later to react against it in radical ways. He graduated in law from Poitiers and then started to travel in Europe. He spent time in army service, but continued his philosophical meditations. In 1619, in a cold room in Bavaria, he conceived the ambitious scheme of alone reconstructing the basis of philosophy. He travelled widely in Europe after leaving the army in 1619. A Dutchman, Isaac Beeckman, introduced him to the precision and completeness of mathematical ways of thought, and this interest Descartes developed throughout his life.

The understanding that mathematics brought made Descartes aware that the metaphysics he had learnt from the Jesuits was flawed because its foundations were open to doubt. His recognition of the importance of the scientific observations and methods of Galileo confirmed his view that the logic of mathematics should set the agenda for philosophical inquiry. At the same time, the condemnation of Galileo by the Congregation of the Holy Office in 1633 disturbed Descartes, and influenced his own decisions on publication of material which might have run counter to conventional theology.[159] The profound scepticism of Montaigne about the scope of human reason probably also had a significant influence on Descartes.[160]

Descartes settled in Holland in 1628, and lived there for most of the rest of his life. In 1643, Cartesian philosophy was condemned by the University of Utrecht. In 1644, he returned to France, and was awarded a pension by the King of France in 1647. In 1649, he moved to Sweden on the invitation of Queen Christina. He died of pneumonia in Stockholm in 1650.

This very bare account of his life gives no measure of his achievement, nor of his influence. We need to inquire further about the intellectual context of the times and the ways in which Descartes rejected and refashioned it.

The intellectual context

Descartes was quite clear in stating the ambitions of his project. He found philosophy in a state of confusion and weakness, particularly the scholastic philosophy he learnt from his Jesuit teachers at La Flèche. In a letter to Mersenne, he wrote:

> I do not think that the diversity of the opinions of the scholastics makes their philosophy difficult to refute. It is easy to overturn the foundations on which they agree, and once that has been done, all their disagreements over detail will seem foolish.[161]

This is a useful starting point from which to examine the discourse that Descartes developed, because it has to be seen in this context of rejection. What follows must necessarily be incomplete and fragmentary, and does little justice to the richness and complexity of major thinkers and intellectual movements.

Galileo and the new science

Galileo Galilei epitomises the scientific challenge to theological authority in the late sixteenth and early seventeenth centuries. He lived between 1564 and 1642, and expressed the new interpretation of nature that came from observation and experiment, rather than reliance on the systems of received philosophy. He challenged the authority of Aristotle by claiming that mathematics lay at the heart of natural science or physics. He championed Copernicus' heliocentric theory. He was also a convinced atomist, a point of view that was seen by the Church to be incompatible with the doctrine of the divine presence during the Eucharist. His letter to the Grand Duchess Christina of Tuscany sets out in blunt terms the distinctions that he sees between theology—the 'Queen of the Sciences'—and the physical sciences.

> I think that in discussions of physical problems we ought to begin not from the authority of scriptural passages, but from sense-experience and necessary demonstrations.[162]

It is quite clear that Descartes knew and approved Galileo's work, although his reference to it in 'The Discourse on the Method' is guarded.

> I will not say that I accepted this theory, but only that before their condemnation I had noticed nothing in it that I could imagine to be prejudicial either to religion or to the state, and hence nothing that would have prevented me from publishing it myself, if reason convinced me of it.[163]

In this very brief and incomplete overview, I have tried to introduce the background to Cartesian thinking, which, for various reasons, needs to be seen in its historical context if we are to understand its impact and its shortcomings.

What is Cartesian thinking?

The method which Descartes evolved for the physical sciences can be seen as a reversal of the process suggested by Francis Bacon. For Bacon, the scientific method involved the derivation of general laws by inductive ascent from less general relations. The Cartesian process is one of descent from foundational certainty to conclusions deduced from this secure proposition. Such a method presupposes a commitment to the Aristotelian ideal of a deductive hierarchy of propositions, but at the same time it can be seen as the foundation of scientific modernity.

Descartes published widely. His most enduring works are 'Rules for the Direction of our Native Intelligence', 'Discourse on the Method', 'Meditations on First Philosophy', 'Objections and Replies', 'Principles of Philosophy', 'Comments on a Certain Broadsheet', 'The Passions of the Soul', 'Geometry and the Optics'. Most of these are published in *Descartes: Selected Philosophical Writings*, translated by Cottingham, Stoothoff and Murdoch,[164] and the page numbers mentioned in the footnotes refer to this edition, unless otherwise specified. A complete collection of the works in three volumes is also available from the same translators,[165] but I have been sparing in my references to it because it is less readily available.

Descartes was determined to reform philosophy, and he was determined to achieve the reform by himself, feeling that one man could produce a more coherent and functional system than could many men. Because Descartes had come to distrust what he had learned from the Jesuits, and perhaps because he was influenced by Montaigne's scepticism, he developed his 'method of doubt.' It is worked out at some length most explicitly in the 'First Meditation' in 'Meditations on First Philosophy'.[166] Descartes begins by admitting that everything that he experiences may be part of a dream or even a deception planned and perpetrated by God. Worse still, sense experience may be the deception of a malicious demon, whose stratagems are deliberately designed to ensnare the judgment. There can be no proof that these arguments are false, so that sense experience cannot provide a foundation for a philosophy. In order to do that, Descartes proposed to clear away from his mind all the knowledge and beliefs accumulated over his lifetime, and to find a certainty from which to build anew. This process anticipated Husserl's similar method of phenomenological reduction, by which conventional views, judgments and values are systematically 'bracketed' and removed from the object of examination, and Husserl acknowledges the debt.[167]

But on what could Descartes depend? His solution came from recognising the experience of thinking. The person thinking has proof of his own existence. No matter how distorted the thinking might be made by malicious demons, the act of thinking proved that the thinker existed —*Je pense, donc je suis*, or *Cogito ergo sum*.[168] This was, for Descartes, a certainty and a starting point from which to build a system. But it still did not guarantee that sense perceptions were not the product of a malicious demon, and something more was needed. The turn which Descartes took to find a way from subjective certainty to a scientific system depended on the existence of a good and benevolent God, who would guarantee the truth of reason and perception. Very briefly, Descartes fashioned this proof of God's existence from finding that he had ideas of perfection beyond his own attainments, and that he saw some truths 'clearly and distinctly.'[169] These ideas and recognitions must come from somewhere, and presumably from a being that can only be God. Furthermore, since God is the sum of all perfections, and existence is a perfection, God must exist.[170] With these proofs, Descartes hoped to establish God as guarantor of the truth of sense experience. He hoped, in short, to establish, with his foundationalist *Cogito* and his benevolent God, a method of proceeding with rational thought, based upon a rule 'that everything we conceive very clearly and distinctly is true.'[171] But how was the philosopher to proceed from this base? The answer to this, Descartes thought, lay in mathematics.

The influence of mathematical thinking

Mathematical process seemed to Descartes to offer something therapeutic to philosophy. In 'Rules for the Direction of Our Native Intelligence', for example, he writes:

> I came to see that the exclusive concern of mathematics is with questions of order or measure and that it is irrelevant whether the measure in question involves numbers, shapes, stars, sounds, or any other

object whatever. This made me realise that there must be a general science which explains all the points that can be raised concerning order and measure irrespective of the subject-matter, and that this science should be termed mathesis universalis . . .[172]

And in 'Discourse on the Method' he writes:

Those long chains composed of very simple and easy reasonings, which geometers customarily use to arrive at their most difficult demonstrations, had given me occasion to suppose that all the things which come within the scope of human knowledge are interconnected in the same way.[173]

We can see that Descartes' method involves both foundationalism and rationalism. The reasoning that was to lead from the undoubtable foundations was to be linear and reductionist. The reductionist program was clearly stated in the rules set out in 'Discourse on the Method of Rightly Conducting One's Reason and Seeking the Truth in the Sciences':

The first was never to accept anything as true if I did not have evident knowledge of its truth: that is, carefully to avoid precipitate conclusions and preconceptions, and to include nothing more in my judgments than what presented itself to my mind so clearly and distinctly that I had no occasion to call it into doubt. The second, to divide each of the difficulties I examined into as many parts as possible and as may be required in order to resolve them better. The third, to direct my thoughts in an orderly manner, by beginning with the simplest and most easily known objects in order to ascend little by little, step by step, to knowledge of the most complex, and by supposing some order even among objects that have no natural order of precedence. And the last, throughout to make enumerations so complete, and reviews so comprehensive, that I could be sure of leaving nothing out.[174]

In a strict sense, Descartes could be seen as setting out to derive physical laws from metaphysical principles. His scientific methodology was a variety of the hypothetico-deductive method, as Losee has pointed out.[175] It had, as we shall see, many shortcomings as a method for the physical sciences, but made a major contribution to abstract mathematical thinking. Gaukroger writes that Descartes:

provide[s] us with the first explicit epistemological and metaphysical basis for a mathematical physics in the history of philosophy, and in many ways its role in Descartes' thought is more central than even the *Cogito*.[176]

The program for the physical sciences and its problems

Descartes' new program for the physical sciences began with his conception of the tree of knowledge, a model which claimed metaphysics as the roots, physics as the trunk and the applied sciences, like medicine, as the branches.[177] Central to his program was his understanding of matter as whatever has extension. Matter in these terms became *res extensa*, which could be entirely accounted for by specifying size, shape and the motion of its particles. This was clearly a reductionist and atomistic conception of the ontology of matter. Physical existence must be mathematically expressible, and for this reason mathematics must be central to any theories of physical existence. The Cartesian system is generally deemed to be the paradigm of rationalism, of deductive reasoning from a metaphysical certainty.

Descartes revealed a marked preference for analytical thought over synthetic thought, and we will encounter this preference later. While it is certainly true that Descartes worked by deduction from his metaphysics, it is also true that he saw the value of observation and experiment. Further, he saw that empirical evidence became more important the further the rationalist program progressed. In the Discourse, for example, he wrote:

> I also noticed, regarding observations, that the further we advance in our knowledge, the more necessary they become.[178]

Faced with a realisation of the indeterminacy of explanatory hypotheses in science, he seems to anticipate some aspects of the modern experimental method. He writes, for example, that the choice of hypothesis must be made:

> by seeking further observations whose outcomes vary according to which of these ways provides the correct explanation.[179]

At this point, he seems to come close to the positivist theory of verifiability as criterion of truth. Descartes was an early champion of Harvey's theory of the circulation of the blood, and obviously respected the way in which that theory had been tested by observation and experiment.[180]

It is also clear that he carried out dissections and observations himself. His description in 'Discourse Five of the Optics' gives explicit instructions for the performance of dissection of

> the eye of a newly dead person (or failing that, the eye of an ox or some other large animal) . . .[181]

in order to conduct an experiment to demonstrate the function of the lens of the eye in producing an image of external objects on the back of the eye.

Descartes was determined to banish certain Aristotelian concepts and terms. These included the substantial forms, real qualities, vegetative and sensitive souls and vital powers which Aristotle invoked to explain the nature of existence and the phenomena of life. Descartes' views were strictly positivist in the domain of physical matter. Bodies, including human bodies, were made of res extensa, and that was all. He dismissed material falsity 'which occurs in ideas, when they represent non-things as things.'[182] The vegetative and sensitive souls he claimed to be able to explain mechanistically.

But materialism of this kind posed many problems. Setting aside the difficulties it contained for physiology and psychology, there remained serious objections in the domain of the physical sciences. By insisting on the centrality of extension as defining substance, Descartes seemed to be denying any force or power in matter in and of itself. God became a necessary part of Descartes' system as the 'primary cause of motion', and motion became essential to Cartesian physics:

> All there is in body is extension, and the only way that bodies can be individuated from one another for Descartes is through motion.[183]

And motion for Descartes meant local motion from one place to another and every place between, rather than the motion accepted by the scholastics, which covered every type of change in place, shape or time. Descartes motion was motion in a straight line, and it was determined by the total amount of motion God had given to the totality of matter at the Creation. These metaphysical and physical principles were, of course, to be challenged radically by people like Newton, Leibniz and Hume in the next century. We shall not consider his physics further, except insofar as we need it to examine some of the thinking he produced about the way that humans function in both their physiology and psychology.

The dualism of mind and body

To animate the substance which was the animal body, Descartes needed a second principle—the soul. Mind and spiritual soul are not clearly separated in this model. Soul is to be seen as an antithesis to material body. Body is extended, spatial and divisible. Soul must therefore be unextended, indivisible and non-spatial. It can only be conceived as incorporeal and self-existent, capable of existing without body. The difficulty for this dualistic conception of the relationship between mind and body lies in explaining how corporeal and inert matter can be moved by incorporeal, unextended soul. This is the problem highlighted by Gilbert Ryle's famous term 'The ghost in the machine.'[184] Descartes was able to explain that the nerves, which were considered all to be both afferent and efferent, could produce physical effects on the motor arm and conduct sensory impulses on the sensory side. This he managed by postulating hydraulic transmission, and 'animal spirits' that were moved with the transmitted fluids.[185] The motive power in the brain was the pineal gland, whose movements caused the fluids to move. But this still did not explain how the insubstantial soul could actually interact with body. This problem was never satisfactorily resolved. It led to the development of occasionalism, particularly at the hands of Malebranche, who postulated that all causation was divinely mediated, God producing the cause on each occasion by his intervention. Despite the logical and conceptual difficulties, mind-body dualism has remained influential to the present, and we will return to its problems when we consider specifically the impact of Cartesian thinking on medical thinking.

The influence of the Cogito

Cogito ergo sum is so familiar that few people stop to consider what it implies beyond its simple existential statement. It legitimises the subjective. Montaigne had turned to himself as a source of experience and doubt, and shown that his ruminations could engage thoughtful readers. But he was not a systematic philosopher. Descartes, on the other hand, turned inward to establish his foundation in certainty, and then built a system from a slender metaphysical base. But this manner of proceeding has its paradoxes. The conscious world is still private, and self-reflection is not seen to have the certainty of physical science. Nor can we be absolutely sure that it is possible to communicate subjective experience, although Wittgenstein would say that we can in ordinary language,[186] and Husserl has dwelt at length on the possibility of achieving intersubjectivity.[187] Further, Descartes spent a good deal of time explaining how uncertain subjective experience could be, and denying that it could be used as a reliable source of belief.[188] This ambivalence toward the validity of the subjective has persisted to our day, and we will discuss it further.

The dualism of facts and values

Descartes' insistence on measurement and mathematics, on strict reductionist method and on the simplicity of matter led to another dualism, between facts and values. In this particular sense, he can be seen as a powerful influence on the British empiricist movement. We know, for instance, that Locke was influenced by Descartes, although he disagreed strongly with many details and principles.[189] This same dualism can be seen in the work of the Viennese school of logical positivism, which held that mathematics and science were epistemically valid because their material was studied objectively and their conclusions were 'verifiable'. Metaphysics and ethics, in this belief, were not worth discussing because their contents could not be tested in the same way. The logical positivists also held that analytical statements (those whose truth is contained in the terms used) were the most powerful statements to be made, and that synthetic statements (those which are inductively true by virtue of the way the world is) could at least be confirmed or denied by objective observation. Descartes also preferred analysis to synthesis. This preference is clearly stated in the 'Objections and Replies':

> Synthesis . . . is not as satisfying as the method of analysis, nor does it engage the minds of those who are eager to learn, since it does not show how the thing in question was discovered.[190]

While Descartes' usage of these terms is probably somewhat idiosyncratic, his drift is clear, and he certainly held that in his mathematical method, solutions to problems were all that mattered, without further comment or deductive inference. Indeed, it seems that he actively opposed deductive inference, on the grounds that it could never have epistemic value.[191] By taking this stance, as Leibniz was to point out, Descartes cut himself off from a major source of enrichment because:

> in the synthetic or deductive presentation of results in mathematics we set in train a systematic structuring of and extension of knowledge which enables gaps, difficulties, flaws, etc. to be recognised, precisely identified and solved.[192]

This insistence on excluding deductive inference from the realm of abstract mathematics, on the methods of which Descartes proposed to develop his philosophy, seems strange when we read in the 'Rules for the Direction of our Native Intelligence' that:

> Deduction . . . remains as our sole means of compounding things in a way that enables us to be sure of their truth.[193]

Whatever Descartes may have meant by these apparently contradictory statements, his influence within the fact-value dichotomy has been powerful and enduring.

The Cartesian legacy in medicine

The Cartesian program was explicitly anti-Aristotelian. It was designed to remove the need to postulate the nature of man as composed of the four elements of earth, fire, air and water and expressed as the four humours of bile, black bile, phlegm and blood. It could not, however, eliminate concepts like 'animal spirits', a term that Descartes uses frequently in 'The Passions of the Soul'. The program was meant to be therapeutic in ridding philosophy of speculative forces and ideal forms. But there is far more to Descartes' program than the mere elimination of outmoded concepts. Physicalism (or materialism) is the first enduring Cartesian legacy. Hatfield remarks that:

> Considered systematically, Descartes' aim was to mechanize virtually all of the functions that had traditionally been assigned to the vegetative and sensitive souls.[194]

The vegetative soul had been supposed to govern growth, nutrition and reproduction; the sensitive soul sensation, appetites and movement. The rational soul had to be saved as the source of intellect and will. The rational soul allowed to the human—but to no other animal—a capacity to choose and to accept or reject the promptings of the vegetative and sensitive souls. The mechanisation of the vegetative and sensitive souls had profound implications. Certain types of behaviour and response to stimuli left the domain of the soul and became part of the domain of matter and the mechanical body. In 'The Passions of the Soul', Descartes writes:

> Thus every movement we make without any contribution from our will —as often happens when we breathe, walk, eat and, indeed, when we perform any action which is common to us and the beasts—depends solely on the arrangements of our limbs and on the route the spirits, produced by the heat of the heart, follow naturally in the brain, nerves and muscles ... Having thus considered all the functions belonging solely to the body, it is easy to recognize that there is nothing in us which we must attribute to our soul except our thoughts.[195]

It required little for this assertion to become the credo for behaviourism.

Mind-body dualism has been immensely influential and persistent in psychological thinking. The concept of mind as something unextended and privately contained within a material body lies at the centre of the metaphysics of the behaviourist psychologists. If the mind is private and inaccessible, then all that we can do is to record and theorise about what we can objectively observe in human behaviour. This metaphysical view was perhaps most marked in the work of Skinner[196] and his followers, but has persisted at least as far as the work of Bruner[197] and Miller.[198] An acceptance of the inaccessibility of the mind is also present in the work of Freud, although in a different form. For Freud, the mind is also inaccessible to the owner of the mind, until he seeks help to interpret what is buried in that mind.[199] There is an increasing realisation that such models are too restrictive, and that personal development within language by experience and interpretation of modes of discourse may give a better picture, but argument persists to this day.[200]

The second legacy is reductionism. Reductionism may be seen to exist at three levels. Ontological reductionism is concerned to reduce explanatory entities to a minimum. In doing away with vegetative and sensitive souls, Descartes was clearly trying to work parsimoniously. Similarly, his insistence on matter and soul as the only elements necessary for an explanatory system indicates the same devotion to reduction. Methodological reductionism seeks reduction to the smallest possible explanatory unit, to genetic explanations. In describing his method, Descartes repeatedly emphasises the value of splitting complex problems into constituent parts, and seeking to explain the parts. Finally, there is theory reductionism, which claims that old theories can be accounted for—as it were, deductively deduced—from new theories. Thus, Descartes claimed to account for the actions of the vegetative and sensitive souls in Aristotle's model with his mechanical theory of bodily functions.

The Cartesian program is very strongly reductionist in its orientation at all three levels, and reductionist science can be seen as stemming from his program. Reductionist methods have also dominated medical practice and research for more than 200 years. Indeed, in medicine, the conception of illness as disorder of one part of the bodily machine still dominates thinking.

There can be no better example of reductionist thinking than the huge international effort to map the human genome. This program is thought to hold the promise for a unified model which will reconceptualise human disease, its prevention and treatment. It represents reductionism at all three levels—ontologically, by promising a fundamental particulate origin of health and disease; methodologically, by providing truly 'genetic' explanations of human functioning and malfunctioning; and at the level of theory by explaining everything that older theories sought to explain.

There are other medical conceptions that may owe much to Cartesianism. The medical desire to rely only on those things that can be 'clearly and distinctly' perceived is evidenced by the conviction that objective tests are better than subjective impressions, even when the impression seems to tell us something important.

We tend to dismiss complaints of pain if we can find nothing in the material body to explain the subjective sensation of pain. We assume that this is a disorder of the 'soul' or the psyche as we might call it today. The status of suffering is problematic in the Cartesian system. Suffering must be done by the soul, but only the body can become sick. Dualism of this kind allows us easily to justify ignoring suffering on the grounds that fixing the machine will fix the suffering. Oddly, Descartes seems to have recognised that this was not always so, and he quotes with interest anecdotes of phantom limbs,[201] whose presence the person continues to feel after the limb has been amputated. The fact-value dichotomy has spilt over into many areas, and the weakening of a concept of soul, with its overtones of divinity, has had many implications for medicine. The preferred status of 'organic' illness, the devotion to a material model of human health, the high status of research which draws on the physical sciences and the suspicion with which value-laden judgements are greeted, all owe their existence to the Cartesian preference for reductionism, analytical thinking and mathematical abstraction.

The last 200 years have seen medicine move from its base in the wisdom of its best practitioners to the science of the Cartesian tradition. It hardly needs saying that the science of medicine has brought great richness and genuine progress in the understanding and treatment of disease, as Descartes said it would:

> It is true that medicine as currently practised does not contain much of any significant use; but without intending to disparage it, I am sure that there is no one . . . who would not admit that all we know in medicine is almost nothing in comparison with what remains to be known, and that we might free ourselves from innumerable diseases, both of the body and of the mind, and perhaps even from the infirmity of old age, if we had sufficient knowledge of their causes and of all the remedies that nature has provided.[202]

The rhetoric of this claim has remained a part of the rhetoric of medicine from Descartes' day to ours.

The Cartesian shortfall

Descartes' work attracted critics even during his own lifetime.[203] The critiques need not concern us too much. It is enough to say that there were those who recognised the logical problems of God's existence which was fundamental to Cartesian metaphysics; those who attacked him on theological grounds; others, like Hobbes and Gassendi, who criticised his resort to dualism. Spinoza and Leibniz felt that Descartes' foundationalism had failed. Leibniz was particularly critical of the Cartesian criterion of truth (that which I perceive clearly and distinctly) which he took to be meaningless unless clarity and distinctness could be defined. He was also strongly critical of Descartes' physics, which was indeed full of errors. Locke attacked Descartes for his dogmatism.

In modern terms, however, many of these criticisms have little relevance. We may be less concerned with the theological implications of the Cartesian program and the detail of his physics; but we are the direct inheritors of some aspects of the method of doubt, and of Cartesian dualism, materialism and reductionism. The method of doubt still underpins modern scientific method. Merton, in his examination of the sociology of science, concluded that 'organised scepticism' was one of the norms which defined scientific endeavour.[204] This implied that scientists will accept only that which can be objectively confirmed, which will, in other words, satisfy the current criteria for clarity and distinctness. Even our statistics are governed by scepticism. We test the null hypothesis, designing our studies with the sceptical idea that our hypotheses are most likely to be wrong. Type II statistical errors acknowledge that this sceptical premise may lead us into error when the hypothesis is falsely disproved. This may be mathematically sound, but it enshrines scepticism, and commits investigators to a negatively critical view of their own work and the work of others.

Dualism and materialism

Dualism in modern thought permeates much of what we do. The mechanistic account of body allows powerful science and objective observation into medicine, but sequesters the mind to another domain. 'Proper medicine' and psychiatry are, in many minds, divorced from one another. The weakening of the concept of soul leaves mind as another entity, and the behaviourists have attempted to model the mind as an almost wholly determined function of material body. Mind, in their view, was inaccessible to study. Its manifestations in behaviour were observable and provided the only key to the mental processes. Behaviourism is losing its influence today, but it has been powerful, and there are still those who distrust 'qualitative' research which depends on judgment and other subjective phenomena. Further, there is still a tendency to objectify illness, and to define it in material terms by images and measurements, rather than by the suffering it causes to individuals. There is another subtle way in which dualism influences our patterns of thought and action. Descartes recognised the need for something other than body to account for intellect and will, and he used soul to solve his problem. His reasoning about soul was characteristically dualistic. If material body was extended, bounded and solid, then soul must be all the things that body is not—that is, it must be unextended, unbounded and insubstantial. This dichotomous reasoning still dominates Western dialectic.

An imperfect state of health has perfection as its counterpole, rather than a better state of health. The WHO definition of health, as 'a state of complete physical, mental and social well-being, not merely the absence of disease or infirmity' expresses this polarity. Since up to 95 per cent of adults experience symptoms in any two week period,[205] the definition seems to express an unattainable, even transcendental, conception based on dichotomous or dualistic thinking. Dualism implies black or white, not shades of grey, and it is shades of grey which actually describe the human condition.

Reductionism

Of all Descartes' achievements, reductionism has been the most influential and persistent in science and the applied sciences. It is a foundation of much modern scientific method, and is still strongly influential in medical thought. Ontological reductionism is expressed in the devotion to the structural explanation of disease; methodological reductionism by the search for further explanations at the level of the molecule and the gene; and theory reductionism by the way in which we assimilate teleological explanation into genetic explanation—for example, the way we assimilate classical descriptions of inflammation into the cellular and subcellular levels of infection. Medicine in practice and in research is reductionist, and reductionism has enabled the extraordinary developments of scientific medicine over the last 200 years.

But reductionism has its weaknesses. Reductionism in science assumes 'bottom-up' causation—that is, it assumes that ultimate causes can be found at the lowest levels of physical structure, the molecule, the fundamental particle. Putnam and Oppenheim have proposed a hierarchical model of reductionism in six layers, with Level 1 the most fundamental, Level 6 the most integrated.[206]

6. Social groups
5. Multicellular living things
4. Cells
3. Molecules
2. Atoms
1. Elementary particles

Popper has proposed an extended version of this structure, which includes a level for sub-sub-elementary particles as yet unknown.[207] He also expressed his reservations about the reductionist assumption of 'bottom-up' causation.[208] He pointed out that there are scientific phenomena that are explained only by a holistic account of structure. The way in which some crystals work on photons to produce polarised light provides one such example. Lasers, masers and holograms similarly require non-reductionist explanation, while machines created to serve an end (or telos) could not be understood by considering their fundamental constituents in isolation.

The same reservation applies even more strongly to accounts of social systems and human bodies. Human death, for instance, can only be understood holistically. After death has been established by conventional definitions, many cells continue to live for some time. Medawar, in his critique of reductionism, pointed out that the higher levels of the hierarchy could best be seen as enrichments of the lower levels.[209] In this sense, there was no level which possessed pre-eminent virtue. All levels were worthy of study.

Others have argued from other directions that something more is needed in modern thinking than the reductionist program. In 1970, Dubos wrote:

> A sophisticated form of ecology will have to complement Democritus' atomism and Descartes' reductionism;[210]

and Putnam, in a discussion of the science-ethics dichotomy, wrote:

> Instead of trying once again to discover some deep truth contained in positivism—in the fact-value dichotomy, or in non-cognitivism, or in the verifiability theory of meaning—we should break the grip of positivism in our thinking once and for all.[211]

A Cartesian account of suffering

Given the strength of reductionism and its manifest contributions to medical progress, it is difficult to establish its shortcomings. We may, however, gain some measure of its limiting effects by considering the nature of suffering, using Cartesian concepts as we understand them and have inherited them. Cassell has argued that suffering:

> is experienced by persons, that it is provoked by a perception of impending personal destruction and that suffering can occur in relation to any aspect of the person.[212]

It is not to be equated with pain, which may provoke suffering, but which is by no means the only cause of suffering. The term 'person' in our times has gained many associations. 'Mind', 'individuality', 'autonomy' and 'self' are all bundled into the concept 'person'. The Cartesian soul-body dichotomy has been translated in modernity to a person-body dichotomy. The person (who suffers) presents with a body which causes the suffering because of a defect of structure or function. Medicine, in its Cartesian mould, undertakes willingly the cure of the body, but not of the insubstantial, immaterial, unextended and uncomprehended soul which has now become the person. Within the modern version of the Cartesian system, suffering is a separate issue to the central one of sickness. If the sickness (cancer, rheumatoid arthritis, HIV infection) cannot be cured, then the best that we can offer will be some form of symptom control. The person, with his mind, his lost autonomy and threatened selfhood, must fend for himself in that territory of insubstantiality. Anatole Broyard, dying of prostate cancer, wrote:

> There's a physical self who's ill, and there's a metaphysical self who's ill. When you die, your philosophy dies along with you. So I want a metaphysical man to keep me company.[213]

Toombs, suffering from MS, wrote

> an empathic understanding is available to all . . . The lifeworlds of physician and patient . . . provide the starting point for mutual understanding.[214]

These pleas from the ill are largely unanswerable from within the modern version of the Cartesian framework, because they are seen as separate issues from those that relate to the 'legitimate' material domain of the body.

Making good the Cartesian shortfall

Reductionism and dichotomous thinking have worked to disengage medicine from its foundations. The whole health endeavour is justified in Western societies by the high valuation we place on human life. But it is the whole human whose health we defend or restore, not her liver or heart alone. The justification for the existence of health workers of any kind is to be found in this core value. The distaste for the medical profession, which is publicly expressed by newspapers, television and radio, by litigation and legislation, at least in part reflects public unease at the gap that has grown between the science of medicine and its function of caring. Until we do more than pay lip service to caring for the ill who suffer, rather than simply for their diseases, it is unlikely that the pressures on medicine and health will subside. Similarly, we will never be at peace within the health care professions until we stop the dichotomous thinking which opposes medicine to public health. Both ends of this scale are justified by the same value—a high valuation placed on human life. What therapies might there be to rescue the health endeavour? Holism is much misunderstood. It has become equated, as holistic medicine, with 'New Age' theories and the rejection of rationalism. In reality, it has far more secure grounding. Holism demands that the object of study should be studied as a whole. This does not deny the value of examining the constituent parts of the whole organism, but it does demand that the results of the examination should be restored to their context within the whole being. In this respect, it accords closely with the hermeneutic project, which aims to find explanations by examining the constituent parts, and to find understanding by restoring the explained parts to their context in the whole work.[215] For the hermeneutist, understanding and explanation are linked in a circular process, the one enriching the other. Further, hermeneutics began as the interpretation of biblical text, and it has methods of approaching interpretation which are relevant to the understanding of what people say to one another in circumstances like the medical consultation.[216,217] Finally, the ethical movement in medicine promises some help for a medicine which is entrapped in reductionist science.[218] By reminding the profession that it is dealing with individuals, not simply possessing legal rights, but with more fundamental human rights to respect and a sensitive hearing, the movement has restored something of personhood to the threatened and therefore reduced human who is the patient.

Further, the discourse ethics of Habermas contain much that is relevant to the medical process, by proposing an ethics which is evolved by consensus in a discourse that adheres to guidelines.[219] All of these understandings offer new modes of thought that might help to refresh the medical paradigm which, powerful though it has been, is now leading the profession away from its justification—the suffering of individual humans.

Summary

Descartes came to a philosophical world dominated by Aristotelianism, Thomism and scholasticism. It was his avowed intent to sweep all of this away, and to begin again. What he produced was a towering and enduring structure, based in foundationalism, and rationalist in its structure. From the metaphysics of the *Cogito* and proof of the existence of God, he proceeded to erect a materialist ontology coupled to a dualist concept of mind as distinct from matter. He described a reductionist method of great power for dealing with complex matters. He saw the power of mathematics, and his contribution to abstract mathematical thinking was of central importance. His physics was often flawed, but his influence on both the method and the content of philosophy and physical sciences has been enduring. Cartesian thinking, particularly in the realms of mind-body dualism and reductionism, continues in medicine. Its effects are not always good. Mind-body dualism has been challenged strongly, but materialism and reductionism continue to influence both clinical and research medicine. Both have tended to separate person from body, and have caused the health professions to invest more in the cure of bodies than the cure of persons. The gap between the grounding value of medicine and its reductionist practice has reached a critical stage, and it is time to think again about the priorities to be assigned within practice, teaching and research. We need to deploy holism, hermeneutics and new appreciations of ethics to re-examine what we are doing, and to refresh the fundamental value which justifies our existence as a profession—the unique valuation we place on human life.

REFERENCES

157. Russell B. *History of Western philosophy*, 3rd impression. London: Allen and Unwin, 1948, p583.
158. Hatfield G. Descartes' physiology and its relation to his psychology. In: Cottingham J (ed). *The Cambridge companion to Descartes*. Cambridge: Cambridge University Press, 1992, p362.
159. Descartes R. Discourse on the method of rightly conducting one's reason and seeking the truth in the sciences (part VI). In: Cottingham J, Stoothoff R., Murdoch D (trans). *Descartes: selected philosophical writings*. Cambridge: Cambridge University Press, 1988, p46.
160. Koyrc A. Introduction. In: Anscombe E, Geach PT (trans). *Descartes: philosophical writings*. Edinburgh: Nelson, 1954, ppxiii–xvii.
161. Descartes R. Letter to Mersenne. In: Cottingham JG, Stoothoff R, Murdoch D, Kenny A. (eds and trans). *The philosophical writings of Descartes, vol III*. Cambridge: Cambridge University Press, 1991, p156.
162. Galileo Galilei. On theology as the Queen of the Sciences. In: Baumer F le V. (ed). *Main currents of Western thought*. New Haven: Yale University Press, 1978, p327.
163. Descartes R. Discourse on the method of rightly conducting one's reason and seeking the truth in the sciences. In: *Descartes: selected philosophical writings*, ibid, p46.
164. Descartes R. In: Cottingham J, Stoothoff R, Murdoch D (trans). *Descartes: selected philosophical writings*. Cambridge: Cambridge University Press, 1988, ibid.
165. Descartes R. In: Cottingham J, Stoothoff R, Murdoch D (trans). *The philosophical writings of Descartes*, vols I and II. Cambridge: Cambridge University Press, 1987; vol III, same translators with Kenny A, 1991.
166. Descartes R. Meditations on first philosophy. In: *Descartes: selected philosophical writings*, ibid, pp76–9.
167. Husserl E. *The crisis of the European sciences and transcendental phenomenology*. Evanston: North Western University Press, 1970, pp73–84.
168. Descartes R. Discourse on the method. In: *Descartes: selected philosophical writings*, ibid, p36; and Meditations on first philosophy: second meditation, ibid, pp80–6.
169. Descartes R. Meditations on first philosophy. In: *Descartes: selected philosophical writings*, ibid, p92.
170. Descartes R. Meditations on first philosophy. In: *Descartes: selected philosophical writings*, ibid, pp105–10.
171. Descartes R. Discourse on the method. In: *Descartes: selected philosophical writings*, ibid, p39.
172. Descartes R. Rules for the direction of our native intelligence, rule four. In: *Descartes: selected philosophical writings*, ibid, p5.

173. Descartes R. Discourse on the method. In: *Descartes: selected philosophical writings*, ibid, p29.
174. Descartes R. Discourse on the method. In: *Descartes: selected philosophical writings*, ibid, p29.
175. Losee J. *A historical introduction to the philosophy of science.* Oxford: Oxford University Press, 1993, pp79–82.
176. Gaukroger S. The nature of abstract reasoning: philosophical aspects of Descartes' work in algebra. In: *The Cambridge companion to Descartes*, ibid, p111.
177. Descartes R. Preface to the French edition of Principles of Philosophy. In: *The philosophical writings of Descartes*, vol I, ibid, p186.
178. Descartes R. Discourse on the method. In: *Descartes: selected philosophical writings*, ibid, p48.
179. Descartes R. Discourse on the method. In: *Descartes: selected philosophical writings*, ibid, p49.
180. Descartes R. Passions of the soul. In: *Descartes: selected philosophical writings*, ibid, p220.
181. Descartes R. Optics. In: *Descartes: selected philosophical writings*, ibid, p63.
182. Descartes R. Meditations on first philosophy: third meditation. In: *Descartes: selected philosophical writings*, ibid, p93.
183. Garber D. Descartes' physics. In: *The Cambridge companion to Descartes*, ibid, p303.
184. Ryle G. *The concept of mind.* Harmondsworth: Penguin Books, 1978, p17.
185. Descartes R. Passions of the soul. In: *Descartes: selected philosophical writings*, ibid, pp221–2.
186. Wittgenstein L. In: Anscombe GEM, Rhees R (eds). *Philosophical investigations.* Oxford: Blackwell, 1953.
187. Husserl E. In: Gibson WRB (trans). *Ideas: general introduction to pure phenomenology.* London: Collier Books, 1969.
188. Descartes R. Meditations on first philosophy, meditation one. In: Gibson WRB (trans). *Descartes: selected philosophical writings*, Collier Books, London, 1969, pp76–9.
189. Jolley N. The reception of Descartes' philosophy. In: *The Cambridge companion to Descartes*, ibid, pp416–18.
190. Descartes R. Objections and replies. In: *Descartes: selected philosophical writings*, ibid, pp150–1.
191. Gaukroger S. The nature of abstract reasoning: philosophical aspects of Descartes' work in algebra. In: *The Cambridge companion to Descartes*, ibid, p106.
192. Gaukroger S. The nature of abstract reasoning: philosophical aspects of Descartes' work in algebra. In: *The Cambridge companion to Descartes*, ibid, p106.
193. Descartes R. Rules for the direction of our native intelligence. In: *Descartes: selected philosophical writings*, ibid, p16.
194. Hatfield G. Descartes' physiology and its relation to his psychology. In: *The Cambridge companion to Descartes*, ibid, p343.
195. Descartes R. Passions of the soul. In: *Descartes: selected philosophical writings*, ibid, p225.
196. Skinner BF. *Beyond freedom and dignity.* Harmondsworth: Penguin Books, 1971.
197. Bruner JS. *Beyond the information given: studies in the psychology of knowing.* New York: Norton, 1973.
198. Miller GA, Johnson-Laird PN. *Language and perception.* Cambridge: Cambridge University Press, 1976.
199. Freud S. An outline of psychoanalysis. *International Journal of Psychoanalysis* 1940, 21: 27–84.
200. Harré R, Gillett G. *The discursive mind.* Thousand Oaks, California: Sage Publications, 1994.

201. Descartes R. Meditations on first philosophy. In: *Descartes: selected philosophical writings*, ibid, pp113–14.
202. Descartes R. Discourse on the method. In: *Descartes: selected philosophical writings*, ibid, p47.
203. For an account of these critiques, see Jolley N. The reception of Descartes' philosophy. In: *The Cambridge companion to Descartes*, ibid, pp393–419.
204. Merton RK. The institutional imperatives of science. In: Barnes B (ed). *Sociology of science*. Harmondsworth: Penguin Books, 1972, pp65–79.
205. Wadsworth M, Butterfield W, Blaney R. *Health and sickness: the choice of treatment*. London: Tavistock, 1971.
206. Oppenheim P, Putnam H. Unity of science as a working hypothesis. In: Freigh H, Scriven M, Maxwell G (eds). *Minnesota studies in the philosophy of science*, vol II. Minnesota: University of Minnesota Press, pp3–36.
207. Popper KR, Eccles JC. *The self and its brain: an argument for interactionism*. New York: Springer-Verlag, 1981, p17.
208. Popper KR, Eccles JC. *The self and its brain: an argument for interactionism*, ibid, pp14–21.
209. Medawar PB. A geometric model of reduction and emergence. In: Ayala FJ, Dobzhansky T (eds). *Studies in the philosophy of biology*. London: Macmillan, 1974, pp57–63.
210. Dubos R. *So human an animal*. London: Rupert Hart-Davis, 1970, p27.
211. Putnam H. Objectivity and the science-ethics distinction. In: *The quality of life*. Nussbaum MC, Sen A (eds). Oxford: Clarendon Press, 1993, p155.
212. Cassell EJ. *The nature of suffering and the goals of medicine*. Oxford: Oxford University Press, 1991, pp32–3.
213. Broyard A. *Intoxicated by my illness*. New York: Fawcett Columbine, 1992, p40.
214. Toombs SK. *The meaning of illness. A phenomenological account of the different perspectives of physician and patient*. Dordrecht: Kluwer Academic, 1992, p87.
215. Ricoeur P. In: Blamey K, Thompson JB (trans). *From text to action: essays in hermeneutics*. Evanston, Illinois: Northwestern University Press, 1991.
216. Little JM, Leeder S. Logic, hermeneutics and informed consent. *European Journal of Surgery* 1996; 162: 3–10.
217. Little JM. *Humane medicine*. Cambridge: Cambridge University Press, 1995, pp141–159.
218. Little JM. *Humane medicine*, ibid, pp89–121.
219. Habermas J. In: Lenhardt C, Nicholsen SW (trans). *Moral consciousness and communicative action*. Cambridge: Polity Press, 1992.

CHAPTER SEVEN

Reason and Emotion in Medical Ethics: A Missing Element

PAUL M. MCNEILL

Introduction

Of all the professions, medicine offers a unique opportunity to experience other people at moments of great challenge. Doctors are privileged to receive what is most personal, most intimate, most basic, most joyful, and most scary from people they may have just met.

Not all encounters between a doctor and patient are intimate in this sense. The patient may simply want a health check-up, or a cream for an irritation on the skin. Yet when my mother was in hospital, possibly dying, it was the doctor I wanted to talk to, before the nurse, or the social worker. When it was me lying on a stretcher, still in shock from an accident on the road, it was a doctor I wanted to care for me, not only to deal with my injuries, but to tell me whether the numbness in my arm was an indication of something seriously wrong, or something that would pass. At the birth of each of my daughters, I wanted a doctor to be there.

It is likely, at high points, and even more likely at low points, in my life (and yours) that a doctor will be there as a welcome and trusted professional and as a fellow human being. How will this doctor respond to me when I am in ecstasy, when I am crying, when I am fearful about the meaning of this or that change in my body, or when I am in pain, in shock, or grieving a loss more terrible than I know how to bear?

A missing element

Earlier this year I went with a friend, Marion, to see a doctor. She had been experiencing headaches and indications of a growth, possibly a brain tumour, in the centre of her brain. Friends had been called back from overseas, her son thought she might die within the week, and Marion was very frightened. She had X-ray pictures of her brain, MRI images, a radiologist's report and an appointment to see a neurologist. The pressure in Marion's head made it difficult for her to think clearly. She was too upset to be able to formulate the questions she needed to ask and wanted help to decide on the best option to follow. So she asked me to come with her to see the neurologist, to support her, and ask any questions on her behalf that she might forget. The neurologist studied the X-ray pictures of her brain, MRI images, and the radiologist's report and concluded that it was probably a non-malignant growth in the brain, a cyst, or sac of fluid that could be drained. Only an operation would confirm the diagnosis. Yes, it was serious and the operation needed to be done within days. It would take between 5 and 8 hours but the long-term outlook was very promising and the risks were minimal. If the diagnosis was correct, there would be a full recovery and a return to normal life.

What struck me, as an observer of this interaction between my dear friend and her highly commended medical specialist, was his aloofness. He was cold, almost robotic in his manner. Minimal in both movement and speech. He gave no indication of recognising Marion's obvious fright and fragility. The message, as I received it, was:

'This is straightforward. Marion is fortunate that there is a clear diagnosis and we have the surgical procedures that can rectify the problem.'

If it had been Marion's car, his manner would have been understandable. But this was her brain. For Marion it was her life. Even the need to protest feels strange: as if he was from another planet and from a species with no understanding of human feeling, like Mr. Spock from Star Trek.

Yes, it was good news, relative to what we knew of brain tumours and their likely fatal consequences, but the manner in which the diagnosis was given and the treatment recommended lacked common human feeling and was disturbing.

There were other complaints too. He had not communicated some of the major consequences of the operation without being pressed. For example, until asked, he had not told Marion that she could expect intense headaches for several days after the operation. One of his responses to a question was:

'I have already answered that question.'

Maybe he had and maybe this is just an example of his cold formality. But it was also a discouragement to ask any further questions.

Any textbook on communication would have told him that a distressed patient may well need to have information repeated. The message I took was 'There is no need to worry, simply turn up for the operation and all will be well.' It was subtle, hard to identify the many ways in which open communication was restrained, yet the restraint was palpable. I am trained to ask questions both as a researcher and a lawyer, yet I felt inhibited. I imagine most people would simply acquiesce.

Is this an isolated example? A doctor on a bad day with a head cold or having had an argument with his lover? In either circumstance I could understand, see him as human and excuse his non-caring as an occasional lapse. I suspect not, however. My suspicion is that he treats most of his patients like that.

Medical ethics has emphasised giving sufficient information to allow patients to exercise their rights to decide for themselves. In Australia, as in the United States, this principle has been upheld by the courts, whose decisions have challenged accepted practices within the profession.[220] A concern with autonomy and 'disclosure of information' is not the main focus of this chapter, however. Whilst it is important to inform patients and allow them their rights to decide for themselves, my major concern is with a lack of understanding and openness to the fragility and vulnerability of a person in crisis and a lack of respect for normal emotional responses.

This lack stems in large part, I will maintain, from a poor estimation of the emotions themselves and a mistake about the influence of emotions on our ability to make decisions. It is a non-recognition of an essential aspect of our humanity which has its roots in the myth of science and objectivity and in a limited approach taken to philosophy and ethics which can be traced to the early Greek philosophers.

It is likely that you, the reader, know what I am writing about from your own experience. In case you need further persuasion I refer you to an excellent book by a surgeon, who draws on criticisms of the medical profession made by non-medical writers (like myself) and from the accounts of doctors of medicine who became patients and were similarly 'disappointed' by their treating doctor's 'impersonal manner.'[221] Fortunately there are many doctors who retain their human warmth in interacting with their patients, but it is a general condition of lack of openness to the other and to their suffering that I wish to explore.

Ethical decision-making in a medical context

There are important principles and rules that capture changes in attitudes and expectations in the community towards doctors. From a perspective of clinical medicine, however, there is a concern about how useful these principles are in helping doctors (and other health professionals) to act ethically. It is not sufficient, I claim, to teach ethics only in terms of principles. The problem is: what does a doctor do when a patient is in need of urgent medical attention? Should the doctor stop to consider: 'autonomy, beneficence, non-maleficence, and justice'? What if the patient states that she is a Jehovah's Witness and will not accept a blood transfusion on the basis of her religious beliefs? The question might be 'How should the doctor weigh ethical principles alongside a (felt) imperative to treat this person and with knowledge of how easy it would be to save this person's life?' Jonsen, Siegler and Winslade suggest a practical approach. They assert that:

> The ethics of any case arises out of the facts and values imbedded in the case itself. Ethics is not added to a clinical case by imposing on it some alien principles or values. Clinical ethics is a discipline that provides a structured approach to decision making that can help a doctor identify, analyse, and resolve ethical issues in clinical medicine.[222]

They recommend that four factors be considered whenever a decision is made about a patient. The four factors are:

1. Medical indications
2. Patient's preferences
3. Quality of life
4. Contextual features.

Power of the profession

In his book *The Healer's Power*, Howard Brody argues that everything that has been written on medical ethics skirts a basic issue. The reality is that doctors wield power and the ethical issue is how to use that power responsibly. His central argument is that 'medical ethics is about power and its responsible use.'[223]

He described three kinds of power: Aesculapian power which is the 'power the physician possesses by virtue of her training in the discipline and the art or craft of medicine'; charismatic power which is 'based on the physician's personal qualities such as courage, decisiveness, firmness, and kindness'; and social power which 'arises from the social status of the doctor.'[224] In his view the:

> skilful use of charismatic and social power kept medicine successful over the centuries when Aesculapian power was relatively empty of effective interventions.[225]

Brody states that the ethics of medicine derives from the obligation to use power (in all three senses) to support the interests of the patient and particularly in the interest of the patient in getting better. Doctors have 'considerable power to alter the course of an illness. But this same power can, with only subtle redirection, be used against the patient instead of against the disease on the patient's behalf. The problem is to empower physicians for the performance of their essential tasks while protecting the patient from the potential misuses and abuses of power.'[226]

Brody's approach is important, especially from the perspective of outright abuse of power. In New South Wales, as in many other jurisdictions, a number of disciplinary cases brought against medical practitioners has highlighted a need for this recognition. These cases have included sexual abuse of patients, defrauding of public funds though false claims for medical services, scientific fraud, and gross abuse of obligations to diagnose and treat. Doctors, charged with disciplinary offences, have been surprisingly naïve about their power in relation to a patient and their responsibility to use that power only for the benefit of patients. (This observation is based on my experience as a lay member of the Medical Tribunal and Professional Standards Committees which are established in New South Wales to consider complaints against doctors.) Whilst I agree that the power of doctors (for good or ill) is important to recognise, I am also aware that the majority of health professionals fulfil their obligations diligently and endeavour to act ethically. An acute awareness of their power may assist them in this process but is insufficient, on its own, to assist in deciding on the best, most ethical course in each situation.

Ethics and philosophy

Up to this point my discussion of bioethics has been within the traditions of Anglo-American philosophy. The question is whether ethics, as discussed within these traditions, is sufficient to redress the unfeeling and detached manner in which medicine is practised too often. Bioethics, as a reaction to the paternalism of medicine, was still a development within a tradition of rationalist, analytical philosophy. This is true whether the approach was deontological (duty-based) following Kant or consequentialist following Bentham, Mills and others. The principles of Beauchamp and Childress[227] which (as they have said themselves) can be justified either in deontological or consequentialist terms, are in this tradition of Anglo-American rational, analytical philosophy. Other approaches discussed above are also within these traditions. They simply operate at a different level. For example, the approach of Jonsen et al is concerned with practical ways of incorporating concerns about autonomy, beneficence and quality of life within medical decision-making. Brody has argued that power is the important factor which has not been given sufficient attention. Yet his approach is also rational and analytical and leaves unquestioned the philosophical basis on which his analysis of the role of power proceeds. Whilst these approaches deal with important ethical issues, they do not fundamentally address the concerns about the cool detachment and lack of responsiveness I raised at the outset of this chapter. They are necessary but not sufficient.

My concern is with a practice of medicine that is deficient in its recognition of important aspects of our humanity including emotion and feeling. This is *more* than a question about style of practice. The cool and detached manner of doctors can be understood as founded on a belief in the value of detachment. It is true that many medical practitioners believe they should not allow themselves to become emotionally involved with the suffering of their patients. This belief in detachment, as a psychological necessity, is open to challenge. In the midst of crises it *is* possible to function effectively as a concerned and caring human being. However I suggest that these beliefs are resistant to challenge because they have their roots in a prejudice. The prejudice (prior judgment) consists of a view that emotions and feelings in a human being are of little value, or worse, that they are a source of distortion and error. As Callahan puts it:

> The working model of moral conflict has been that of emotion warring against reason, with only reason's mastery offering trustworthy guidance.[228]

This is a prejudice that can be traced back to the Greek philosophers, an argument I develop (subsequently) by reference to the work of Nussbaum.

Furthermore, I claim that the high value given to detachment in medicine is bolstered by undue faith in the standing of science and the faith given to an objective view of what is *real*. Medicine gained its ascendancy in power and prestige by identifying with science. Even today, in discussion of the relative merits of medicine and alternative therapies (the names for the alternatives are problematic), representatives of modern medicine base their arguments for medicine's superiority on its foundation in science. Whilst empirically medicine may prove to be more effective in treating some conditions, its value is still open to question in each circumstance. An appeal to its scientific methodology does not end the argument for all cases, unless you share a fundamental faith in the value of science as the ultimate arbiter. There is a naïve realism implicit in a defence of medicine as 'scientific'. A fundamentalist faith in the value of science, as the arbiter of what is real and what can be known, ignores limitations in science itself.[229,230]

Science is blinkered in its approach to what can be known by assumptions of objectivity. By definition, these assumptions exclude subjectivity and biases (so-called) which are peculiarly human. An objective (or non-subjective) view, relies on an abstract idealised position. It is a perspective viewed from a platform outside of ourselves: the 'view from nowhere' as it has been called.[231]

It is acknowledged that the assumption of objectivity has proved to be extraordinarily effective. In part its effectiveness is due to a reduction in the complexity of the field of inquiry. This reduction is an instrumental device of great merit. Just as the simple assumptions of Newtonian physics gave a basis for a multitude of solutions to practical problems, so too the simple assumptions, on which much of medicine is based, have led to remarkable discoveries and cures for a multitude of ills. To press the simile further, we still rely on Newtonian physics to solve practical problems whilst recognising the limitation of a Newtonian mechanical picture of the universe. A similar recognition is needed in relation to any ontology (any view of human beings or the world) arising out of medicine. A set of simple assumptions which treat the body as a machine, and leave out important aspects of our being (including consciousness and feeling) can easily be justified on pragmatic grounds, but they have very obvious limits when applied to what is *real* or *true* and any picture of human beings based on them will be limited and suspect.

Nowhere is this more apparent than in ethics. Yet our ethics is unduly swayed by the style and methodology of science and the biases of a philosophy that give little recognition to human feeling.[232]

Postmodernism

Science and philosophy have recently come under attack from postmodernist writers.[233,234] The effect of their critique is to call into question faith in science as the arbiter of what is real. Postmodernism, to quote Charlesworth, is:

> more of a diffuse mood than a unified movement, more a climate of thought than a philosophical system.[235]

It is best understood as a reaction to the assumptions of 'modernism'.[236,237] The German philosopher Jürgen Habermas defined modernity as:

the efforts to develop objective science, universal morality and law and autonomous art according to their inner logic.[238]

In philosophy this project was both epistemological in defining legitimate approaches to knowledge and ontological in defining the nature of reality. Only an objective view of reality, stripped of any subjective bias, was legitimate. A comparable program to provide a solid basis for ethics was that of Immanual Kant whose system was founded on a principle of universality and whose 'categorical imperatives' functioned something like the laws of nature.

Postmodernism is critical of this approach. For example Lyotard, a French philosopher, identified the 'meta-narratives' which guided the project of modernity. Included in these meta-narratives are 'two great myths' of the enlightenment: the speculative unity of all knowledge and the liberation of humanity. He defined postmodernity as incredulity toward all such 'meta-narratives'.[239]

Charlesworth has identified 'two main forms of postmodernism'. One of these is the reaction to science, technology and instrumental reason which:

subjects Enlightenment rationality to radical criticism, and redirects us to the beliefs and values which modernity denies. It refuses to see science as some kind of supreme model or meta-narrative.[240]

As Havel (the Czechoslovakian playwright turned president) put it:

We have to abandon the arrogant belief that the world is merely a puzzle to be solved. A machine with instructions for use waiting to be discovered, a body of information to be fed into a computer in the hope that, sooner or later, it will spit out a universal solution.[241,242]

The other 'stricter sense of postmodernism' is essentially a critique of René Descartes and the resultant view of the world as separate from the conscious or knowing subject. The foundation of all knowledge, for Descartes, was the thinking subject ('I think therefore I am'). The self, in the Cartesian model, is a transcendent reference point, separate from the world of objects. Descartes' duality consisted of a mind, capable of universal knowledge, and a world (including the human body) which is best known in terms of mathematics and mechanical principles. To put it simply, Cartesian duality became a platform for the development of science, philosophy and ethics. Charlesworth makes the point that, although Descartes himself did not develop an ethical system, his epistemology is essential to the subsequent philosophies including that of Kant. The emphasis of Kant on the value of autonomy:

clearly derives from the Cartesian idea of the conscious subject pre-existing the external world and other conscious subjects, and independent of them.[243]

Postmodernism calls into question Cartesian dualism and the resultant system of knowledge, based as it is on the assumption of an autonomous, separate self. Foucault, for example, portrays 'self' as a construct which owes its existence to powerful social and cultural factors including language.[244,245]

Some postmodernist writers claim that our models of the universe have no direct contact with the external world and consist of textual statements that refer only to themselves.[246,247,248,249] A realist response is that entities really exist, we can trust our perceptual processes, our powers of reason, and our scientific instruments and methodology to establish the truth about them.[250]

In ethics the concomitant view is that there are values in the real world that matter, such as the worth of sentient human beings, and such values are not relative to particular cultures or a construction of language.[251] These claims however are tenets of faith. There is no way of asserting them that will establish their validity beyond demonstrating their effectiveness in an instrumental sense.

A defence of the realist position is to point to the successes of science and technology in the modern age. It was science, built on assumptions of the Enlightenment (including objectivity and rationality) that, for example, put a man on the moon. But these successes have been counter-weighted by notable failures including the poisoning of our environment, undermining of indigenous cultures everywhere in the world, an increase in the sense of individualism and a consequent isolation of individuals and breakdown of community, 'the divorce between technology and moral values' and 'the denial of the validity of "local knowledge" or tradition.'[252] Faith in reason and objectivity, which was the basis for optimism in the Enlightenment, has not led generally to the elevation of human kind. Whilst there has been a rise in the level of well-being and material wealth of a minority on the planet, the majority of human beings has been pushed further into poverty, disease and starvation. The Second World War, including its death camps, inhumane scientific experimentation and destruction of Hiroshima and Nagasaki by atomic weapons, spelt the end of faith in reason and rationality as guiding principles of enlightened progress for humankind.

My difficulty with the picture of the world given to us by realists and those with an absolutist view of ethics, is with large omissions from their world view. Their view, based on a philosophical system of universal truths and methods of reductionism, is dismissive of cultures and philosophies which do not fit. It values reason as opposed to emotion, and the material as opposed to the aesthetic. Consequently we live in societies that substantially reward those who work in the material world of commerce, construction and knowledge, and generally undervalue the work of artists, musicians, actors and poets. In medicine, a realist view is at the core of materialist approaches to health and illness and a failure to recognise and adequately respond to the experience of illness, trauma and suffering. Cassell suggests that the problem is a desire for certainty and a consequent fascination with technology. He advocates a 'return to focus on persons sick and well and on their suffering.'[253]

Accepting a postmodernist critique is not destructive of science. What is lost is the dogmatic certainty that a simple concrete view of the world exists or is attainable. The picture is more complex and subtle than modernism led us to believe. Most of us know that anyway. What science offers is, at best, a perspective which may be more useful and appropriate in some circumstances. The recommendations for treatment, for example, arising from careful research might be preferred to those of a witch doctor on pragmatic grounds: they may be shown to work better. However ontological claims arising from that research have no privileged status. Even without accepting a postmodernist perspective, Kuhn's work on paradigms, Gödel's theorem, and studies showing the limitation of our perceptual processes have undermined assumptions implicit in the modernist program.[254,255] To treat objectivity as the only valid view is a form of fundamentalism, a belief, which is as pernicious as any other fundamentalist belief. It is likely that:

> 'truth' in all spheres involving human beings (including medicine) will be seen as multi-faceted, culturally determined, and the result of a process of negotiation. [256]

Similarly in ethics, a system based on reason and universal principles may, in the end, be seen for what it is: an abstract idealised picture devoid of the nuances, quirkiness and experience of human beings. It is a perspective which takes insufficient account of the customs and integrity of particular social groups and traditions, and insufficient account of the experience of individuals.

A major concern for realists is what will happen if we give up our certainty about the world out there. This is the same fear that motivates a tenacious holding to religious beliefs in the face of challenge. One expression of that fear is that postmodernism would lead us to a world of relativity where no values could be questioned on the ground that all values are equal. More specifically there is a fear that writers such as Rorty, Williams, Derrida and others will 'demolish philosophy, theology and ethics simultaneously in full capitulation to the Nietzschean legacy' which is the idea that 'one Truth' is an illusion.[257] The reaction is often very strong as is seen in the description of postmodernism and deconstructionism as a 'philosophical virus'.[258]

The ethics of 'deconstruction'

The writings of Nietzche, Levinas, Derrida and others *are* a turn against (a 'deconstruction' of) the ontological approach taken in Western philosophy and ethics. Yet this deconstruction, for Levinas and Derrida, is prompted by an ethical concern (although they are cautious in using the term 'ethics'). It is an ethics understood in a radically different way as 'the relation of myself and the Other'.[259] Levinas and Derrida use the terms 'self' and 'other' in their singular and particular sense before any universalisation or generalisation.[260] There is an immediacy in this relation, an opening, or 'scission of Being', that cuts across complacency and makes a demand of the self prior to any reflexive thought.[259] Critchley comments that:

> The paradigmatic ethical moment is that of being pre-reflexively addressed by the other person in a way that calls me into question and obliges me to be responsible.[261]

He raises the objection, as does Derrida, that 'such an ethics is no ethics at all' although this 'ambiguity' does not undermine the project to reposit or 'displace ethics and think it anew by locating its condition of possibility in the relation to Other'. This is a view of ethics (or 'ultra-ethics') that supports a position I wish to develop. It emphasises the individuality of this particular 'subject' relating to this particular 'other' before any generalisations.[260] In the medical context it challenges the doctor to be present to this particular patient (as 'other') free from (prior to) analysis and any need to comprehend. Implicit is a respect for 'otherness' and avoidance of *comprehending* in the sense of taking hold (*prend*) as a possession or acquisition.[262] It pricks the conceit of knowing as if 'other' can be known as 'self.' Such an approach to ethics and to medicine is clearly antagonistic to the detached, aloof and knowledgable attitude of doctors which is of primary concern in this chapter.

The objection could be made that I am advocating a position more clearly developed by an ethics of virtue. I have chosen not to rely on that tradition on the ground that a deeper critique is needed. Virtue ethics leaves unchallenged the basic ontological approach of Western philosophy on which medicine is founded. It has been my concern in this chapter to pursue an approach, suggested by postmodernism and deconstructionism, that radically challenges this ontological approach and leaves a doctor free from its constraints to find and validate new ways of being in the presence of suffering. This is not to suggest that the virtues advocated by Pelligrino and others are not worthy of practising. It is simply to prefer a radical critique of premises which support an objective (and objectifying) approach to medical practice, and a detached and aloof professionalism in the face of suffering.

There is still a place for the virtues, and for a more conventional ethics of principles, policies and procedures. However I am reluctant to accept any external point of reference that would establish the values of conventional ethics *a priori*. The relative merit of different perspectives is dependent on an attribution of value that we have to decide for ourselves as a community. Such an approach is suggested by Habermas in terms of 'discourse ethics' whereby those with legitimate interests resolve ethical issues and reach consensus by discussion.[263,264,265] In some areas such discourse already proceeds: for example in the use of committees to develop ethical policy for a hospital and committees to decide on the ethical soundness of proposals for research.[266,267,268] There are problems and the approach is open to a charge that ethics, without recourse to principles, would become a matter of consensus and populism. Whilst these problems are acknowledged, I will not attempt to develop the position here beyond suggesting that a traditional and conventional domain of ethics is still available, but free of any illusion of foundation in absolute principles, and unsupported by any single ideology.

Critique of a philosophy devoid of emotion

Throughout this chapter I have referred to the work of Martha Nussbaum, and particularly her essays in *Love's Knowledge*, to question assumptions in philosophy that reason, in the absence of emotion, can be trusted as a base for establishing what is true, and especially for establishing what is good or right.[269] Nussbaum challenges the view that emotion is a corrupting influence that would sway and bias judgment. The theme throughout her essays is that Anglo-American philosophy has followed a tradition which negates emotion. The tradition goes back as far as Plato, the Stoics and its development by Spinoza. A central purpose of Nussbaum is to call into question the view that emotions lead to irrationality and to suggest:

> with Aristotle, that practical reasoning unaccompanied by emotion is not sufficient for practical wisdom: that emotions are not only not more unreliable than intellectual calculations, but frequently more reliable.[270]

She attacks two of the bases for the exclusion of the emotions—firstly that:

> emotions are blind animal reactions, like or identified with bodily feelings, that are in their nature unmixed with thought, undiscriminating, and impervious to reasoning.

Her response is that this is an 'impoverished view of emotion that cannot survive scrutiny.'[290] The second reason for dismissing the emotions is, not because they are irrational but that the 'judgments on which the major emotions are based are all *false*.'[271]

In response to the view that emotions are devoid of thought and 'impervious to reason' Nussbaum demonstrates that emotions have a cognitive element. This element includes beliefs about facts and beliefs about the way things ought to be. For example anger rests on a belief that 'one has been wronged or damaged in some significant way by the person toward whom the anger is directed.'[272] Grief presupposes 'a family of beliefs about one's circumstances: that a loss has taken place: that the loss is of something that has value.' She goes on to say that 'Love, pity, fear, and their relatives—all are belief-based in a similar way: all involve the acceptance of certain views of how the world is and what has importance.'[273] For Nussbaum:

> emotions are not simply blind surges of affect, recognized, and discriminated from one another, by their felt quality alone; rather they are discriminating responses closely connected with beliefs about how things are and what is important.[270]

If something, which is believed, is shown to be false (for example, the loved one did *not* die, or the precious vase was in fact *not* precious at all but a cheap imitation) then grief or anger may well dissipate. Similarly if a belief about what ought to have occurred is challenged (for example the belief that 'children ought not to have been playing near the precious vase' by being told 'they had permission to play there') then the anger may be mollified. Hunger and other body sensations are not amenable to changes of belief in this way.

The second reason that emotions were dismissed from philosophy is that they were said to lead to false conclusions. This is a more sophisticated objection: the emotions leave us in an incomplete and needy position as 'hostages to fortune'.[274] This perspective is associated with 'aspirations of transcendence' so as to be above all those influences that deprive a person of full mastery and self-control. It follows the views of Plato, and the Stoics, was developed by Kant and has been the predominant influence in Anglo-American philosophy and ethics. The problem with the emotions, from the perspective of transcendence is, *not* that they are irrational but, that they involve a rationality that includes

'false and pernicious reasoning.'[275] Essentially 'they are an acknowledgment of the importance of things that have no true importance.'[276]
A consequence of this view is that:

> The person who aims to live a godlike life, transcending his or her humanity, must do away with [the emotions]. . . . A self-sufficient and complete person, in short, has nothing to fear, nothing to grieve for, nobody to love in the usual human sense, the sense in which love implies incompleteness and the absence of control.[277]

A view of emotions as irrelevant is at odds with a life of engagement in the world.[278] However, if we are 'not so enamoured of the pursuit of transcendence' then this second argument against the involvement of the emotive quality of our humanity is not persuasive.[279]

On the contrary, we are likely to have strong feelings about issues of importance to us. An emotional response should be taken into account and be seen as a necessary element in an appropriate ethical response. Nussbaum put it this way:

> Because the emotions have this cognitive dimension in their very structure, it is very natural to view them as intelligent parts of our ethical agency, responsive to the workings of deliberation and essential to its completion.[272]

When emotion is left out, a response may be irrational. As she puts it:

> On this view, there will be certain contexts in which the pursuit of intellectual reasoning apart from emotion will actually prevent a full rational judgment—for example by preventing an access to one's grief, or one's love, that is necessary for the full understanding of what has taken place when a loved one dies.[272]

Clearly this has implications for the practice of medicine. A doctor acting in the traditional manner of cool professional detachment is at risk of acting unethically and inappropriately for the reason that he, or she, has lost the means for understanding his or her patient's experience.

Abstract philosophy v storytelling and emotion

What is the antidote to this condition? Cassell argues that there is no point in medicine turning away from a scientific perspective. What is needed is an added focus on the subjective experience of individuals and the idiosyncratic meanings they attribute to their experience.[280]
Nussbaum characterised philosophy as:

> abstract, detached from one's immediate context and from the bodily senses, concerned with universals, deductive and mathematical in its form.[281]

This was the style adopted by philosophers, including the philosophers of the natural sciences. It was the predominant mode of ethical inquiry and it was the style which has been most influential in medicine. Those who fail to adopt it are judged as lacking. In this hierarchy of values, reason and objectivity are the means for establishing what is true and good. Universal and abstract principles are preferred over the particular, and the emotions are of little (or negative) value. A consequence is that the detail, the individual story, and the passion are all reduced to irrelevance.

Medicine, influenced by a cool detachment and universal approach, has ceased to be interested in people's stories—except so far as they are relevant to a logico-deductive methodology concerned with diagnosis and treatment. Listening in this way is to do 'violence' to their story.[282,283] What is needed is open listening to subjective experience, not to reveal the patient's reasons for their actions as Cassell advocates, but simply to listen and appreciate that person's story.[284] From this perspective the nuances of each person's life and the emotional component are important elements in their story. Without them, individual experiences, the richness, poetry, pleasures, pathos and tragedy are gone.

Nussbaum concludes that 'If detached, purely intellectual, abstract, deductive reasoning about universals was the winner in this transcendence-oriented tradition, it is easy, too, to see who the losers were. The losers were stories, and the storytelling imagination and emotions.'[285] This suggests that a simple stratagem is to be interested, as a human being, in other people's stories: to take an interest in their lives and be open to being affected by their emotion.

Inviting their stories

I am writing this chapter during the Christmas holidays and have just spoken to my friend Peter, a specialist in intensive care. His holidays were interrupted by emergencies and he has shared in the grief of two different families. In one family, Peter informed young parents that their child had an inoperable tumour and was unlikely to live much longer. Two years earlier, they had lost their other child to a tumour. In another family a woman lost her partner of 57 years. They had been travelling together on a tour bus when he had a heart attack. I asked Peter how he had responded. He said that in the past, when faced with hopeless situations in which nothing could be done medically, he had wanted to find some way to take the pain away. He had wanted to mollify their suffering. In the last few years he has learned that this is not possible. With these people he had simply encouraged them to talk. He had asked the young parents to tell him about their son. They told him the story of his illness, his life and their love for him. And the woman spoke of her husband, her life with him and her grief.

This openness makes sense as good preventive medicine. Evidence suggests that unresolved grief can be a factor in developing a subsequent medical condition and that giving people an opportunity to talk is important in the process of coming to terms with grief. Whilst this may be true, such instrumental reasoning is not relevant to the predominant concern in this paper. The concern in this chapter is with cool, unemotional medical practice and lack of openness to the experience of the other. It is expressed by the patient saying 'He exhibited no interest in me as a person'.[286] (This was said by a patient, also a medical practitioner, of his treating doctor). The obvious counter to this cool detachment is a humane interest and concern for people's lives. An invitation to tell their stories offers a simple yet profound means for expressing this interest.

What I have advocated is listening, or 'open relating', before any analysis or need to comprehend. It is based on an ethic, suggested by Derrida and Levinas, that allows the other person to be present in the moment with his/her experience, emotional expression and story, without interrupting and without defending myself against the possibility of being affected by that person and without attempting to comprehend his/her story in a way that makes it known as an acquisition of mine. (I am not suggesting that Levinas or Derrida would support this extrapolation of their ideas and take responsibility for this 'reconstruction'.) It is an act of courage in being open to, and affected by that person. It is an openness that is *not* (in those moments) about diagnosis, or medicine in its scientific, definitive and reductionist sense. It requires a recognition and avoidance of the 'seductive power' of medicine to 'lure' the doctor

> away from the richly textured world of particulars to the lofty heights of abstraction . . . to a world made more simple and schematic.[287]

It is a privilege to be open to, to receive, and yield to intense human experiences. I acknowledge that is easier to say than to put it into practice. Anyone experiencing the suffering of another human being needs to find ways of being open to that person, being emotionally available to listen to his/her story, without being undermined by it. Yet this is possible. What may be needed is a different understanding of detachment. There is a difference between a detachment that is warm and supportive and a detachment that is cold, aloof and cut-off. The former is founded in respect for another (as 'other') in the midst of his/her life and confronted by his/her difficulties. While I can be moved by that person's story and can share to some small extent in it, he/she is a separate person from me with the capability, in time, of making sense of these terrible circumstances and being richer and deeper for them as a human being. A detachment that is cold, aloof and cut-off, however, is based on fear—fear that 'I may not be able to cope if I let you touch me, as a feeling human being, in the midst of your suffering'. It is also based on a mistake about the role of objectivity, the emotions and a belief in a need for a cool, scientific detachment.

Science and objectivity have their place as does the process of calm, logical and deductive reasoning required of a doctor. Science, objectivity and reason on the one hand, and a warm human responsiveness on the other, are compatible. The two views on which they are based may not be reconcilable, but reason and passion might co-exist in a 'dynamic tension between two possible irreconcilable visions.'[288] Sidney Callahan advocates a:

> mutual interaction of thinking and feeling in ethical decision making and a personal equilibrium in which emotion and reason are both activated and in accord.[289,290]

It is demanding to ask this degree of maturity of a doctor: to incorporate a capacity for cool, clear-headed science and warm humanity, yet this is the challenge. Medicine is a profession requiring both art and science, reason and passion. A philosophy, based on non-recognition of the importance of feeling, is a severe disadvantage to anyone attempting to find themselves as a professional and as a human being in this role. In an ethics of care, emotion must be recognised and allowed to coexist in equilibrium with reason.

REFERENCES

220. Rogers v Whittaker, High Court of Australia, Australian Health and Medical Law Reporter, para 77–061, NSW Court of Appeal, (1991) 23 NSWLR 600; Canterbury v Spence, United States Court of Appeals (for the District of Columbia), 464 F 2d. The court restated the principle 'fundamental in American jurisprudence' that '[e]very adult human being of adult years and sound mind has a right to determine what shall be done with his own body . . .'
221. Little, JM., *Humane medicine*. Cambridge: Cambridge University Press, 1995, pp2–12, and p6.
222. Jonsen AR, Siegler M, Winslade WJ. *Clinical ethics: a practical approach to ethical decisions in clinical medicine*, 3rd edition. New York: McGraw-Hill, 1992.
223. Brody H. *The healer's power*. New Haven, Yale University Press, 1992, p13.
224. Brody H. *The healer's power*, ibid, pp16–17.
225. Brody H. *The healer's power*, ibid, p19.

226. Brody H. *The healer's power*, ibid, p36.
227. Beauchamp TL, Childress JF. *Principles of Biomedical Ethics*, 4th edition. Oxford: Oxford University Press, 1994.
228. Callahan S. *The role of emotion in ethical decisionmaking.* Hastings Center Report, 18: 9–14.
229. Little JM. *Humane medicine*, ibid, 34–6.
230. Cassell EJ. *The sorcerer's broom: medicine's rampant technology.* Hastings Center Report, 1993, 23: 32–3.
231. Nagel T. *The view from nowhere.* New York: Oxford University Press, 1986.
232. Nussbaum MC. *Love's knowledge: essays on philosophy and literature.* New York and Oxford: Oxford University Press, 1990, p19.
233. Anderson WT (ed). *The truth about the truth: de-confusing and re-constructing the postmodern world.* New York: Jeremy P Tarcher/Putnam, 1995.
234. Bertens H. *The idea of the postmodern: a history.* New York: Routledge, 1995.
235. Charlesworth M. *Postmodernism and theology.* The Way: Contemporary Christian Spirituality, July 1996, 188–202.
236. Harvey D. *The condition of postmodernity: an enquiry into the origin of cultural change*, Cambridge: Basil Blackwell, 1989, p27.
237. Taylor C. *Two theories of modernity.* Hastings Center Report, 1995, 25: 24–33.
238. Habermas, J., *Modernity: an incomplete project.* In: Foster H(ed). *The anti-aesthetic: essays in post modern culture.* Washington: Bay Press, 1983, p9.
239. Lyotard J-F. In: Bennington G, Brian Massumi B (trans). *The postmodern condition: a report on knowledge.* Manchester, UK: Manchester University Press, 1984 and 1991.
240. Charlesworth M. *Postmodernism and theology*, ibid, 190.
241. Havel V. The end of the modern era. *New York Times*, March 1992, pE15, quoted in: Anderson, WT. *The truth about the truth*, ibid, p161.
242. Havel V. The search for meaning in a global civilisation. In: Anderson WT. *The truth about the truth*, pp232–8.
243. Charlesworth M. *Postmodernism and theology*, ibid, 191–3.
244. Foucault M. The subject and power. In: Dreyfus H, Rainbow P (eds). *Michel Foucault: beyond structuralism and hermeneutics.* Chicago: University of Chicago Press, 1983, p208, as discussed in: Charlesworth M. *Postmodernism and theology*, ibid, pp194–5.
245. Foucault M. In: Hurley R (trans). *The history of sexuality: an introduction.* London: Penguin, 1979.
246. Rorty R. *Philosophy and the mirror of nature.* Princeton, NJ: Princeton University Press, 1979.
247. Rorty R. *Contingency, irony and solidarity.* New York: Cambridge University Press, 1989, pp4–5.
248. Critchley S. *The ethics of deconstruction: Derrida and Levinas.* Oxford, UK and Cambridge, USA: Blackwell, 1992.
249. Madison GB. Coping with Nietzsche's legacy: Rorty, Derrida, Gadamar. *Philosophy Today* 1992; 34: 3–19.
250. Armstrong D. *Universals and scientific realism.* Cambridge: Cambridge University Press, 1978.
251. Gaita R. *Good and evil: an absolute conception.* Basingstoke, UK: Macmillan, 1991.
252. Charlesworth M. *Postmodernism and theology*, ibid, p190.
253. Cassell EJ. *The sorcerer's broom: medicine's rampant technology*, ibid, p39.
254. Kuhn TS. *The structure of scientific revolutions*, 2nd edition. Chicago and London: Chicago University Press, 1970.
255. Hofstadter Douglas R. *Gödel, Escher, Bach: an eternal golden braid.* Hassocks, UK: Harvester Press, 1979.
256. McNeill PM. *Science as negotiation*, in press.
257. Pelligrino ED, Thomasma DC. *The virtues in medical practice.* New York and Oxford: Oxford University Press, 1993, p191.

258. Franklin J. Casting about for the philosopher's stone. *Sydney Morning Herald*, 31 December 1996, p9.
259. Levinas, quoted in: Critchley S. *The ethics of deconstruction: Derrida and Levinas*, ibid, p17.
260. Critchley S. *The ethics of deconstruction: Derrida and Levinas*, ibid, p18.
261. Critchley S. *The ethics of deconstruction: Derrida and Levinas*, ibid, p48.
262. Critchley S. *The ethics of deconstruction: Derrida and Levinas*, ibid, p6.
263. Habermas J. In: Christian L, Christian S (trans). *Moral consciousness and communicative action*. Cambridge, Massachusetts: MIT Press, 1990.
264. Brand A. *The force of reason: an introduction to Habermas' theory of communicative action*. Sydney: Allen & Unwin, 1990.
265. Callahan D. *Bioethics: private choice and common good*. Hastings Center Report, 1994, 24: 28–31.
266. McNeill PM, Walters J, Webster IW. Ethics decision making in Australian hospitals. *Med J Aust* 1994; 161: 63–5.
267. Minogue B. *Bioethics: a committee approach*. Boston, London and Singapore: Jones and Bartlett, 1996.
268. McNeill PM. *The ethics and politics of human experimentation*. Melbourne: Cambridge University Press, 1993.
269. Nussbaum MC. *Love's knowledge: essays on philosophy and literature*. New York and Oxford: Oxford University Press, 1990.
270. Nussbaum MC. *Love's knowledge: essays on philosophy and literature*, ibid, p40.
271. Nussbaum MC. *Love's knowledge: essays on philosophy and literature*, ibid, p42.
272. Nussbaum MC. *Love's knowledge: essays on philosophy and literature*, ibid, p41.
273. Nussbaum MC. *Love's knowledge: essays on philosophy and literature*, ibid.
274. Nussbaum MC. *Love's knowledge: essays on philosophy and literature*, ibid, p387.
275. Nussbaum MC. *Love's knowledge: essays on philosophy and literature*, ibid, p388.
276. Nussbaum MC. *Love's knowledge: essays on philosophy and literature*, ibid, p388.
277. Nussbaum MC. *Love's knowledge: essays on philosophy and literature*, ibid, p387.
278. Nussbaum MC. *Love's knowledge: essays on philosophy and literature*, ibid, p371.
279. Nussbaum MC. *Love's knowledge: essays on philosophy and literature*, ibid, p389.
280. Cassell EJ. Changing uses of the subjective in medical practice. In: Cassell EJ, Siegler M (eds). *Values in medicine*. USA: University Publications of America, 1979, pp151–166.
281. Nussbaum MC. *Love's knowledge: essays on philosophy and literature*, ibid, p385.
282. Poirier S, Brauner DJ. Ethics and the daily language of medical discourse. Hastings Center Report, 1988, 18: 5–9.
283. Elliott C. *Where ethics comes from and what to do about it*. Hastings Center Report, 1992, 22.
284. Cassell EJ. *Changing uses of the subjective in medical practice*, ibid, pp163–6.
285. Nussbaum MC. *Love's knowledge: essays on philosophy and literature*, ibid, pp385–6.
286. Little JM. *Humane medicine*, ibid, p6.
287. Nussbaum MC. *Love's knowledge: essays on philosophy and literature*, ibid, p238. Nussbaum refers to philosophy in her text and not to medicine as I have suggested here.

288. Nussbaum MC. *Love's knowledge: essays on philosophy and literature*, ibid, p190.
289. Callahan S. *The role of emotion in ethical decisionmaking*, ibid, p9.
290. Carson RA. *Sensibility and rationality in bioethics.* Hastings Center Report, vol 24, no 3, May/June 1994, pp23–4.

CHAPTER EIGHT

The Politics of Bioethics

MAX CHARLESWORTH

From the mid 1970s until the present there has been a quite extraordinary growth of interest in the ethical issues raised by the new biotechnologies—in vitro fertilisation, genetic screening and manipulation, new ways of postponing death and so on. The increasing public debate about these radically novel and unprecedented issues, as the community has tried to come to terms with them, and the setting up of an array of institutions (both governmental and non-governmental) to cope with them, is a major socio-cultural phenomenon which deserves study in its own right. Some time ago I made a rough list of the Australian institutions concerned with just one area, the new reproductive technologies, and I was astonished at the number of those institutions and their fecundity, so to speak, in terms of the numbers of reports, position papers, symposia etc., they generated.

There are now signs that bioethics as a discipline—or the model of bioethics that has been adopted for the last fifteen years or so—is losing its original impetus. Even the name 'bioethics' has become suspect (at least in some European countries) because of its association with certain bioethicists' views on embryo experimentation and euthanasia. Thus, the Council of Europe's bioethics committee recently decided to change its name to 'Committee on Human Rights and Biomedicine'. This was, it appears, motivated by German and Austrian representatives objecting to the term 'bioethics' because of pressures from domestic right-to-life groups.

Again, there is a good deal of questioning about the method of bioethics with criticisms of what is now seen as naive ethical deductivism or 'principlism', where bioethics is seen as the business of the application of certain general principles—personal autonomy, justice, benevolence, the 'sanctity of human life'—to particular cases. One critic has in fact referred to 'the tyranny of principles' in bioethical discussion.[291,292]

116

Modern committee structures

There has been much disenchantment with bioethics committees and institutions and with the early utopian idea that these committees would bring about a national or community consensus on crucial bioethical issues. In the USA the major governmental bodies set up in the 1970s and early 1980s have mostly collapsed because of political wrangling, mainly due to conflicts between pro-abortion and anti-abortion lobbies and pro- and anti-foetal transplant advocates in the US Congress. The National Commission for the Protection of Human Subjects of Biomedical and Behavioral Research (1974–1978); the Ethics Advisory Board (1978–1980); the President's Commission for the Study of Ethical Problems in Medicine (set up by President Carter and dominated by Carterite representatives: 1978–1983); and the Biomedical Ethics Board and its adjunct the Biomedical Ethics Advisory Committee (1985–1989) have all foundered. At the same time, it must be recognised that both the National Commission and the President's Commission (under the direction of the distinguished legal academic Professor Alexander Capron) produced an astonishing quantity of high class reports in a brief time: thus the National Commission issued ten reports between 1975 and 1978, and the President's Commission published ten reports between 1981 and 1983.[293] These are set out in Table 8.1.

However, from 1983 until 1996 there was no Federal advisory committee on bioethical issues in the USA. Happily, a new National Bioethics Advisory Commission has now been set up, in July 1996, by President Clinton.[294] In passing, it is worthwhile mentioning a 1995 report, 'Society's Choices', by the Committee of the Institute of Medicine of the US National Academy of Sciences, on the Social and Ethical Impacts of Developments in Biomedicine. Among other things, the report proposes criteria by which national bioethics bodies could be assessed— intellectual integrity, sensitivity to democratic values, effectiveness.[295]

In Australia, the National Bioethics Consultative Committee, set up in the late 1980s (on the model of the US President's Commission and the French National Committee on Ethics in the Life and Health Sciences) during the high tide of interest in bioethical issues, has been redirected and renamed. It is now the Australian Health Ethics Committee and has been incorporated into the complex and conservative structures of the National Health and Medical Research Council. The story of the founding and brief career of the NBCC, and its transformation into the AHEC, is an extremely instructive one and full of lessons for the student of the politics of bioethics. For one thing, when it first

Table 8.1 Major reports of two US ethics bodies 1975–1983

Reports of the US National Commission for the Protection of Human Subjects of Biomedical and Behavioral Research and the President's Commission for the Study of Ethical Problems in Medicine and Biomedical and Behavioral Research			
National Commission Reports		*President's Commission Reports*	
Research on the foetus	1975	Defining death	1981
Research involving prisoners	1976	Protecting human subjects	1981
Research involving children	1977	Compensating for research injuries	1982
Psychosurgery	1977	Making health care decisions	1982
Research involving those institutionalised as being mentally infirm	1978	Whistle-blowing in biomedical research	1982
		Deciding to forego life-sustaining treatment	1983
Institutional review boards	1978	Implementing human research regulations	1983
The Belmont Report	1978		
Ethical guidelines for the delivery of health care	1978	Securing access to health care	1983
		Splicing life	1983
The special study (implications of advances in biomedical and behavioural research)	1978	Summing up	1983
Research involving prisoners	1981		
Disclosure of research information under the FOI Act	1982		
Counselling for genetic conditions	1983		

began the NBCC was desperately anxious to establish itself as a new body and, in a sense like an over-achieving child, it tried too hard to please its political parents. I remember a senior health bureaucrat saying to me:

> You (the NBCC) produced too many reports too quickly. We had no sooner got to grips with your report on the rights of children to know their biological parents, when we were hit by your report on surrogacy, and then the report on access to reproductive technology, and so on. It was too much for the ministers of health and their advisers to assimilate.

In other words, the NBCC made the mistake of being too efficient and successful!

The AHEC appears to be mainly concerned with the monitoring of the work of institutional ethics committees and with the preparation of guidelines on issues like in vitro fertilisation and genetic counselling, and it is not as concerned with promoting the public debate on bioethical issues in the way its predecessor, the NBCC, saw its main role. In the UK, after a long period of inaction following the celebrated Warnock Committee Report, the *Human Fertilisation and Embryology Act* was passed in 1990 and the Human Fertilisation and Embryology Authority set up. However, a national body, the Nuffield Council on Bioethics, was established in 1991 by the independent body, the Nuffield Foundation, to investigate more general bioethical issues. The membership of the Nuffield Council on Bioethics is so prestigious and the quality of its reports so exceptional that one may think that an independent national committee of this kind, relatively free of political pressures, is the way to go in the future. Being a statutory body has undeniable advantages, but having links to government also has its costs.

At all events, the growth of bioethics in Australia is worth study in its own right as a significant socio-cultural phenomenon as the Australian community tries to get to grips with the issues and problems raised by the new biotechnologies. In many ways the debate in Australia has been at a very high level and compares favourably with what has been happening in the USA and Europe and the UK.

Different concepts

Some years ago I wrote, with three collaborators, a book on how science was produced in a scientific institute, the Walter and Eliza Hall Institute of Medical Research.[296] The book, *Life Among the Scientists*, was an attempt to use an anthropological/ethnographic method to understand how scientific knowledge (in this case immunology) was produced in a typical context or sub-culture (in this instance the Walter and Eliza Hall Institute) within the wider sub-culture of contemporary biological science which has been dominated by molecular biology. Through this anthropological understanding we hoped to be able to throw some light on some of the apparent contradictions in modern science, for example, the ambivalence between a highly competitive and individualistic (winner takes all) approach, memorably exemplified in James D. Watson's book on the discovery of DNA,[297] and the nineteenth century ideal of scientific knowledge as publicly and freely available knowledge to be shared disinterestedly with everyone. We also hoped to show that the ideology of scientific positivism, which has been parasitic upon modern science, was a 'construct' that prevented scientists from recognising the role of 'subjectivity' in their work.

In my view, we need some such method to investigate the emergence of bioethics as a socio-cultural phenomenon. There have, of course, been social historical and some sociological studies of the emergence of the new reproductive technologies (especially by feminist scholars), but those approaches screen out most of the idiosyncratic and unpredictable factors which play such a large part in public and social life. They also, for the most part, neglect what have been

called 'the political processes that are an essential part of the management of rivalries among communal values.'[298]

Philip Pettit has reminded us of Oliver MacDonagh's illuminating study,
written in 1958, of the explosion of regulative legislation and statutory
committees in the UK between 1825 and 1875 concerning social issues
such as public health, children employed in factories, workplace safety
and the condition of prisons.[299,300] In each case, MacDonagh argues, a
common pattern emerges. (I cite here Pettit's useful summary). There
is first,

> an evil to be dealt with by policy, usually an evil associated with the
> industrial revolution and the results of that revolution for the organ-
> isation of social life. Second, this evil is exposed, usually in the more
> or less sensational manner of the developing nineteenth century news-
> papers; the exposure of the evil may be triggered by some catastro-
> phe or perhaps by the work of a private philanthropist or fortuitous
> observer. Third, the exposure of the evil leads to popular outrage.
> Fourth, the popular outrage forces government to react by introduc-
> ing legislative or administrative initiatives designed to cope with the
> evil.[301]

This fourth phase involves:

> the putting in place of a regulative bureaucracy, concerned with
> monitoring, reviewing and intervening in the activities where the ori-
> ginal evil arose . . . We now have rule by officials and experts; we have
> the appearance of a new area of bureaucracy.[302]

I would call the factors in MacDonagh's analysis—recognition of an
evil, exposure, public outrage and legislative and bureaucratic reaction—'political' factors in that they involve competing interest groups
in the shaping of public policy, and they are roughly of the kind I have
in view in attempting to understand the extraordinary growth of the
bioethics 'industry'. However, I do not think that MacDonagh's evolu-
tionary schema is of general application since there are, as I noted
before, all kinds of contingent and idiosyncratic facts, large and small,
which have to be taken into account. We must, as I argued, take a more
modest 'anthropological' approach, attempting to see the emergence
of biotechnology within its sub-cultural contexts—first, in the context
of medical science in general and contemporary biology in particular;
second, in the context of modern technological society where the
emphasis is on technological 'fixes' and where science is industrialised
and promises immense financial rewards to those who control it; third,
in the context of the modern hospital system where the benefits of
biotechnology are delivered to people in IVF, cancer treatment, and
the treatment of genetic diseases; then in religious and ethical contexts where ideas and attitudes about the human body, illness, death

and dying, human nature, fertility etc., are formed; and finally, in socio-political contexts where liberal values of autonomy and equality are central, or supposed to be central.

One could discuss at length this complex cultural context within which biotechnology has emerged, but I will single out for brief comment one of the sub-cultures I have mentioned, the modern high technology hospital. The hospital, as we know it, is a recent arrival in our culture, being no more than 150 years old. If we looked at the emergence of the modern hospital with an anthropological eye we would see it as an historically contingent phenomenon appearing at a particular moment in Western culture in response to a complex set of socio-cultural factors. This was not just as the institutional expression of 'scientific medicine' that became established in the nineteenth century but also as the expression within European culture of a socio-cultural process that the French thinker Michel Foucault calls 'renfermement' or 'enclosure' or 'sequestration'. For Foucault the emergence of the hospital is linked with the emergence of the asylum, the factory, the modern prison, the school, even the modern family—all forms of institutional 'enclosure' which he connects with the dramatic increase of state 'surveillance' and control from the eighteenth century onwards.[303]

Again, the American medical sociologist, Elliot Mishler, has claimed that the introduction of the machine model into medicine, the professionalisation of medicine and the coming into being of the modern hospital all went hand-in-hand. As he says:

> a machine model of the body is central to the way the profession of medicine entered the twentieth century.[304]

Mishler also notes that the celebrated Flexner Report (1910) redefined the nature of medicine in terms of technology:

> Medical curricula and practice were shaped around what was easily standardised and defined in technological models. To work appropriately and to claim expertise in the late nineteenth and early twentieth centuries was to work with standardised objects defined in isolation from their social context. The body became a standardised object, and the medical curriculum organised around standardisable skills.[305]

As a result, death was transformed from a human and religious phenomenon into a 'problem of bodily function'. Attention was directed to the body and—as with so many aspects of nature—it became a machine susceptible to repair and intervention. From this redefinition of health, illness and death, and from the professionalisation that it led to, the institution of the hospital as we know it developed.[306,307]

I cannot discuss all the elements of the socio-cultural context within which biotechnology has developed and I restrict myself to mentioning three topics which have come up in my experience on various governmental committees—the Victorian Standing Review and Advisory Committee on Infertility in the 1980s, the Federal National Bioethics Consultative Committee in the late 1980s and its successor the Australian Health Ethics Committee, now a principal committee of the National Health and Medical Research Council.[308]

In 1984 the *Victorian Infertility (Medical Procedures) Act* was passed by the State government after the report of the Waller Committee. Under that Act a Standing Review and Advisory Committee (SRACI) was set up to interpret the Act for the Minister of Health, to receive applications from IVF scientists to carry out procedures governed by the Act, to keep records, and in general to make decisions about the control of IVF and allied matters. Curiously, SRACI owed its existence to the National Party which was opposed to the Minister having unfettered power to administer the Act. But right from the beginning the work of the Committee was considerably affected by the brute political fact that the then Labor Government did not have a majority in the Upper House, so that great caution had to be exercised in introducing discussions about sensitive issues, for example, the micro-injection of sperm into ova, embryo experimentation, IVF assisted surrogacy etc. Explaining to committees of the various parliamentary parties the mysteries of human conception and making fine and delicate distinctions between an 'ovum in the process of fertilisation' up to the point of syngamy (characterised by 'the alignment of chromosomes on the mitotic spindle') at twenty hours, a fertilised ovum postsyngamy, and an individual human embryo, was a rather daunting business! For most politicians (and a large section of the media) the whole area of IVF and reproductive technology was fraught with political danger, despite the fact that most of the polls and surveys showed that the Victorian community was generally in favour of the new technology. Politicians are usually thought to be acutely sensitive to public attitudes but on these kinds of issues they were often quite astray.

These attitudes of politicians were political factors, in the most literal and vulgar sense of 'political', which affected discussion about IVF and biotechnology in Victoria. But there are other less obvious, though important, factors that I would call 'political'. For example, the role of bureaucracies in the health care field is often neglected, although they can play a major part (both negatively and positively) in the shaping of policy. Thus, the National Bioethics Consultative Committee was set up in 1988 to advise the Federal and State Ministers of Health on bioethical issues, but there was already in existence a very powerful sub-committee of health bureaucrats and ministerial advisers who clearly saw the NBCC as usurping their functions and taking over their territory. Almost every time that the NBCC issued a report this sub-committee made an accompanying, and usually contrary, report of its own. I remember a member of this sub-committee saying to me: 'You (meaning the NBCC) can produce your reports but I'm the one who tells my minister what they mean and what he should do about them'. This bureaucratic territoriality is, of course, totally to be expected, but it is something which is not often taken into account. Some years ago, my then colleague Professor Weston Bate arranged a very interesting symposium on Royal Commissions. He invited a number of people—Dick Scotton, William Wentworth, Ronald Henderson and others—who had been involved in various Royal Commissions and asked them to speak about how their commission had been set up, whom they had addressed their report to, whether they felt that they had been used by the government for purely political purposes, whether their report had any real effect and so on. Almost all of the former Royal Commissioners complained about the lack of research and infrastructure support and the role of unsympathetic ministerial advisers in 'killing' politically unwelcome reports. For the most part they regretted their own lack of attention to the bureaucratic reception and 'spin-doctoring' of their reports.

In parenthesis, I might mention that the bureaucratic role is, of course, not always an obstructive or territorial one and that good bureaucratic support can produce good results. In the mid 1980s I was involved in a report of the Victorian Government's Social Development Committee on 'Options for Dying with Dignity' (March 1986) which resulted in the *Victorian Medical Treatment Act* allowing patients to refuse life-sustaining medical treatment. The secretary of the Social Development Committee, a young Victorian public servant, managed the process of consultation extremely well. He arranged the publication of a discussion paper presenting a range of options for 'dying with dignity' and generally brought the whole matter to a very successful conclusion. I have often thought about how valuable it would be to have a reflective account of the whole process from the young departmental secretary's point of view which, despite the sensitive and contentious nature of the issues, resulted in a worthwhile piece of legislation, the *Victorian Medical Treatment Act* 1988. Unfortunately, Australian bureaucrats tend not to publish their memoirs.

The second topic I wish to highlight is the different cultural or sub-cultural styles of the members of bioethics committees. Philosophers, 'ethicists', theologians, lawyers have played a major part in the work of these committees, and members from a broadly feminist background have made an important contribution.[309] These various groups all have their own distinctive professional styles and approaches and 'cultures':

thus philosophers tend to see the function of bioethics committees as the initiation of a quasi-theoretical community debate about the issues under scrutiny in the hope of reaching some kind of community consensus about them and they are often willing to leave their conclusions open-ended. On the other hand, lawyers typically see their role to be the formulation of practical guidelines for coping with the ethical issues arising from medical research and clinical practice and they tend to be critical of the philosophers' 'on the one hand, on the other hand' approach.

Philosophers and public policy

In an American 'Symposium on the Role of Philosophers in the Development of Public Policy', the lawyer Alan J. Weisbard notes that the former President's Commission for the Study of Ethical Problems in Medicine and Bioethical and Behavioral Research used the services of academic philosophers 'to an unprecedented extent'.[310] However, Weisbard claims that the Committee philosophers were not only incapable of translating theory into practice but also used standards of proof and justification that were completely out of touch with the real world of political decision-making. Taking as an example the issue of compensation for injured research subjects, Weisbard says that:

> at the level of macro-policy . . . philosophical analysis tended to invoke standards for justification that few real-world policy initiatives could meet.

And he continues:

> Which, if any, of the social welfare functions of the modern state could survive the type of philosophical scrutiny applied to the proposal to compensate injured research subjects.[311]

A philosophical formation, Weisbard alleges, prevents one from recognising 'the art of the possible' that is necessary in translating theory into practice. No doubt, he concludes, there is a role for philosophy, but it is 'as a critical rather than as an immediately constructive force'.[312] Weisbard admits that his criticism of committee philosophers is made from the pragmatic point of view of the lawyer.

However, much the same kind of criticisms are echoed by a philosopher, Dan W. Brock, who was also a member of the President's Commission. In a contribution to the same symposium Brock argues that the policy maker is inescapably concerned with the likely consequences of any policy that is put in place whereas the philosopher must be concerned with 'an unconstrained search for truth whatever the consequences'.[313] When philosophers join government committees and 'move into the public domain, they must shift their primary commitment from knowledge and truth to the political consequences of what they do'. For Brock then, philosophy is inevitably compromised when it is enlisted in the process of governmental decision-making. The philosopher can, no doubt, contribute to the public debate on issues of concern, but from the outside, so to speak. Thus Brock concludes:

> Philosophers' forays into the world of policy should at best be limited and temporary, not full-time and permanent. The philosophical virtues that enable philosophers to make effective, valuable and distinctive contributions to the policy process are probably best maintained if their primary base and commitment remain in academic philosophy.[314]

I do not, myself, completely agree with Weisbard's or Brock's criticisms of the Committee philosophers but there is no doubt that the difference of professional style and approach and culture of the various committee members is an important consideration in understanding the career of the bioethics movement. In Australia the influence of lawyers, both practical and academic, has been central—one thinks of Mr Justice Kirby, Professor Louis Waller, Russell Scott, Keith Mason, Robin Layton, Don Chalmers and most of the chairpersons of the various state biotechnology enquiries. In his survey of US bioethics commissions Bradford Gray contrasts the National Commission's staff, dominated by career governmental employees, and the President's Commission's staff (appointed mainly by Capron) which was dominated by people from outside government who had professional commitments, in law, medicine, sociology, etc. The members of the President's Commission evaluated its reports in terms of their scholarly quality, while:

> the National Commission was clearly more interested in finding a set of recommendations that they could agree upon than in laying out a rigorous line of reasoning how they got there.[315]

Ethics committees and consensus

The third topic I wish to discuss briefly is the function of bioethics committees in promoting community consensus on the ethical issues raised by the new biotechnologies. There is no doubt that at the beginning of the bioethics movement there was a utopian over-estimation of what is possible in ethical reflection and decision-making, and unrealistic expectations were excited as though the new committees could produce instant and unambiguous solutions to every problem and as though ethical dilemmas and ambiguities were rare and anomalous and not part and parcel of everyday life. Some sociologists have argued that the explosion of interest in bioethics and the emergence of the new committees was due in large measure to the fact that they provide symbolic assurance to the community that some sense can be made of the volatile, bewildering and dangerous scene in modern technology.

This is, so these sceptical sociologists argue, the real social function of bioethics and bioethics committees and has very little to do with the question of whether they have any real and effective role at the practical level. The *Victorian Infertility (Medical Procedures) Act* of 1984 was enacted to ensure that the field of reproductive technology was subject to regulation and control, as though grave moral and social dangers and abuses would occur if it were left unregulated by the law. But the successive governments of New South Wales have refused to follow the Victorian example and there is still no legislative control in the state of New South Wales of reproductive technology (save for prohibition of IVF assisted surrogacy). In my view, it would be difficult to argue that the situation in New South Wales, without the benefit of legislation, is in any way more ethically dubious than in Victoria where there has been quite draconian legislation prima facie at odds with Federal anti-discrimination legislation. From this point of view, one might argue that the real function of the Victorian legislation is largely symbolic, that is, it warns the community that the field of reproductive technology is ethically volatile and that we must maintain surveillance over it.

In parenthesis, one might remark that there is a connection between the method of ethical reflection favoured by a committee and the way it sees its role. I do not want to suggest that the methodology of ethics can be determined by the social role that ethical reflection plays in a particular context. However, the deductive view of ethics which sees ethical decision-making as the application of clear-cut universal principles (personal autonomy, justice, beneficence and non-maleficence) to particular cases and situations, chimes in nicely with the view I have been speaking about, that is as providing symbolic reassurance that the new and potential dangers of biotechnology can be coped with.

When the US Congress established the National Commission for the Protection of Human Subjects in 1974, it required the Commission 'to identify basic ethical principles that could be applied to biomedical and behavioral research'. In 1978 this commission issued its final report, known as the Belmont Report, in which, as one observer has put it, the Commission 'dutifully identified three basic principles: autonomy, beneficence and justice'. It also defined a 'basic ethical principle' as:

> a general judgment that serves as a basic justification for particular prescriptions and evaluations of human actions.[316]

The Commission seems to have assumed that these three basic ethical principles would never come into conflict with each other so that we would never have to decide, for instance, between the claims of personal autonomy and the claims of justice or beneficence. It would, it seems to have been supposed, be relatively easy to reach some kind of minimum community consensus about bioethical issues. As has been remarked, the main purpose of the basic principles and of the whole approach and methodology that went with them was 'to articulate common values and foster consensus about biomedical advances in the face of cultural and religious heterogeneity'.[317] The American philosopher Albert Jonson was a member of the Commission that composed the Belmont Report, and some years after it appeared Jonson wrote as follows: 'As a Commissioner I participated in the formulation of the [Belmont] Report. Today, I am sceptical of its status as a serious ethical analysis. I suspect that it is, in effect, a product of American moralism, prompted by the desire of Congressmen and of the public to see the chaotic world of biomedical research reduced to order by clear and unambiguous principles'. Jonson sees the historical sources of American moralism's fascination with clear and unambiguous ethical principles in secularised versions of Calvinism and Puritanism and Irish Catholic Jansenism and 'rigorism'.[318]

As I have already said, the bioethics committees of the 1970s and 1980s all had the utopian hope that it would be possible to formulate a minimum community consensus and no attention was paid to the ethical pluralism of modern multicultural and liberal societies.[319] Now, in the late 1990s we realise that a community consensus of this kind is both practically impossible and—in a liberal and ethically and religiously pluralist society—ethically and socially undesirable. One of the Victorian ministers under whom I served often spoke of 'the Victorian community': 'The Victorian community wouldn't stand for such and such', the Minister would say. When I asked a ministerial minder on one occasion how one could possibly determine what 'the Victorian community ' was and who spoke for it and what it would and wouldn't stand for, the minder patiently explained to me that what the Minister really meant was that he had a dozen letters from a lobby group on his desk opposing, for example, embryo experimentation, IVF surrogacy or access to IVF for unmarried couples.

A critic of the Warnock Committee's report in the UK has observed that the fact that the Committee, chaired by a professional philosopher, Dame Mary Warnock, tended to raise in some people's minds false expectations as to the nature of the final report. They expected the Committee's recommendations to be backed up by rigorous philosophical argument. In the event, we are given, in the Warnock Report, arguments for and against various positions, and we are given conclusions. But the relationship between the two often remains obscure; we are not always told by which arguments the Committee was persuaded and why. The reason for this, as Mary Warnock has explained, lies in the sheer diversity of views represented on her Committee. 'Every sentence', she has said, 'had to be argued over. To reach agreement on conclusions was difficult enough. To have arrived at an agreed line of argument would have been impossible'.[320]

In similar vein, Stephen Toulmin, who was a staff member with the US National Commission for the Protection of Human Subjects of Biomedical and Behavioral Research in the early 1980s, has pointed out that although commissioners usually agreed on recommendations, they could rarely agree on the principles and arguments on which those recommendations were supposedly based.

> When the eleven individual commissioners asked themselves what 'principles' underlay and supposedly justified their adhesion to the consensus, each of them argued in his or her own way: the Catholics appealed to Catholic principles, the humanists to humanist principles, and so on. They could agree; they could agree what they were agreeing about; but, apparently, they could not agree why they agreed to it.[321]

Much the same view has been taken by Patrick Verspieren, a member of the French National Consultative Committee on Ethics in the Life and Health Sciences established by President Mitterand in the late 1980s.[322] Verspieren (who is a Roman Catholic theologian) rejects the idea that we can formulate some kind of 'common ethics' or 'minimal ethics' for our society. This is to neglect the fact that Western societies are pluralistic, that is characterised by 'the coexistence of diverse philosophical, spiritual and religious options'. On certain matters to do with the origins and the end of human life (for example, procreation and the care of the terminally ill) there are fundamental differences that cannot be negotiated. The best we can do here is to promote enlightened public debate 'where all the families of thought are able to have their say'; then we must 'discover where the most irreducible divergences are located, appreciate the depth of the convictions that are expressed, perceive the values to which the different ethical tendencies are most attached, identify the practices which most deeply offend certain members of society'. Verspieren sees this as the main task of national and other public bodies in the field of bioethics.

That conception of bioethics and of bioethics committees is also of course a 'political' one, in that it is bound up with the politics of the liberal society—a society that is ethically and religiously pluralistic, with a certain view of the relationship between morality and the legal order—many things may be thought to be *immoral* but that does not mean that they should therefore be made *illegal*; and with a novel idea of the relationship between the state and the civic community—many issues should be debated and negotiated within the civic community (abortion, death and dying, reproductive technology, multicultural issues) which, as US experience shows, cannot appropriately be debated and decided at the formal state level.[323,324]

But that is another story, and another argument.

REFERENCES

291. Toulmin S. *The tyranny of principles.* Hastings Centre Report, 1981, 11: 31.
292. Devettere R. *Practical decision making in health care ethics: cases and concepts.* Washington, DC: Georgetown University Press, 1995.
293. For an excellent overview of the US bioethics commissions see Gray Bradford H. Bioethics commissions: what can we learn from past successes and failures? In: Bulger RE, Bobby EM, Fineberg HV (eds). *Society's choices: social and ethical decision making in biomedicine.* Washington DC: National Academy Press, 1995, pp261–306.
294. Spicker SF. Government and bureaucratic bioethics: addressing moral issues in the service of ideology. *The Journal of Medicine and Philosophy* 21, 1996; 113–19.
295. Bulger RE, Bobby EM, Fineberg HV (eds). *Society's choices: social and ethical decision making in biomedicine,* ibid.
296. Charlesworth M, Farrall L, Stokes T, Turnbull D. *Life among the scientists: an anthropological study of an Australian scientific community.* Melbourne: Oxford University Press, 1989.
297. Watson JD. *The double helix: a personal account of the discovery of the structure of DNA,* 1st edition. New York: Atheneum, 1968.
298. Moreno JD. Ethics consultation as a moral engagement. *Bioethics* 5, 1991; 54.
299. MacDonagh O. The 19th century revolution in government: a reappraisal. *Historical Journal* 1, 1958.
300. Pettit P. Instituting a research ethics: chilling and cautionary tales. *Bioethics* 6, 1992; 2: pp89–112.
301. Pettit P. Instituting a research ethics: chilling and cautionary tales, ibid, p90.
302. Pettit P. Instituting a research ethics: chilling and cautionary tales, ibid, p91.
303. Foucault M. *Punir et surveiller.* Paris: Presses Universitaires de France, 1975.
304. Mishler EG, AmaraSingham LR (eds). *Social contexts of health, illness and patient care.* Cambridge: Cambridge University Press, 1981.
305. Mishler EG, AmaraSingham LR (eds). *Social contexts of health, illness and patient care,* ibid, p232.
306. Mishler EG, AmaraSingham LR (eds). *Social contexts of health, illness and patient care,* ibid, p239.
307. Charlesworth, M., *Bioethics in a liberal society.* Melbourne: Cambridge University Press, 1993, pp55–60.
308. Charlesworth M. Bioethics in Australia: 1989–1991; Bioethics in Australia: 1991–1993. In: Lustig BA (ed). *Regional developments in bioethics.* Dordrecht, Holland: Kluwer Academic Publishers, 1992 and 1995.
309. Charlesworth M. Whose body? Feminist views on the reproductive technologies. In: Komesaroff Paul A (ed). *Troubled bodies: critical perspectives on postmodernism, medical ethics and the body.* London: Duke University Press, 1995.
310. Weisbard A. In: Weisbard A, et al. Symposium on the role of philosophers in the development of public policy 1987, *Ethics* 97, (4).

311. Weisbard A. *Symposium on the role of philosophers in the development of public policy*, ibid, p87.
312. Weisbard A. *Symposium on the role of philosophers in the development of public policy*, ibid, p787.
313. Weisbard A. *Symposium on the role of philosophers in the development of public policy*, ibid, p786.
314. Weisbard A. *Symposium on the role of philosophers in the development of public policy*, ibid, p791.
315. Gray BH. Bioethics commissions: what can we learn from past successes and failures? In: Bulger et al (eds) *Society's choices,* ibid, p269.
316. Devettere RJ. Washington: *Practical decision-making in health care ethics.* Georgetown University Press, p22 and chapter 14.
317. Devettere RJ. *Practical decision-making in health care ethics,* ibid, p25.
318. Jonson A. American moralism and the origin of bioethics in the United States. *Journal of Medicine and Philosophy* 1991; 16: 115–29.
319. Charlesworth. M. *Bioethics in a liberal society,* ibid.
320. Cited in Michael Lockwood. *The Warnock Report: a philosophical appraisal.* In: *Moral dilemmas in modern medicine.* Oxford: Oxford University Press, 1985, p155.
321. Toulmin S. The tyranny of principles. *Hastings Centre Report,* 1981, 11: 31–9.
322. Verspieren P. Appréhension des problèmes de la bioéthique. *Après-Demain* 266, 1984; pp37–8.
323. Grant L. Fertile grounds for debate. *Guardian Weekly,* 13 October 1996. In a recent comment on the UK Human Fertilisation and Embryology Authority Grant claims that there is a feeling 'that we should create stronger laws over the bodies of women in case they make decisions we don't approve of'. The HFEA, she says, 'has been given the power to decide questions . . . which the combined forces of the world's departments of philosophy have failed to resolve over 2000 years. Perhaps we are not asking too little of the HFEA, but too much—and too little of ourselves in surrendering to the state control over the most personal of dilemmas'.
324. Pfeffer N. *The stork and the syringe.* London: Polity Press, 1993.

CHAPTER NINE

Judgment Difficult

Eric J. Cassell

'Life is short, and the art long; the occasion fleeting; experience fallacious; and judgment difficult. The physician must not only be prepared to do what is right himself, but also to make the patient, the attendants, and the externals co-operate.'

(The first aphorism of Hippocrates.)[325]

Rose Gonzalez lived in the apartment building above a physician's office. Her son called during office hours to say that his mother was very sick and could he bring her down immediately. The secretary, impressed by the fear in his voice, said yes without asking the physician. Her son half carried, half dragged his mother into the office and, with help, put her on an examining table. Mrs Gonzalez was dry, cachectic, febrile, her eyelids were retracted and her eyes sunken, she barely moved and answered questions after long pauses in a coarse whisper. She was obviously close to dead.

She said she did not know how long she had been sick, but that she, 'hadn't been eating right for a long time'. She was not in pain, but could contribute no more history. A quick examination revealed a heart rate of 120/min, rales in both lungs, and a distended abdomen with an enlarged liver and multiple hard masses. Her lower legs were grossly swollen.

The physician and son conversed away from the mother. The son explained that he had tried to get her to a physician for months, but she had adamantly refused. Away for two weeks, he was shocked when he came to visit this afternoon. The physician said that his mother was going to die very shortly, maybe even today or tomorrow. She appeared to have metastatic cancer. She could go to the hospital or be cared for at home, what did the son want to do? Her son became belligerent, insisting that his mother get the best care money could buy, he wanted her life saved at all costs, and he didn't like the idea that the physician was 'giving up on her'.

An ambulance was called, after Mrs Gonzalez agreed, and she was brought to an emergency department. The physician called the emergency department chief to tell him about the case and the son's behaviour. She died during the night.

This is a straightforward case, yet many decisions and judgments were made in the brief time that this patient was in the physician's office. This chapter is about how such judgments are made. Almost three decades ago, in the book, *Clinical Judgment*,[326] Alvan R. Feinstein examined how judgments are made in clinical medicine. He argued that each case is like a scientific experiment that starts from a certain point, is acted on, and leads to outcomes. Unlike laboratory science, however, there are no controls against which to measure the results of interventions. Instead, the clinician's experience provides the background against which the case must be compared. The problem is that the clinician's previous experience will not count for much, nor will the present case, unless the physician is able to develop 'measures'[327] for the many features and experiences presented by each clinical happening that will allow comparisons between cases and between different periods in the same case. In a recent paper, Dr Feinstein expressed his disappointment that in the years since the publication of *Clinical Judgment*, the field of clinical epidemiology that had evolved from his work stressed quantitative mathematical models on which to base decision-making, rather than having to come to terms with the necessarily qualitative nature of the information in most clinical situations.[328] Something else happened. The word 'judgment' was replaced by the term 'decision-making'. Decision-making allows for rules; formulas for arriving at things like specificity, sensitivity, positive predictive value, likelihood ratios, and such like. These, as we all know, can be very useful in deciding, for example, in what general circumstances a positive test result is most useful, or when the addition of another test will add little or no more useful information.[329] So useful, in fact, that every clinician should be comfortable and conversant with the concepts and methods of clinical epidemiology and their use in clinical situations.

Clinical judgment versus clinical epidemiology

Understandings of judgment are an essential aspect of the classical field of logic. For John Dewey,

> Judgment . . . is a continuous process of resolving an indeterminate, unsettled situation into a determinately unified one, through operations which transform subject matter originally given.[330]

According to Bernard Bosanquet, a famous logician of the late nineteenth century,

> Judgment . . . is the intellectual function that defines reality by significant ideas, and in so doing affirms the reality of those ideas. I use the term 'define', because to define implies something given which is to

be defined; and it is an essential of the act of judgment that it always refers to a reality which goes beyond and is independent of the act itself.[331]

Let me go a step further to clarify the relationship between the methods of clinical epidemiology and what this chapter is about.

Take this case, for example:

Bertha Turner is a 74-year-old, high-strung woman whose symptom is exertional dyspnoea. For the past month she has noted shortness of breath walking on the street. It is not consistent. On one occasion it happened after walking a block, while on another it took three blocks to develop. She believes that it is worse after eating—it both happens more quickly and is more severe. She never has to stop because of the symptom. She has no chest pain but feels the shortness of breath substernally. She does not have orthopnoea. She has never had the symptom previously. Her husband had angina for many years and recently had a successful coronary artery bypass. Physical examination is normal. So are her chest X-ray, EKG, pulmonary function studies, CBC, and screening blood chemistries.

Is her symptom angina and does she have ischaemic heart disease? What else could it be? There is no evidence that she has pulmonary disease (a judgment) and there are no evident aetiologies (a judgment). Heart failure is equally unlikely (a judgment). It might be psychogenic. However, it is unlikely that she would develop a new psychologically determined symptom at her age (a judgment). On the other hand, she might interpret something that is quite common for her in a new manner that would make it seem like a new symptom. Several approaches to the diagnosis present themselves. We might ask her to pay more attention to her shortness of breath and return in a week with a symptom diary. Or, one might suggest that she take sublingual nitroglycerin prior to the circumstances in which she usually becomes dyspnoeic as a diagnostic trial. Both approaches were common years ago. Making the diagnosis either way presumes a prior judgment that she is not immediately threatened by her symptom or its underlying illness and thus can wait for a definitive diagnosis. In the present era it would be usual to recommend that she have an exercise test to determine if she gets EKG changes or develops her symptom with measured exercise. On the basis of published (validated) criteria for ST changes, the test would be considered positive or negative.

There are established levels of sensitivity, specificity, and positive predictive value of treadmill exercise tests depending on whether you believe that the patient belongs in a population for whom the diagnosis of ischaemic heart disease would be probable or improbable. If the test is positive, the next judgments concern the necessity (or lack thereof) for further studies to determine the nature and extent of her possible coronary artery disease and whether she should have an angioplasty or coronary artery bypass surgery. If not, what medications should be prescribed and whether exercise and diet will be part of her treatment. As she initially tells the story of her exertional breathlessness, all these judgments raise their head. All of them are influenced by who she is (demographically and individually), by the nature of the disease believed to be present (or absent), by the current state of the diagnostic and therapeutic art, and by the diagnostic and therapeutic goals that have been established specifically for her. Because of all of the elements that enter into the judgment about Bertha Turner's care, I believe it is safe to say that judgment is not decision-making in the fashion described by clinical epidemiology. Judgment is, by definition, an opinion arrived at by applying general information (whether from experience or scientific evidence) to a specific circumstance—defining that situation. There can be, therefore, no set rules, formulae, or quantitative methods for arriving at a judgment. This is the reason it is said that judgment cannot be taught, but only learned by experience. So how can it be that I am writing a chapter about how to make judgments? Because it is possible to understand the elements of judgments, what enters into them, what kind of thinking leads to better judgments, and what kind to unreliable opinions.

Let us return to the opening case. See the number of different areas in which judgments were made. The secretary decided to tell the patient's son to bring her down immediately 'because of the fear in his voice'. Physicians' secretaries learn to make such decisions so that the sick are not turned aside nor the healthy allowed to jump the queue. The physician quickly estimated the severity of her illness, recognising classic Hippocratic facies:

> In acute diseases the physician must conduct his inquiries in the following way. First he must examine the face of the patient and see whether it is like the faces of healthy people, and especially whether it is like its usual self. Such likeness will be the best sign, and the greatest unlikeness will be the most dangerous sign. The latter will be as follows. Nose sharp, eyes hollow, temples sunken, ears cold and contracted with their lobes turned outward, the skin about the face hard and tense and parched; the colour of the face as a whole being yellow or black. If at the beginning of the diseases the face be like this, and if it be not yet possible with the other symptoms to make a complete prognosis, you must go on to inquire whether the patient has been sleepless, whether his bowels have been very loose, and whether he suffers at all from hunger. And if anything of the kind be confessed, you must consider the danger to be less. The crisis comes after a day and a night if through these cause the face has such an appearance. But should no such confession be made, and should a recovery not take place within this period, know that it is a sign of death.[332]

as a sign of terminal illness as well as the weakness, and virtual inability to answer questions. Then a judgment was made on the basis of physical findings, that she probably had metastatic cancer. A prognostic judgment was made about the nearness of death. Possible dispositions were offered—the hospital or home. Mrs Gonzalez was asked what she wanted—it was the physician's opinion (judgment) that she still had the capacity to participate in the decision. When her son became aggressive, the physician judged it not to be truly related to the physician's actions but to something within the son (guilt, perhaps, or fear). A decision was made to send her to the emergency department rather than directly to a hospital room for terminal care. And to warn the physician there to treat her as though it might be possible to save her life so the son would know 'that everything had been done'. Diagnostic, therapeutic, prognostic, filial, social, psychological, and political arenas were all considered.

Medical judgments are not merely personal opinions

We need another case:

> A 42-year-old white derelict lying on a stretcher in the Bellevue emergency ward said that an hour earlier he had been walking on the street when he suddenly became severely short of breath and could not walk. He leaned against a building for a long time until he gradually felt better. His extreme anxiety did not subside, however, so he came to the hospital. There had been no previous similar episodes and he considered himself 'a healthy drunk'. He had not previously come to the emergency room and had last seen a physician years earlier. His blood pressure was 220/130. There were no other findings of note except for his general filthiness, tachycardia, and cut and bruised legs.
>
> An hour later the resident asked the intern why nothing had been done. Where was the chest X-ray, EKG, blood gases? Only blood had been drawn and an IV started, and those by the nurse. The intern explained that the man was a bum and had only come into the ER because it was cold outside, and besides, there was nothing to find on examination. Spurred on by a very angry resident who had taken his own history and warned how sick the patient was, no matter what he looked like or who he was, the studies were completed just before the patient went back into pulmonary edema.[333]

Both the intern and the resident had made clinical judgments; one was wrong and the other was right. Not simply because the resident knew more medicine, although that is partly the reason. Their judgments were about different things. The resident formed an opinion about why an otherwise healthy white man with a blood pressure of 220/130 would suddenly become very short of breath and then, just as suddenly, feel well again but remain frightened and come to a hospital. He probably thought that pulmonary oedema had been the source of the dyspnea. I doubt if he consciously thought about all the steps in the unusual chain of events that led to the patient's appearance in the emergency ward. Did he actively consider the pathophysiology involved in a white man who did not go to doctors and was an alcoholic and had such an elevated blood pressure, who probably had heart disease—hypertensive heart disease, or maybe cardiomyopathy? More likely is that he was answering the consciously expressed question, 'why is this particular man here at this time with this history?'

The intern had formed an opinion about drunks and winter time. Since he had not had much experience with derelicts it was probably not his own opinion, but a bias he had learned from others. A stereotype, if you will, in which the opinion is not formed on the basis of first hand experience. It did not answer a question posed by the appearance in the emergency ward of this particular derelict, it could have been the answer about any other Bowery alcoholic who showed up in that ward. Because it was a judgment about any derelict in winter time, it stood a good chance of being wrong from the beginning. And it was. The judgment was about the wrong particular.

This intern's judgment was simply his own opinion. It is a common saying that everyone is entitled to his or her own opinion. An opinion is a judgment, so, by extension, everyone is entitled to his own judgment. Or put another way—just to exaggerate—a judgment is a personal opinion that may be right or wrong, but is a personal matter. Idiosyncratic. This is one of the criticisms that has been levelled against teaching judgment. In this view, not only is judgment the application of a general truth to a particular situation (so there can be no set rules to guide it), but, because it is a personal opinion, it is like taste. Taste, the saying goes, is not a matter of dispute because it is individual. This next case may help.

> Evan Lynch is a 24-year-old man who developed what seemed to be a cold two days ago. Yesterday he had a headache, was tired, and had difficulty concentrating. This morning his headache became terrible and unremitting, he had a temperature of 104° F and vomited. He called his doctor and seemed somewhat confused. The physician asked him to try touching his chin to his chest. The manoeuvre caused severe neck pain. The physician told him to go to the emergency room immediately. The emergency room was alerted to the probability that he had meningitis and needed an emergency lumbar puncture and prompt treatment with antibiotics.

It is not a surprise that the physician made the diagnosis. The patient's symptoms were typical and the stiff neck was a strong confirmatory demonstration. Were the physician's judgments her personal opinion? Yes. On the other hand, almost any physician would have come to the same conclusion. Thus, while the judgment was a personal opinion, it was not idiosyncratic, it was not whimsy, nor based on information pulled out of thin air. It was grounded in the *shared* knowledge that makes up medical science, in the skills common to clinicians, and, crucially, in the shared values of professional responsibility. While the clinician's judgment was her opinion, it wasn't merely a private matter. What would you have thought if she told the patient that he probably had a cold and shouldn't worry? You would probably, in common with virtually all clinicians, believe that she had made a life-threatening error. Why? A temperature of 104° F does not happen with a cold. Neither do terrible headaches, confusion, or a stiff neck. The implications of these facts are part of shared medical knowledge, public knowledge, if you will. The doctor in this case is aware that other people have the same knowledge and that they would criticise her if she acted incorrectly. Where did she get that idea? From the earliest days of their training, physicians are publicly criticised for their errors. There are many circumstances—for example, case conferences, morning reports, or bedside rounds—where mistakes are openly discussed. The intent of such public reproach is to have physicians acknowledge to themselves and others when they make a mistake. Another consequence is that for the remainder of their professional lives, physicians know that even private medical judgments have an internalised audience. The internalised social group is a powerful force for maintaining behaviour, in all aspects of life, not just medicine.

Medical opinions are not just technical judgments

The physician in the preceding case did not just make a technical decision regarding the probable diagnosis of meningitis. She also decided that the patient's life was in danger and required immediate action. That is a moral judgment. You may believe that it is self-evident, physicians are meant to save life above all. That may be true, but the decision in this case helps clarify why medicine is not merely a technical profession, but a moral profession as well. It has to do with the welfare of its patients—what is good and right for them, as well as what is technically correct. In this instance, we know that the patient shares the physician's values in this regard or he would not consent to go to the emergency ward.

To make the point, let me change the case. Suppose that this patient had end-stage non-Hodgkin's lymphoma. All treatments had failed to arrest his disease and he was clearly dying and being cared for at home in a hospice program. He had expressed the wish never to return to the hospital. In this instance, his physician, just as aware that he had some type of meningitis, might have ensured that he received adequate pain relief for his headache and made no suggestion about the emergency ward or antibiotics. Here the moral context has changed and the need to accede to the patient's wishes and provide a comfortable death are the dominant values in coming to an opinion about the right thing to do. Virtually every medical judgment has a value component and it is necessary to identify the values at issue in order to take them into account. Sometimes, as in the case above, they are obvious, but on other occasions they can be troubling.

In order that values enter appropriately into medical judgments, they must be identified and given suitable weights. For example, out of vanity many people do things to and with their bodies that may, from a physician's point of view, endanger their health or life. Making clear the danger is usually sufficient to change the behaviour. There are very few people who would rather be dead than unattractive to others. Yet the strength of vanity as a value may be enormous and very different from the value structure of the physician.

It is necessary in making judgments to clarify which are the patient's values and which are the physician's values. Here is a brief case that shows such a conflict:

A 36-year-old single childless professional violist had recurrent carcinoma in the same breast after both lumpectomy and radiation to the breast. The most potent chemotherapeutic regimen had a high probability of producing peripheral neuropathy in her fingers that might end her career. In conjunction with the patient, an alternate regimen was chosen. This judgment, although requiring up-to-date technical knowledge, was based on a difficult calculus of values, especially in view of the probabilistic nature of all the possible outcomes.

It is in end-of-life decisions that physicians have the most difficulty factoring in the multiple competing values. In the face of inevitable death, when should treatment be changed from an attempt at cure to primary relief of symptoms? When should the dying patient be removed from the respirator? Our difficulty with these judgments reflects our inadequate training in eliciting patients' values and our seeming inability to give them equal weight with technical values in the process of making judgments. We know that physicians are aware of the importance (another word for value) of personal matters in the care of the sick by how they behave in their own or their family's illnesses. In this short section I cannot do justice to the difficulties inherent in factoring values into making judgments. It is merely necessary to point out that there are very few value-free judgments and that the field of bioethics and the bioethicists, now members of many hospital staffs, specifically address this issue.

Family and society

The judgments made in the case of Rose Gonzalez that opened this chapter required thought about the nature of relationship among family members. It is also necessary for the physician to understand how society views the obligations of children to their parents. The son, who says that he had tried for weeks to get his mother to a doctor, returns after a two week absence to find her desperately ill. Is it true that he advised her to seek medical care? We do not really know and the son is aware that we might doubt him. Any question we have about his attention to his mother would be the equivalent of criticism because of the social rules that guide the obligations of children to their parents. Perhaps he feels guilty that he abandoned her in these last two weeks when she really needed him. One way or another he is going to have feelings about his behaviour at the time of her death and these feelings and thoughts will last for years.

We might also feel guilty in similar circumstances. We are aware of other possibilities—perhaps he hated her and this is his chance to get even for the injuries of infancy. How do we know? These are part of the shared facts of the social world and relationships within families. Do physicians have obligations in this regard—should these facts enter their decision-making? Before answering this question it is necessary to understand that it is impossible to make a judgment that will not have one effect or another on the son. For example, the reasonable suggestion that she might be cared for at home during this terminal illness evokes anger in the son. He suggests that it means that we 'are giving up on her'. The physician might say: a) 'There is no sense hospitalising her, she will be dead very shortly and it doesn't matter what anybody does.' Unspoken might be the further sentence, 'If you care so much, why didn't you bring her sooner?' b) 'Why should we hospitalise her just because you can't bring yourself to recognise that she is going to die?' c) 'We'll hospitalise her because you want us to, but it won't make any difference.' Instead, an ambulance was called to bring her to the hospital without any comment to the son. However, the discussion with the attending physician in the emergency department acknowledged the place of the son in the decision-making and the desire to have the son know that 'everything possible was done'. Once it is realised that any judgment will have an impact on the son, then the physician making the judgment has a responsibility for not only the mother, but also the son.

Medical judgments are made in the real world, which means that they are never isolated to include only the patient, or even solely the patient and the family. They always have a wider social force. The next case illustrates this:

> Alston Brook is a 78-year-old man who had a mitral valve replacement in the middle of August. It is now the end of November and he is still in the pulmonary intensive care unit. In early October he was transferred to a rehabilitation facility, but was back in the hospital because of ventilatory failure before 12 hours had elapsed. His physicians believe that he cannot maintain his own respiration because of weakness of his diaphragmatic and other muscles of respiration. For the last two weeks it has been impossible to disconnect him from the respirator. He has a deep sacral decubitus. Although conscious, he now rarely recognises anyone, even his wife who is always at his bedside. None of his physicians—including the house-staff—believe he will live to be discharged from the hospital.

In the past, while well, this patient had frequently expressed abhorrence at the idea of dying on 'machines'. His brother and brother-in-law are physicians. His daughter, 26, is a graduate student in the sciences. The wife and the attending physician agreed some weeks ago that he should be disconnected from the respirator and allowed to die away from the unit. His wife, however, wanted to have general agreement on the subject within the family, including all the doctors. The daughter has been the last holdout. She visits him on weekends and proudly tells the staff about his improvement since the last visit. What to do about him has been the source of disagreement among the staff of the unit. The wife's friends and acquaintances all have opinions—generally in favour of disconnecting the respirator, but not unanimously. It is obvious that whatever decision is made, there is a considerable audience. Most physicians are unaware of the size of the group that is attentive to their judgments. The public, as we all know, has become very knowledgeable about medical matters, and it has opinions about doctors and what they do. Most physicians, when they start practising, do not know that the intertwined networks of their patients make it likely that what they do for one is known by other patients in short order. They soon learn this. Not only the family, then, but a larger social group is affected by the judgments of physicians.

In recent years the audience has enlarged to include third party payers—for example, insurance companies, employers and unions. These agencies examine the acts of physicians in order to determine payment or adherence to payment policies. Managed care organisations audit the records of doctors in a more inclusive manner. Managed care plans may also check to see whether physicians have adhered to clinical practice guidelines. Finally, there are lawyers and the courts. The threat of malpractice looms so large in American medicine in this last generation that doctors may constantly feel the threat even if they have never had a malpractice suit. All of this scrutiny is new in the history of medicine, but it makes clear how public and social the act of medical judgment has become, an act that used to be considered too personal and private to be taught.

Medical judgments are political

When I use the term 'political' I mean it in its old-fashioned sense as the relations between persons in a social group or an institution. Specifically, dealing with the relationships of physicians to patients, other physicians, their institutions, and community. For example, the judgments that made the physician send Rose Gonzalez to the emergency department instead of back upstairs to her apartment and made him call the emergency department chief and warn him of impending trouble were not directly for the benefit of the patient. How was the intern's standing affected by his wrong judgment in the case of the derelict? What did the cardiologist think when Bertha Turner was sent for a stress test but not a consultation? What do the various physicians, nurses, other staff, and family members think of the various judgments made about leaving Alston Brook on the respirator or taking him off it? In other words, what is the impact of a judgment on the physician making the judgment? There can be no doubt that people's standing in their communities are affected by their actions, and a judgment is a public action because it almost always has an audience, even if only in the mind of the person making the judgment.

Some might ask, not denying the political nature of judgments, whether this is really medicine. Bertha Turner was sent for a stress test rather than a consultation so that her attending physician could maintain control of the case. He knows that the cardiologist is more aggressive than he about recommending angioplasty or bypass and he does not want these options discussed with her before he is ready. Is that medicine? I believe that it is medicine in its practice, if not its theory, and the failure to learn these aspects of judgment means that judgments will be made either inadequately or intuitively rather than after searching for the right question and consciously thinking through the options.

On reflection physicians may discover that vanity, pride, or the desire to look good to others, is playing a larger part in their judgments than might be best for their patients. Everyone is motivated by these personal desires, just as they are by the wish to make money. It is the balance between what is in the best interest of the patient, and what is primarily for the benefit of the physician or health care organisation that is often at issue. I am not naive enough to believe that a chapter on judgment can change behaviour that is motivated primarily by greed or vanity—these are issues of character. On the other hand, only by actively reflecting on troublesome problems do physicians (and others) come to control them. Conflicts of interest pervade medicine—for example, financial interests of physicians versus patients, physicians' attentions to their own families and personal lives versus attention to patients, time spent working versus time for themselves. The outcome of these contests are reflected in clinical judgments, therefore it is here that they should be considered.

Practical wisdom

When political factors and conflicts of interest are seen to be part of clinical judgments, there can be no further doubt that we have left clinical epidemiology and 'decision-making' far behind. To find out where we have arrived, we have to go back to Aristotle, a physician himself and the son of a physician (an Asclepiad who probably lived a generation or so later than Hippocrates). Aristotle distinguished what he called practical wisdom (phronesis) from technical proficiency, knowledge and understanding.[334] Knowledge—beliefs about what things are, how they came to be, what becomes of them, and how they work—is what in medicine is called knowing medical science. There is little doubt that to this day, few would consider knowing medical science, even in great depth, to be the equivalent of having good clinical judgment. Understanding, on the other hand, operates on knowledge by questioning and deliberating to produce generalisations that can be brought to bear on issues for which there is insufficient specific knowledge. Good medical scientists use their understanding of their subject matter to design further research or speculate on how things are going to turn out in specified circumstances. GWF Hegel, an important philosopher of the nineteenth century, also distinguished understanding as a step of the intellect beyond reason. Aristotle continues:

> . . . but understanding and practical wisdom are not the same. For practical wisdom issues commands, since its end is what ought to be done or not to be done; but understanding only judges.[335]

Practical wisdom is the quality of mind concerned with things good and right for persons. Because of this goal, it is a moral endeavour which is more often found among the excellent than among those who are morally deficient. Since no one believes that people are born with wisdom, but rather develop it, it is not surprising that the personal excellence necessary to practical wisdom is acquired through understanding the need for it and striving after it in practice.

Clinical wisdom in clinical judgment

This brings us to an uncomfortable conclusion. Clinical judgment, as must be apparent by now, is not merely an issue of technical knowledge, but is something involving what is best for patients with consideration of the personal, familial, social and political issues raised by all but the most trivial judgments. Further, it involves what is best for the physician as well, after the interests of the patient have been given primacy. Why is the conclusion discomforting? Because most people thinking about judgment consider it a personal, private or idiosyncratic operation. Objective medical science was meant to solve exactly this feature of clinical medicine—to surmount the need for the personal opinions of clinicians. Will medical practice rest on a permanent framework of science and objective fact or the chaos of a medicine arising from personal opinions or self-proclaimed authority?

This is not a problem for medicine alone. The end of the nineteenth and the beginning of the twentieth centuries have seen the development of a successful science and a belief throughout our whole society in the power of empirical knowledge. In recent decades there has been an increasingly strong case made for the fact that the concepts of truth, rationality, reality and others must be understood as relative to specific contexts, cultures, societies and conceptual schemes. The claim that it is science, and science alone, that is the measure of reality, knowledge and truth is confronted with the understanding that there are other legitimate sources of knowledge and experience to be found in the classical humanistic disciplines and the tradition of practical wisdom. As the twentieth century draws to a close, a more balanced view seems to be emerging that cannot but help influence medicine.[336]

The recent spate of guidelines for clinical action covering many diseases and states and the new call for 'evidence-based medicine' are current examples of attempts to get around the necessity for the judgment of individual physicians.[337] I have already shown that judgment is not the private and personal thing that most commentators believe it to be. We know this position to be impossible in the face of its inherently public nature. Yet, the problem raised by returning to the example of practical wisdom as described by Aristotle is that good medical judgment—clinical wisdom—would seem to require good physicians. Not merely the cognitive requirement of the knowledgeable or technically proficient, but the moral requirement of good in themselves. To do what is right and good for the patient is really doing what is right and good for a person—in the manner of Aristotle's practical wisdom. The problem to be solved is how clinicians get that way—good in the sense that we say of someone that he or she is a good person?

One way that people try and get around this is to say that most judgments are made about only one aspect of a case and do not involve patients themselves. The choice of an antibiotic, for example, or of a treatment for a leg ulcer. Whether to do an MRI or a CT scan of the head in a claustrophobic patient might be another instance. In all these illustrations, the decision must have some impact on the patient or one would not bother with the decision in the first place. Even in decision-making terms, when considering the positive predictive value of (say) a treadmill exercise study, the issue is not whether the test indicates ischaemic heart disease, but whether the person has ischaemic heart disease. Analogously, when surgeons operate, the patient is frequently draped in such a manner that only the operative field is visible, as though whatever is being done is done only to the bowel (for example). It isn't true, however; the surgery is being done to the whole person. The fact is, one cannot make a judgment about a part of anything without also making a judgment about the whole.

Clinical judgments are meant for the good of the patient. What says that morally deficient clinicians cannot make good decisions? Nothing, except that the sins of clinicians—vanity, pride, greed, deceit, disinterest, laziness, carelessness, untrustworthiness, callousness, insensitivity and overriding self-interest—might interfere with making the good of the patient the primary good. All share in these failings from time to time and to some degree. Becoming a good clinician involves suppressing or keeping these urges within bounds, in order that the patient should come first. Most good clinicians whom I have known work their way over the years to achieving the goodness necessary to their work, generally without thinking of it in those terms. My chairman, Walsh McDermott, once said that as a young physician he thought that he himself did not have the qualities of character that made good clinicians, but that he knew how to behave in the proper manner, so that is what he did. No one can ask for more.

A simple example may help:

> Rose Celli is a 74-year-old woman with a smoking history of almost a lifetime. She developed a carcinoma of the larynx which was operated on in a small hospital in a New York suburb. Within a year she

developed locally recurrent disease manifested by lymph node enlargement in the neck. The radiation oncologist of the hospital directed her treatment. Not long afterward she had flashing lights in one eye and an MRI showed a large craniopharyngioma. The same radiation therapist started treating this tumour and also started her on a course of chemotherapy.

Craniopharyngiomas are uncommon tumours. Should this radiation oncologist in a small hospital with little opportunity to treat such lesions have referred her to a larger cancer centre? Vanity and pride often cause physicians to work beyond their sure knowledge to the detriment of their patients. On the other hand, the oncologist may have had the training, experience and technical equipment to treat her appropriately. Only he can make the judgment. Part of becoming clinically wise, therefore, is learning to honestly examine your own motives to know who is the primary benefactor of your actions. Not easy. As well as its importance to patients clinical wisdom can bring great personal rewards—little wonder that its pursuit is arduous and continuous. Clinical wisdom is another example of a pursuit in life that doesn't have a final harbour, it is the journey that counts.

Interim summary

Judgment, it turns out, is not merely the private, personal, idiosyncratic function it is frequently thought to be. In medicine, diagnostic, therapeutic and prognostic judgments all have social and political impact on the persons who make them as well as on their beneficiaries. They almost always involve conflicting values. Doctors who make judgments almost always have an audience examining their judgments —if not in fact, then in their minds. They are almost always given wider meanings by doctors and patients. Judgments, even though they may seem to be about limited aspects of the patient's circumstances, always influence the whole patient. I should add here that judgments are never solely about a moment in time. They always have an impact on future judgments. When they are about patients, they are inevitably in the moral domain even when they seem to be solely technical because they have to do with the welfare—what is right and good for the patient—the sick or well person. Making sure that interests of the patient remain central to all decisions requires goodness on the part of physicians. I believe that this, in addition to other aspects of the function, moves clinical judgment into the category of clinical wisdom, the medical equivalent of practical wisdom as discussed by Aristotle.[338]

Questions and answers

The time has come to address the question of how judgments should be made. Strangely, the beginning of the answer is found in the widely held belief that one cannot teach how to make a proper judgment. The faculty of judgment cannot be taught, except by demonstration, it is said, because it is the application of general knowledge to a particular situation. Since every particular circumstance is, by definition, different there is no possibility of a set rule for the application of knowledge. That may be, but what makes something particular, individual and unique are the details, the facts of the particularity. Therefore, learning judgment starts with learning how to isolate the subject of the judgment; how to make clear the details of the particular situation.

Here is a simple case to illustrate:

> Rona Grey is a 58-year-old woman who has had intermittent right upper quadrant pain for more than a year. In the last few weeks it has been more constant, sometimes disturbing her sleep. She went to her primary care physician who elicited the above history. The physician's examination revealed no abnormalities. Because an upper GI series and upper abdominal sonogram were normal, a colonoscopy was performed which also showed no disease. When the physician discovered that her husband was very sick, Mrs Grey was reassured that her pain was probably from stress.

The physician made three common judgments (opinions, decisions) in this all too frequent scenario. First, presumably, that she might have demonstrable disease of the stomach, duodenum, gall bladder or pancreas to account for her distress. When this seemed not to be true, that disease might be revealed in the large bowel. Finally, in the absence of discovered disease, that her pain was from stress. Subsequently, extensive questioning revealed this further history. Her appetite was normal and she had not changed her diet recently. The pain was usually dull and occasionally sticking in quality. It was not as much in the right upper quadrant as up under the right costal margin. In relation to her pain or otherwise, she was not nauseated, queasy or bloated, and she did not vomit. The pain was not related to food which neither brought on nor relieved her discomfort. Her bowel habits had not changed and moving her bowels neither aggravated nor relieved the discomfort. On the other hand, the pain was worse after sitting for long periods. A long automobile trip aggravated the pain. On occasion she had discomfort in her upper back at the same time as her abdominal pain. There was no question that it was worse during the very tense periods sitting with her husband in the oncologist's office and in the hospital. Examination revealed tenderness just under the right costal margin where the anterior abdominal muscles attached to the ribs. There was also a very tender muscle 'knot' in the right infraspinatus muscle (but not in other muscles in the area). In the light of the further history and physical findings, the initial physician's judgments appear inadequate. We could rephrase the judgments by saying, 'There is something causing structural change in the stomach or duodenum (or gall bladder, pancreas or large bowel) which is causing this woman's pain but not disturbing the function of these organs sufficiently to cause other symptoms'. They could be rephrased as a question. 'What causes discoverable structural changes in the stomach, duodenum, (or gall bladder, pancreas or large bowel) that causes pain lasting intermittently for more than a year, that is worse during a period of emotional distress, yet does not result in symptomatic dysfunction of these organs?' I know of no pathophysiology or disease that satisfies these criteria. Since that is the answer to the physician's judgments posed as questions, there was no point in doing the diagnostic studies.

Actually, the patient had intercostal causalgia. The superficial nerve is 'pinched' where it goes through the muscle bundle of the infraspinatus muscle that is in spasm. The discomfort is felt at the destination of the nerve—the anterior abdominal wall on the right side at the costal margin, rather than at the point of irritation. The muscle as it inserts on the underside of the costal margin becomes tender because it also goes into spasm secondary to the pain. Since tight muscles play a part in the pathophysiology of her pain, it is not surprising that the pain is worse during emotional tension.

A judgment, which may be phrased as a proposition, statement, opinion or a decision is, as RC Collingwood has made clear, really the answer to a question.[339] In the question lies the statement of particularity, the details that make the situation unique. Did the physician, in the judgments requesting the imaging studies and then the colonoscopy, have the wrong answer. No, the answer was correct, the diagnostic studies were appropriate to the question he asked based on the inadequate history. The problem is that he asked the wrong question.

He asked the question, 'What discoverable structural change causes pain in the right upper quadrant?' Many things—for example, gall bladder disease, duodenal ulcers, gastroesophageal reflux disease, pancreatitis or pancreatic malignancy, inflammatory bowel disease—and the tests that he requested are one way of going after these diseases as the aetiology of the pain. What makes it a poor question is that it has too many correct answers. In the question-answer pairs used in making judgments, there should be only one correct answer to the question. If more than one correct answer is possible, then the question has not been properly asked—it is not detailed enough to catch the particularity of the problem. Bringing to mind, for example, acute appendicitis, you may not accept this. The diagnostic judgment is not highly detailed and particularised, yet it is the correct answer and leads to a specific, detailed and particularised action—an operation on a particular patient by a particular surgeon using a specific technique, and so on.

The question it seems to be answering is general, what is the cause of the patient's right lower quadrant abdominal pain. Yet, a moment's reflection will show you that neither the question, 'Why does this patient have right lower quadrant pain?' nor the answer, 'acute appendicitis', are vague or general. As one asks the questions of the patient and performs the physical examination that leads to the diagnosis, a particular patient marked by a myriad of individual details is being considered. Similarly, the decision to operate on a particular patient implies more than just the judgment, 'acute appendicitis'. The patient's suitability for surgery, the state of the appendix at this time, other diseases, allergies, and many other features have been considered in the judgments leading to action. Thus the words 'acute appendicitis' are a shorthand for the whole long diagnostic statement in the clinician's head that is the answer to the complex and detailed question about this patient with right lower quadrant pain.

The question-answer method is applicable to every clinical setting and every step in the clinical process. Virtually every patient contact with a physician—admission to the hospital, subsequent hospital visits, office visits, home visits, telephone calls—raises diagnostic questions for which answers may be required. Clinical judgment is grounded on the idea that in every presentation of a patient a detailed and particularised question(s) is posed for which there is a detailed and particularised answer(s). Another way to look at this process is to see the question as exposing a knowledge gap which then has to be researched, either with the patient, on physical examination or in the literature. The clinician's task is to discover the question(s) and attempt an answer(s). It would be nice if the answers were true, but that is not of primary importance, instead it is necessary that the answer be right enough to allow the questioning and answering process to continue. When it is realised that the questions posed by patients are always social, political, personal and moral, as well as technical—the question 'Why is this person sick?' is a very different question in 1996 than in 1976 and in New York City than in Sydney, New South Wales—the meaning of 'detailed and particularised' becomes clearer.

If we go back to Hippocrates' *Book of Prognostics*, a perfect example of detailed question and answer pairs is offered, as suitable now as when written. The questions (although not in question form) are the detailed descriptions of the clinical state that allow the prognostic judgments (the answers) to be made. The famous description of the appearance of the face that allows physicians to make a prognostic judgment of impending death is not a few words long, as is often thought. Here it is in its entirety:

> In acute diseases the physician must conduct his inquiries in the following way. First he must examine the face of the patient and see whether it is like the faces of healthy people, and especially whether it is like its usual self. Such likeness will be the best sign, and the greatest unlikeness will be the most dangerous sign. The latter will be as follows. Nose sharp, eyes hollow, temples sunken, ears cold and contracted with their lobes turned outward, the skin about the face hard and tense and parched; the colour of the face as a whole being yellow or black. If at the beginning of the disease the face be like this, and if it be not yet possible with the other symptoms to make a complete prognosis, you must go on to inquire whether the patient has been sleepless, whether his bowels have been very loose, and whether he suffers at all from hunger. And if anything of the kind be confessed, you must consider the danger to be less. The crisis comes after a day and a night if through these causes the face has such an appearance. But should no such confession be made, and should a recovery not take place within this period, know that it is a sign of death. If the disease be of longer standing than three days when the face has these characteristics, go on to make the same inquiries as I ordered in the previous case, and also examine the other symptoms, both of the body generally and those of the eyes. For if they shun the light, or weep involuntarily, or are distorted, or if one becomes less than the other, if the whites be red or livid or have black veins in them, should rheum appear around the eyeballs, should they be restless or protruding or very sunken, or if the complexion of the whole case be changed—all these symptoms must be considered bad, in fact fatal. You must also examine the partial appearance of the eyes in sleep. For if a part of the white appear when the lids are closed, should the cause not be diarrhoea or purging, or should the patient not be in habit of so sleeping, it is an unfavourable, in fact a very deadly symptom. But if, along with one of the other symptoms, eyelid, lip, or nose be bent or livid, you must know that death is close at hand. It is also a deadly sign when the lips are loose, cold, and very white.[340]

The Hippocratic author has laid down the question in exquisite detail to which the prognostic judgment is the answer. It is unfortunate that succeeding millennia of physicians have retained the general prognostic statement but overlooked the detailed method of question and answer employed by our Greek ancestor to reach the judgment.

The physician making the judgment should be thinking about the question he or she wants to answer. What is the particular situation calling for a judgment? When that has been spelled out in sufficient detail, making the judgment that is the answer becomes much easier. To understand what this means in terms of clinical wisdom, it will be helpful to look again at the case of Alston Brook described above. Remember that he is a 78-year-old man who is still in the intensive care unit several months after a mitral valve replacement. The problem at this point is how to take him off the respirator, recognising that he will not survive. Sometimes the judgments in cases like this become impossibly difficult and painful—King Solomon himself would get a headache. On the other hand, if we could see a tally of all the judgments that have been made about his care since he came out of the operating room, it would occupy a lot of space. Most of them have been frankly technical, even rule driven, no different for him than for any other patient. For example, medication changes, laboratory studies ordered, fluid and blood replacement, respirator settings—by this time literally hundreds of interventions large and small have taken place.

I believe that if we could be privy to the thought processes of the physicians and other caregivers making the judgments that led to these myriad actions we would see that the questions that were being answered were usually narrowly technical. Most judgments probably involved responses to changes in the many parameters of physiologic function that are measured in patients such as these. At other times there were treatment decisions for possible infections, changes in the wound, maintenance of the airway, and other similar problems. Each time, I believe, we would see little evidence that the decision for Alston Brook was any different than for another patient who required antibiotics, wound care, respirator adjustment, or the like. Why should these judgments be different for him? The treatment of such patients has been wonderfully effective, with discharge from the hospital usually taking place within seven to fourteen days.

With every passing day after the expected date of discharge, however, this patient became increasingly different from the internalised model on which most such medical judgments are based. Not only was his respiratory function failing to return on schedule, his muscles of respiration were also becoming weaker. This was perceived by his physicians, but apparently invisible was the fact that every other muscle was also becoming weaker through disuse, just as disuse was affecting many of his functions. Not only his physical state, but also his mental life was changing; cognitive alterations characteristic of illness were settling in and transforming his perception of the world,[341] he was becoming depressed, his ability to interact with others was reduced, his self-image changed. Just as things were happening to him, alterations in his wife's life were taking place, as they were with his daughter. The social setting of his care was also transformed by the length of his residence. He became increasingly personalised to the nurses and house staff. The political dynamics of his care were starting to be influenced by the actions of other senior physicians who became interested in the case in addition to those on the unit. Overriding all was the fact that the chance of survival to discharge, or survival with function acceptable to the previously healthy Alston Brook, progressively fell. Weeks before his death, the outcome was virtually certain. There is little evidence that, in such cases, the dynamics of judgments change to meet the challenge of their care. Judgments remain mostly technical decisions, with the larger issues avoided.

I have shown throughout the chapter that judgments in the form of purely technical decisions are inadequate because they do not encompass the moral, social, political and personal issues (for both patients and physicians) which are part of almost all medical judgments. What the case of Alston Brook makes clear is not only the deficiencies of such narrow compassed judgments, but the apparent inability of physicians and other caregivers to pose or answer wider questions. Why, if medicine is a profession where judgment plays such an important part, are physicians lacking in this skill? There are two main reasons. First, the want of wider scope judgments is not apparent in most clinical situations because standard decisions seem to work. A good example are the patients like Alston Brook who are discharged from the hospital after the usual period. Whatever deficiencies there may have been in judgments made about them are overridden by patients' natural ability to recuperate or handle social or personal problems. This is the case throughout medicine where the lack of recognition of problems beyond the technical creates many difficult issues, but does not seem to have an impact on day-to-day medical care or on medical training. In general, stereotypical responses to people and problems and set rules, which provide the basis for many judgments, work well enough to be invisible because stereotypes have some basis in fact. As soon as the medical problem enlarges—as in the case of Mr Brook—their inadequacy becomes apparent.

The second and more important reason that physicians and other caregivers make inadequate judgments is that they have not been taught a better way. In part this failure arises from the belief that doctoring—the skills (including judgment) employed in the application of medical science to the care of individual patients—is only learned through experience and need not be explicitly taught. Medical science and technology have become much too powerful to depend on romantic notions of the art of medicine for their application or to rest on the belief that only the science is necessary. Doctoring has become a foundational body of knowledge and proficiencies that should be a part of the education of clinicians. I hope this chapter's emphasis on the social, political, and value-laden nature of medical judgments has dispelled the notion that they are personal, idiosyncratic affairs that can only be taught by demonstration. Finally, seeing judgments from the perspective of question and answer makes it clear that in the process of judgment, the most attention must be given to spelling out the question in detail. Narrow understandings of medical situations restricted to technical issues alone, or including stereotypical caricatures of patients or other actors lead to inadequate judgments. It is necessary to specify the particular circumstances in great detail and in the widest terms, including the social, political, personal and moral issues involved, in order to reach suitable judgments. This is the beginning of clinical wisdom.

REFERENCES

325. Adams F. *The genuine works of Hippocrates.* Baltimore: Williams & Wilkins, 1939, p292.
326. Feinstein Alvin R. *Clinical judgment.* Baltimore: Williams & Wilkins, 1967.
327. I have put quotes around the word 'measures' to indicate that it is not numbers that we are after—the usual way we measure things—but any way in which comparisons can be made. Scales are an example of a non-numerical measurement. None, mild, moderate, severe is an example of a scale. So is calm, irritated, upset, angry. Another (asked of a patient), 'On this line, where one end is one and the other is ten, where would you put your pain today, where would you have put it yesterday?'
328. Feinstein Alvan R. 1994. Clinical judgment revisited: the distraction of quantitative models. *Ann Intern Med* 1994; 120: 799–805.
329. Sackett DL, Haynes RB, Guyatt GH, Tugwell P. *Clinical epidemiology: a basic science for clinical medicine,* 2nd edition. Boston: Little Brown & Co, 1991.
330. Dewey J. *Logic: the theory of inquiry.* New York: Henry Holt & Company, 1938, p283.
331. Bosanquet B. *Logic, volume I.* Oxford: The Clarendon Press, 1911, p97.
332. Hippocrates. In: Jones WHS (trans). *The book of prognostics. Book II.* Cambridge: Harvard University Press, 1968, p11.
333. Cassell EJ. *Doctoring, the nature of primary care medicine.* New York: Oxford University Press, 1997, ch 4.
334. Aristotle. *Nichomachean ethics. Book VI.* 1143a 10: 10.
335. Aristotle. *Nichomachean ethics. Book VI.* 1143a 10: 7–9.
336. Bernstein RJ. *Beyond objectivism and relativism: science, hermeneutics and praxis.* Philadelphia: University of Pennsylvania Press, 1988.
337. Davidoff F, Case K, Fried PW. Evidence-based medicine: why all the fuss? *Ann Intern Med,* 1995, 122: 727.
338. Aristotle, *Nichomachean ethics. Book VI,* 1140a 24ff.
339. Collingwood RC. *An autobiography.* Oxford: Clarendon Press, 1939, ch V.
340. Hippocrates. In: Jones WHS (trans). *The book of prognostics. Book II.* Cambridge: Harvard University Press, 1968.
341. Cassell Eric J. *The Healer's Art.* Cambridge, MA: MIT Press, 1985, ch 1.

PART THREE

ACHIEVEMENTS OF MEDICINE

CHAPTER TEN

Research and Progress

JUDITH A. WHITWORTH

'Knowledge for diagnosis comes from research, knowledge for treatment comes from research, knowledge for cures comes from research. Medical research is the beginning, the starting point in hope, in efforts to diagnose, treat, or cure the diseases of mankind.'[342]

Mortality data show that in this century alone life expectancy in Australia has increased by 20 years in men and 22 years in women and infant mortality has fallen from 103.6 to 5.9/1000 live births.[343]

Diseases are conquered in a variety of ways. Improvements in living standards have unquestionably made an enormous contribution to disease reduction and increased longevity.[344] Conversely, the continuing premature death rate and high infant mortality in Aboriginal populations is an indictment of previous policies. It has become fashionable to question the role of medicine in conquering diseases. David Weatherall, in his wonderful book *Science and the Quiet Art* points out:

> that advances in medical science usually result from the coming together of knowledge at a particular stage of development in a number of fields. Although one area of research may be well developed—Harvey's concept of the circulation, for example—unless work in related fields has led to a critical level of understanding, there will be no practical results. This is the main reason for our current inability to deal with many of the major killers of Western society; we have some knowledge, but in whole areas our level of understanding remains so primitive that we can do no better than offer our patients increasingly sophisticated patch-up procedures to control their diseases.
> Until the nineteenth century medical science did not make a great impact on the health of society, and many of the improvements over the centuries resulted from higher standards of living, better hygiene, and other modifications of the environment. The picture has changed dramatically in our own century, although there is still considerable controversy about how much we owe to the impact of scientific medicine and how much to improvements in our environment.[345]

155

As the World Health Organization points out, health is far more than the absence of disease. Environmental, agricultural and foreign policy, for example, impact substantially on health, as may social mores e.g., attitudes to birth control.

Conquering disease depends for the most part on research, and on the effective translation of research into practice. The latter is critical— we already have the knowledge to reduce cancer very substantially (by quitting smoking), or to reduce gun shot wounds (by minimising the availability of guns), or to reduce industrial deafness (with ear plugs). Research is only effective if it finds its way into appropriate practice.

Figure 10.1 The determinants of health and disease[346]

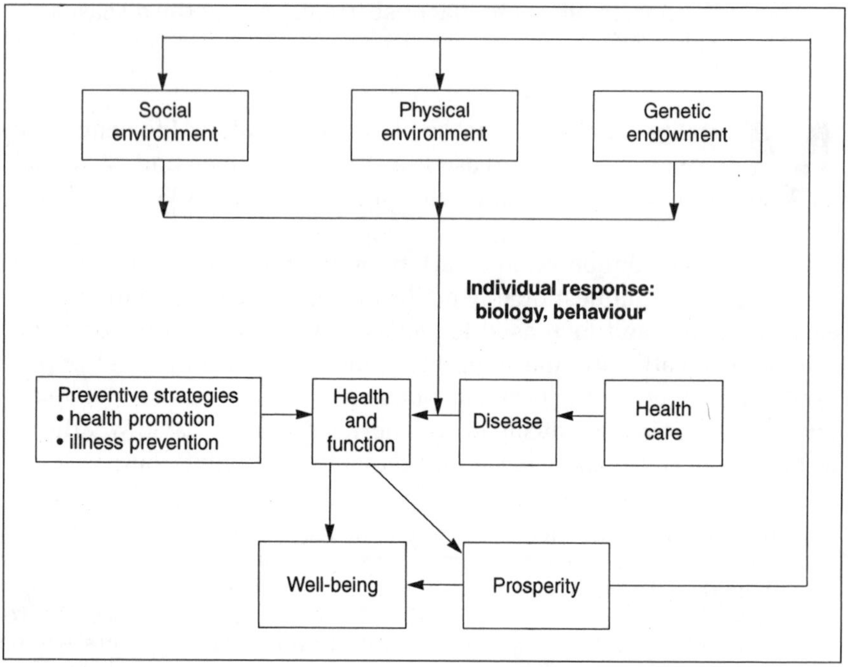

From *Research for a Healthy Society*, PMSEC, 1994.

To quote Weatherall:

> Good clinical research is often initiated by careful and critical observa-
> tion at the bedside, which may be the starting point for work in the
> laboratory encompassing a wide range of disciplines. Or the research
> may remain in the clinic and ward, and involve careful observations
> or measurements carried out directly on patients, or the application
> of statistical methods to assess the value of different types of treat-
> ment. On the other hand, many clinical advances have stemmed from
> curiosity-driven science in completely different fields, whose findings

have often required the insight of clinicians able to see their medical application. Such is the rich and variegated background for our picture of modern clinical research and practice.[345]

Diseases have been conquered by breakthroughs and by incremental advances, by biomedical research, by clinical research and by epidemiological research.

The bicentenary of the demonstration by Jenner that inoculation with vaccinia could prevent smallpox occurred in 1996. Vaccines against diphtheria, whooping cough, tetanus, polio, measles, hepatitis B and Haemophilus influenzae have been extraordinarily effective in prevention of these scourges, and the development of effective vaccines against malaria, AIDS and the diarrhoeal and respiratory infections that kill millions annually in developing countries is a top global research priority.

Surgery and anaesthesia have progressed steadily throughout this century. Arguably, modern surgery was made possible by Lansteiner's curiosity-driven discovery of blood groups and their significance,[347] but incremental technical advances, many of them depending on prior animal work, have collectively revolutionised the discipline. Similarly, since the discovery of x-rays, there have been enormous advances in diagnostic technologies, so that non-invasive imaging can produce extraordinarily detailed information on structure, and more recently, function.

Millions of people worldwide have benefited from epidemiological observations most notably, the link between tobacco smoking and lung cancer. The most definitive evidence that tobacco smoking causes cancer and heart disease came from the long-term British Doctors' studies started in the fifties by Richard Doll.[348-51] The development of randomised clinical trial methodology and meta-analysis has allowed appropriate introduction and evaluation of treatments with relatively small effects which, on a population basis, contribute substantially in reducing disease burden and improving outcomes.

Behavioural and health services research has produced information which is of great practical benefit in conquering disease. Examples here are seat belt legislation in preventing road trauma, legislation to reduce drink-driving and legislation to reduce sales of compound analgesics over the counter.

Most Australians rate good health as their number one priority. The Australian Society for Medical Research ran an opinion poll which showed that the community strongly endorsed the importance of research for health care in Australia.[352] Respondents considered that Australia should do significantly more health and medical research, and they believed that increased government support should be the mainstay of funding in Australia. Research is undertaken to ensure a broad base of expertise in the health care and teaching professions across the board, through biological, clinical, behavioural and social science. Research into Aboriginal health has to be done here in Australia and must be done in partnership with indigenous communities. Melanoma and asthma occur throughout the world but they are particularly common in Australia. Ross River virus and equine morbillivirus may be unique to Australia. We also have a responsibility to contribute to world knowledge, and our four Nobel Prizes in Medicine are one reflection of how this responsibility has been met: Florey, for the development of penicillin, Burnet for his work on immunological tolerance, Eccles for studies of transmission of nerve impulses, and Doherty for recognising how the immune system recognises invading viruses.

We do research here in Australia to obtain the 'seat at the international table' which enables us to share in new knowledge, for example developments in the human genome project. Research done here provides Australia with the expertise needed to evaluate critically new developments for their relevance and applicability to local conditions, and to apply new high technology advances cost-effectively, for example diagnostic ultrasound in pregnancy.

The critical environment engendered by research is essential for the training of the next generation of health care professionals. Neither quality health care nor medical research can be bought off the shelf. Australia needs a highly trained expert research workforce, and as knowledge and technology expand, research training will become increasingly more important. To have multi-disciplinary research, we first need the disciplines. This chapter will consider the past—the role and achievements of medical and health research in conquering disease using some Australian examples, and then in the light of lessons from the past, speculate on some of our possible futures.

The discovery of lithium

The story of the discovery of lithium for the treatment of manic depressive disorder is a fascinating example of the process of discovery itself. Manic depression affects around 200 000 Australians. Untreated, the disorder leads to death in 15 per cent of cases (usually through suicide) and long-term hospitalisation in the majority of the remaining patients. To quote Mogens Schou on John Cade:

> The insatiable curiosity, the keen observation, the willingness to test even the absurdly unlikely hypothesis, and the courage to run the risk of making a fool of himself. The hypothesis which started his work was crude, his experimental design was not particularly clear and his interpretation of the animal data may have been wrong. . . .

Figure 10.2 The interconnection between research, teaching and health practice[353]

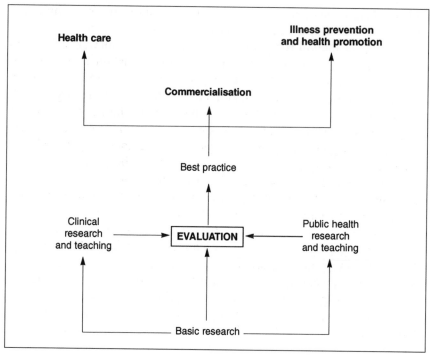

From *Research for a Healthy Society*, PMSEC, 1994.

Nevertheless—and this is the marvel of the thing—a spark jumped in John Cade's questioning mind and he performed that therapeutic trial which eventually changed life for manic depressive patients all over the world.[354]

Cade was keen on the notion of a medical rather than a psychopathological model for manic depressive disorder.[355] It seemed obvious to him as a practising physician and psychiatrist that the patients were truly sick in the medical sense. He reasoned that there was a persuasive parallel in thyroid disease—hyperthyroidism was analogous to mania and hypothyroidism to melancholia, and thus that mania could be due to some metabolic substance circulating in excess, and melancholia the consequence of depletion of that substance. To test if there were differences between manics and depressives, he injected concentrated urine into the abdominal cavity of guinea pigs and compared them with controls. The animals all died but urine from the manic patients seemed to be most toxic. Uric acid was found to enhance the toxic effect of urea but the subsequent experiments proved difficult because the uric acid was relatively insoluble in water. Accordingly, he substituted the most soluble of the uric acid salts, lithium urate. Surprisingly, this appeared to protect rather than enhance the toxicity and in consequence he examined the effects of lithium salts by themselves and found that lithium had a powerful calming effect.

These experimental results prompted Cade to examine lithium salts clinically in mania. In fact, in the best tradition of *primum non nocere*, he took lithium himself before using it on his first patients. His original paper in the Medical Journal of Australia reported 10 case histories of patients with mania treated with lithium with extremely good results.[356] As Cade said:

> I was able to go my own way unhindered by advice, criticism or caution. This is important. I do not think it could happen these days, one would be suffocated by hospital boards, research committees, ethical committees and heads of departments. Instead, I was answerable only to my own conscience and personal drive.[357]

Kirschner and colleagues, writing in *Science* in 1994, calculated that lithium treatment for manic-depressive disorders had saved the USA alone over $145 billion in hospitalisation costs.[358] Extrapolating these cost-benefits to Australia, it is apparent that lithium alone has led to savings well in excess of the cost of our entire national health research effort ever. The non-financial benefits to sufferers and their families are incalculable.

The colony stimulating factors—from basic biology to the bedside

The story of the discovery and development of the colony stimulating factors by Don Metcalf and his colleagues is one of the great epics of Australian medical research, spanning over 30 years work.

Metcalf set out to explore the notion that leukaemia might be due to abnormalities in whatever regulators controlled formation of the white blood cells. This was not a popular idea at the time, even in the Hall Institute where he worked, but Metcalf, supported by a research fellowship from the Victorian Anti-Cancer Council, persisted.

In the mid 1960s Ray Bradley, also working in Melbourne, developed a technique for growing colonies of white cells from mice.[359] These colonies are the clusters of progeny cells formed on a culture plate from single precursor bone marrow cells. Metcalf was excited by the fact that the blood-forming cells could not divide spontaneously in these cultures unless other material, e.g., tissue fragments, was added and that the number and size of colonies developing depended on the amount of such material added to the cultures.

He deduced that the 'colony stimulating factor' (CSF) being detected might be the long sought regulator of granulocytes and macrophages.[360] Some years of effort were required to show that CSF did appear to be this regulator. There followed a 15 year effort to purify the substance, during the course of which it emerged that there were four distinct CSFs and the actions of these were characterised in detail. But the efforts to purify enough CSF to test in even one animal were frustrated by a myriad of technical difficulties. By the mid 1980s the future looked grim. Fortunately, the new techniques in molecular biology came to the rescue, and a variety of mouse and human CSFs were cloned, animal experiments proved positive and two of the materials, G-CSF and GM-CSF, went into clinical trial and rapidly into clinical practice. At the time of writing over 1.5 million patients worldwide have received G-CSF, and haematological and oncologic treatments have been revolutionised. The CSFs augment bone marrow function in production of white blood cells and have been widely used in bone marrow transplantation and to assist recovery from chemotherapy in cancer which can be a fatal side-effect of cancer treatments.

Hypertension research: preventing heart attack and stroke

Australasian contributions to research into hypertension were reviewed in 1988 by two of the doyens of the field, Doyle and Johnston.[361] In the first half of this century there was little effective treatment for high blood pressure. Anti-hypertensive drugs were established in practice by Horace Smirk in Dunedin, New Zealand, who demonstrated dramatic improvements in malignant hypertension with ganglion blocker treatment.[362] Studies in the USA in veterans then showed that drug treatment of moderate to severe hypertension was also effective in reducing stroke and hypertensive heart disease in men.

But most hypertensives (around 15 per cent of the Australian population) have only mild hypertension, and although the risks of heart attack and stroke are higher in the more severe group, the absolute number of cardiovascular events in the mild group is very high.

The Australian Therapeutic Trial in Mild Hypertension (Australian National Blood Pressure Study, ANBP 1) was a large-scale randomised multicentre placebo-controlled intervention study funded jointly by the National Heart Foundation and the National Health and Medical Research Council. This study was the first to show a clear benefit from treating mild hypertension. Around 40 per cent of strokes and 15–20 per cent of heart attacks were prevented, and it is estimated that over 50 000 Australian lives have been saved in consequence.

This represents a net saving in health expenditure of over $100 million a year,[343] in addition to the enormous social benefits to the people whose strokes or heart attacks are prevented. Australian research has also demonstrated the effectiveness of simple dietary changes, such as reduced salt intake, reduced alcohol and a vegetarian style of diet, in reducing blood pressure, together with the efficacy of other life style changes, e.g., exercise.

ANBP 2 is currently in progress and should also prove to be a landmark in hypertension research. It is a multicentre comparative outcome trial of angiotensin-converting enzyme inhibitor and diuretic based treatment of hypertension in the elderly in 6000 subjects, and should define whether or not the newer more expensive angiotensin-converting enzyme inhibitors have any significant advantage over the older cheaper therapy.

Equally important is PROGRESS, a multinational study designed by Australasian investigators to determine the role of blood pressure lowering in preventing secondary stroke, in both hypertensive and normotensive subjects.

Analgesic nephropathy

Between 1959 and 1962 some 100 cases of analgesic abuse-related nephropathy were seen at the Royal Melbourne Hospital. When the disease was at its height, over 20 per cent of all end-stage renal failure requiring dialysis in Australia was attributed to analgesics sold over the counter.[363] Today, the condition is on the way to becoming a historical curiosity, and new cases are a rarity.

The association between chronic interstitial nephritis and analgesic abuse was recognised in Europe in the early 1950s, but it was in Australia that the primary role of renal papillary necrosis as a cause of the chronic interstitial nephritis was first identified.[364] The pathology of the condition was documented and epidemiological studies showed a relationship between analgesic powder sales, the percentage of women taking analgesics daily and the geographic distribution of end-stage renal failure associated with analgesics.[365]

Experimental work in rats showed that, contrary to perceived wisdom in Europe, phenacetin alone was not the only, or even the major culprit, and aspirin and other minor analgesics produced significant papillary damage. But it was the combination of drugs rather than any single drug that was particularly nephrotoxic.

Given the European view that this was 'phenacetin nephropathy' and publicity about the condition, drug companies withdrew phenacetin from their compound analgesic preparations, but with little effect on the development of disease. It was also recognised that analgesic abuse was associated with transitional cell carcinoma of the urinary tract, and with a variety of systemic features, from peptic ulceration to anaemia to decreased fertility and premature aging.

On the basis of local clinical, epidemiological and experimental findings, and the concerted efforts of nephrologists, the Australian Kidney Foundation and the NHMRC, legislation prohibiting the sale of 'over the counter' mixed analgesics was introduced in all states between 1979–1980. From 1983 there has been an inexorable decline in this totally preventable condition. The cost savings are estimated at around $40 million/year.

Helicobacter pylori

The role of Helicobactor pylori in gastrointestinal disease was discovered at Royal Perth Hospital in the early eighties by J. Robin Warren and Barry Marshall.[366] Warren, a histopathologist, had noted what he thought to be curved bacilli in the stomachs of patients with ulcers in 1979. A gastroenterology registrar, Marshall, was given the task of working with him on these organisms in 1981. They were able to demonstrate that the organisms were present in the gastric mucosa from patients with duodenal ulcer, active chronic gastritis and gastric ulcers. The story goes that they were having difficulty in culturing the organism until they left some culture plates unattended in an incubator over an Easter holiday break. Warren and Marshall named the organism Campylobacter pylorodis but it was realised that this was etymologically unsound and for a time it was known as CLO or Campylobacter-like organism until it was finally named Helicobactor pylori. The first report of this work to the Gastroenterological Society of Australia was greeted with substantial scepticism. Most gastroenterologists were happy to accept that the organism was associated with ulcer disease but because of the long-held belief that peptic ulceration was due to excess acid, the notion of a pathogenic role for the organism was very slow to gain acceptance, even though some of the early work in Perth was funded by NHMRC. To demonstrate one of Koch's postulates,[367] Marshall himself drank cultures of the organism and developed transient acute gastritis, which responded to antibacterial therapy.

Helicobactor pylori is now accepted as a Class 1 carcinogen by the World Health Organization, important in gastric cancer and lymphoma of the stomach. The organism is difficult to eradicate and multiple antibiotic therapy is required. This notwithstanding, eradication therapy is significantly cheaper long-term than conventional H_2 antagonists

164 THE TASKS OF MEDICINE

because of the very low relapse rate. It is estimated that the discovery of Helicobactor pylori has saved the United States alone around $600 to 800 million per annum.[358] In 1993–1994 more than 6 million prescriptions for antacids and anti-ulcer drugs were processed under the Australian Pharmaceutical Benefits Scheme at some $163 million, so savings in this country will also be very substantial.

Translating research into practice

From the 1930s to the 1950s, Australia (including this writer) experienced large epidemics of paralytic poliomyelitis. It killed up to 5 per cent of infected children and 30 per cent of infected adults. Many of the survivors were left paralysed, some on iron lungs. The Salk vaccine for polio prevention underwent clinical trials in the USA in 1954, and the excellent results of these trials were published in 1955.[368] Because the Commonwealth Serum Laboratories had a strong scientific base and extensive experience in vaccine production and cell culture research, Australia produced vaccine as early as 1956. We have not had a case since 1970.

The Cochrane collaboration, now active in Australia, is a key element in the synthesis of evidence-based information and its translation into practice and it is becoming an increasingly important source of quality information for health professionals and decision-makers. Professor Silagy, a contributor to this book, is Director of the Cochrane collaboration in Australia.

The future

Everything that can be invented has been invented.[369]

Predicting the future is always difficult, and this is particularly true in research, which by definition explores the unknown. Experts in previous generations failed to predict antibiotics, rockets and space travel, the transistor, the explosion in computer information and communications technology, and a host of other advances which have transformed our lives.

In the near future we will see enormous advances in molecular medicine, particularly in genomics, and bioinformatics. Research will become more multi-disciplinary, e.g., molecular epidemiology, the biochemical basis of behaviour, and the psychology of clinical and administrative decision-making. Molecular genetics will be the foundation for the new public health. Community and ethical considerations will impact research directions and visa versa. Public debate on the ethical and social implications of the explosion in genetic information is only just beginning. Xenotransplantation with genetic engineering of animals using human genes to provide body spare parts will likely become a reality but its application will be shaped by community views. Genetic screening will assist individuals in key life decisions, governments in determination of policy, and industry in design and conduct of drug studies, using much more homogeneous patient populations than is currently possible, but the privacy considerations will be critical. Information technology, and in particular the Internet and its offshoots will do away with the 'tyranny of distance', making national and international collaborations more feasible, increasing access to a host of data bases from the latest quaternary protein structures to the latest genomic sequences, and allowing cheap real time meetings for which travel funds are no longer essential.

Just as AIDS has become a major scourge worldwide in the last decade and just as the influenza epidemic of 1918 claimed 25 million lives, with the world becoming the global village, the explosions in population and travel make new diseases which will decimate populations inevitable. The traditional distinctions between science, medicine, public health and public policy will become increasingly blurred as we endeavour to control new threats, just as they have in the approach to AIDS.

Bigger and bigger groups will do science at all levels. Science will be more expensive. As our knowledge of biology increases and the tools we need become more sophisticated, and the expertise needed covers a range of disciplines, so costs will increase. Long-term longitudinal cohort studies and large scale clinical trials already cost tens of millions of dollars. Our old notions of knowledge as common currency will be outmoded in the context of patent agreements and legal restrictions.

British Telecommunications has produced a timetable for major medical and scientific developments which is Internet accessible.[370] It starts with an artificial pancreas (1998) and moves through artificial blood, as well as records on smart cards (2000) to wearable health monitors (2005), the artificial heart (2010), the individual genome as part of medical record (2015) to a life span of 100 (2020) and artificial eyes (2030). It was recognised that wild card events such as a new worldwide viral epidemic could happen at any time.

We may or may not like this future but to shape it we need to ensure Australia has appropriately trained researchers and adequate research infrastructure. The health and future of Australian research depends on the recognition by all Australians of its importance to our culture and to our development. Australian health and medical research has a star-studded history. It needs a long-term investment and a long-term commitment.

Figure 10.3 Large benefits from a small investment

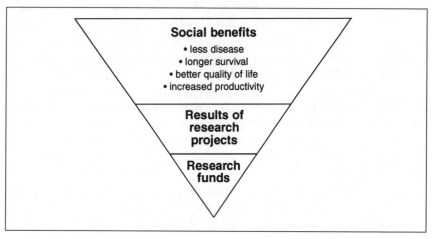

Social benefits
- less disease
- longer survival
- better quality of life
- increased productivity

Results of research projects

Research funds

From *Research for a Healthy Society*, PMSEC, 1994.

REFERENCES

342. Paul Rogers.
343. Australian Institute of Health and Welfare. *Australia's health 1996.* Canberra: AGPS, pp218, 220–1.
344. Baume P, Bauman A (eds). *Public health: an introduction.* Sydney: Eriador Press, 1996, p3.
345. Weatherall D. *Science and the quiet art: medical research and patient care.* Oxford: Oxford University Press, 1995.
346. PMSEC. *Research for a healthy society.* Canberra: AGPS, December 1994.
347. Comroe JH, Dripps RD. The scientific basis for the support of biomedical research. *Science* 1976, 192: 105–11.
348. Doll R, Peto R. Mortality in relation to smoking: 20 years observations on male British doctors. *Brit Med J* 1976; 2: 1525–36.
349. Doll R, Peto R. Cigarette smoking and bronchial carcinoma: dose and time relationships among regular smokers and lifelong non-smokers. *J Epi and Comm Health* 1978, 32: 303–13.
350. Doll R, Gray R, Hafner B, Peto R. Mortality in relation to smoking: 22 years observations on female British doctors. *Brit Med J* 1980; 280: 967–71.
351. Doll R, Peto R, Wheatley K, Gray R, Sutherland I. Mortality in relation to smoking: 40 years observation on male British doctors. *Brit Med J* 1994; 309: 901–11.
352. News Poll Survey. *Attitudes to health and medical research.* Commissioned by the Australian Society for Medical Research, December 1995.
353. PMSEC. *Research for a healthy society.* Canberra: AGPS, December 1994.
354. Schou M. Lithium perspectives. *Neuropsychobiology* 1983; 10: 7–12.
355. Cade JFJ. *Mending the mind: a short history of twentieth century psychiatry.* Melbourne: Sun Books, 1979.

356. Cade JFJ. Lithium salts in the treatment of psychotic excitement. *Med J Aust* 1949; 36: 349–52.
357. Johnson FN. Cade JFJ 1912–1980: a reminiscence. *Pharmacopsychiatry* 1981; 14: 148–9.
358. Kirschner MW, Marincola E, Tersberg EO. The role of biomedical research in health care reform. *Science* 1994; 265: 49–51.
359. Bradley TR, Metcalf D. The growth of mouse bone marrow cells in vitro. *Aust J Exp Biol Med Sci* 1966; 44: 287.
360. Metcalf D. *The colony stimulating factors—discovery to clinical use*. The Burnet Lecture, Proc. Australian Academy of Science (in press).
361. Doyle AC, Johnston CI. Australian contributions to research in hypertension. *Aust NZ J Med* 1988; 18: 245.
362. Smirk FH, Alstad KS. Treatment of arterial hypertension by penta- and hexa-methonium salts based on 150 tests on hypertensives of varied aetiology and 53 patients treated for periods of two to fourteen months. *Brit Med J* 1951; 1: 1217.
363. Australian and New Zealand Dialysis and Transplant Registry (ANZDATA).
364. Kincaid-Smith P. Analgesic nephropathy. *Aust NZ J Med* 1988; 18: 251–4.
365. Senate Standing Committee on Social Welfare. *Drug problems in Australia—an intoxicated society*. Canberra: AGPS, 1977.
366. Marshall BJ, Warren JR. Unidentified curved bacilli in the stomach of patients with gastritis and peptic ulceration. *Lancet* 1984; 1: 1311–15.
367. Hoerr NL, Osol A. *Blakiston's new Gould medical dictionary*, 2nd edition, New York: McGraw-Hill, p653.
368. Salk J. Considerations in the preparation and use of poliomyelitis virus vaccines. *J Amer Ass* 1995; 158: 1239.
369. Charles Duell, Commissioner, US Patent Office, urging President William McKinley to abolish his office, 1899.
370. Dobson R. Researchers try crystal ball gazing to predict future. *Brit Med J* 1996; 313: 706.

CHAPTER ELEVEN

Advances in Disease Treatment

RICHARD LARKINS

The last two or three decades have seen the most astonishing advances in health care in the developed world. All disciplines of medical research have been utilised and these have been allied with technological advances arising from research in physics and engineering to revolutionise the prevention and management of disease. No greater justification for expenditure on basic and applied research in the biological and physical sciences can be provided than the startling improvement in all indices of health in society. No matter whether global indicators of health care such as average life expectancy[371] or perinatal mortality rates are examined, or more specific outcome data such as survival rates in leukaemia[372] and many other forms of cancer, or age adjusted mortality rates[373] from myocardial infarction[374] or stroke,[375] spectacular improvements in outcomes have been documented. Incurable inherited diseases such as haemophilia and cystic fibrosis are now compatible with prolonged survival with reasonable or good quality of life, and chronic acquired diseases such as diabetes mellitus, hypertension, rheumatoid arthritis can now be much better controlled with improved quality of life and less morbidity and mortality. In this chapter, an arbitrary judgment of the most important advances in medical care will be undertaken. The role played by research (basic scientific, technological, clinical and population-based) in enabling these advances will be emphasised. The chapter will conclude by contrasting the enormous dividends being enjoyed in the developed world with the very limited benefits so far being experienced in most developing countries, and an assessment of the remaining challenges and threats.

Randomised clinical trials, evidence-based medicine and clinical practice

This may seem a surprising topic to list first, but without improved ability to evaluate proposed new methods of treatment, we would not be in a position to assess whether altered clinical practice really represented an advance. Small controlled clinical trials using highly selected patient groups under closely supervised conditions have been in use for many years. However, these have often been limited in their significance by the lack of ability to generalise the conclusions to the population at large and by an inability to judge the magnitude of the effect if the intervention were generally applied. The enormous, multi-centre studies of interventions in the management of acute myocardial infarction altered the approach so that superadded effects of drug interventions could be detected in the 'real life' situation of a relatively unselected group of patients with myocardial infarction, already receiving a variety of different medications and with different severity and extent of coexistent disease. The effectiveness of beta adrenergic receptor blocking drugs, aspirin, angiotensin-converting enzyme inhibitor drugs and acute thrombolytic therapy were proven in such studies, and a beneficial role of calcium channel blockers disproven. The management of acute myocardial infarction is now an active process with a number of pharmacological interventions of proven effectiveness combined with the technology of sophisticated monitoring and early treatment of cardiac arrhythmias. These improvements have led to a reduction in the in-hospital mortality of patients with acute myocardial infarction from about 18 per cent to about 9 per cent.[376]

Other applications of large, multicentre randomised clinical trials with significant clinical consequences have included the early studies of the effectiveness of hypotensive medication in preventing stroke, several studies of the role of lipid lowering drugs in the secondary prevention (i.e., in those who have had a previous myocardial infarct) of myocardial infarction and mortality in those with hyperlipidaemia,[377] the demonstration of the reduction in strokes by the use of anticoagulant therapy in subjects with atrial fibrillation (a cardiac irregularity predisposing to throwing off clots into the circulation)[378] and the demonstration of the effectiveness of adjuvant (i.e., additional) chemotherapy in those with breast[379] or colon cancer[380] treated by surgery. There are many other examples in cancer treatment, and indeed all forms of cancer therapy are now evaluated in this way. The Diabetes Control and Complications Trial, a multicentre study of intensive diabetes treatment conducted in North America has finally resolved the controversy about the effectiveness of such therapy in preventing the complications of diabetes.[381] Not only did the study demonstrate that the rate of complications affecting the eyes, kidneys and nerves was reduced by 50 per cent or more, but it also allowed quantitative evaluation of the risks of such therapy. Quality of life data can also be incorporated into such studies.

Techniques have also been developed for combining the results of several different trials, each of which may have produced statistically insignificant results or some of which may have been conflicting. Those studies fulfilling defined criteria of validity are combined in a process known as meta-analysis. This process has allowed several equivocal issues regarding efficacy of drugs or procedures to be resolved definitively and more quickly and economically than the mounting of a trial of the size and duration necessary to answer the question in a single study.

The proliferation of randomised clinical trials and meta-analyses has produced an explosion of information. Even with the ability to review medical publications rapidly using computerised searches of electronic data banks, it is difficult to obtain a balanced view of the state of evidence in particular fields. The Cochrane Collaboration[382] is an international network of academic centres based at Oxford University, which evaluates and summarises the best available information garnered from randomised clinical trials in a variety of clinically important areas. This will facilitate the application of evidence-based decisions into clinical practice, which will continue to transform clinical practice over the next few years.

Technological advances in our ability to image the human body

Over the last three decades, technological developments have led to enormous refinement and increase in our ability to determine structure and function of the human body using non-invasive or minimally invasive techniques. Two decades ago, one of the most common surgical procedures was the exploratory laparotomy—the opening and exploration of the abdominal cavity for diagnostic purposes. This procedure is rarely necessary now, as computerised tomographic radiological scans, ultrasound, nuclear medicine techniques or magnetic resonance imaging, accompanied by radiologically or ultrasound guided needle biopsy allows precise diagnosis before surgery (or indicates that surgery is not necessary).

The brain was extremely difficult to image. The only techniques available were the highly invasive, uncomfortable technique known as pneumoencephalography, where air was injected into the space around the brain to enhance contrast on subsequent x-ray, or the hazardous and indirect methods of injecting dye into the blood vessels (angiography) or cerebral ventricles (ventriculography). Nuclear medicine techniques, introduced in the 1960s allowed large tumours or blood clots to be identified, but were very insensitive and imprecise.

Computerised tomography in the 1970s and magnetic resonance imaging in the 1980s and 1990s have revolutionised neurology and neurosurgery, allowing precise diagnosis where this was previously impossible. Small brain tumours or malformations, previously extremely difficult to diagnose, can now often be cured, and unnecessary surgery for inoperable conditions avoided. Even differences in composition of parts of the brain, such as occur in multiple sclerosis, can be identified by magnetic resonance imaging, allowing easier diagnosis of this highly variable condition. Positron emission tomography, although not yet widely available, allows tissue metabolic activity as well as the morphology (shape) to be determined.[383] Characteristic changes are being identified in the metabolism of areas of the brain in stroke and even in some forms of psychiatric disorders, again leading to greatly improved diagnostic ability.

Although these new technologies are very expensive, they have greatly reduced unnecessary surgery and admission to hospital for more invasive diagnostic procedures and they have led to more accurate diagnosis and more appropriate treatment.

Minimally invasive interventional radiology and laparoscopic surgery

Many conditions previously requiring major surgery and prolonged hospital admission can now be treated using minimally invasive techniques without hospital admission or as day or overnight stay patients. Some of these techniques are based on radiologically guided interventional procedures, and others depend on fibreoptic direct visualisation of the area of procedure. Examples of the former include balloon angioplasty procedures, whereby open cardiac or arterial surgery is replaced by inserting a small catheter into a cardiac or cerebral or peripheral artery (usually reached via insertion of the catheter through the skin into an artery in the groin) with subsequent filling of the balloon to dilate the narrowing. Removal of stones from the kidneys or ureter is now commonly achieved by radiologically guided percutaneous techniques without open surgery. Techniques of obliterating aneurysms (bulges of the arteries likely to burst) and malformations in the cerebral blood vessels are now being introduced, replacing some major and dangerous brain surgery.

Fibreoptic guided procedures are now used to inject bleeding ulcers, or to diagnose and treat stones in the duct carrying bile from the liver and gall bladder to the intestine. Precancerous lesions of the colon are identified and removed by colonoscopy. Many abdominal operations, previously requiring major surgery can now be performed through tiny

holes, guided by the laparoscope. These include gall bladder operations and gynaecological surgery. However, the tradeoff for less post-
operative discomfort and scarring and a much shorter hospital stay is
often a longer and more technically difficult operation, sometimes with
a higher complication rate. Each new application of 'key hole' surgery
needs to be carefully evaluated.

Overall, the need for major, open operations in almost all fields of
surgery has been greatly reduced by these new, minimally invasive
techniques, with obvious benefits for the patient and cost savings for
the community.

Joint replacement surgery

It has been argued that the single most significant advance in medical
care in recent decades as judged by ability to relieve pain and suffering
has been joint replacement surgery, more particularly, total hip replacement. Osteoarthritis of the hip is an extremely common disorder of
older people caused by the destruction of cartilage on the surface of
the bones forming the ball and socket joint. This leads to secondary
inflammation, great discomfort with use, and major limitation of movement. Otherwise healthy people became semi-invalids. The major form
of therapy was pain-killing and anti-inflammatory drugs, which were
incompletely effective and had possible side-effects such as bleeding
from the stomach and kidney damage. The development of artificial
joints made of space-age metals, plastics and glues, that have enormous
durability combined with surgical techniques to allow their insertion
has completely changed the picture. People with severe pain and limitation can be restored to health and mobility. So successful is the operation, and so numerous the people who can benefit, that it has thrown a
major stress on the health system, contributing significantly to waiting
lists in public hospitals.

Although often not so completely successful in relieving symptoms
as hip replacement, total knee and shoulder replacement surgery is
now also common, and a major advance in management of osteoarthritic
joints. In the less common but more disabling condition, rheumatoid
arthritis, replacement of multiple joints can be performed, with removal
of diseased and inflamed tissues producing at least partial relief of
symptoms.

Organ transplantation

Although it may be intuitive to suggest that solid organ transplantation is the most significant advance in our ability to treat disease, in

terms of burden of disease treated and the suffering relieved, it probably ranks below the other advances already referred to. Availability of donors limits the number of people who can be treated, and the need for ongoing immunosuppression to prevent organ rejection after transplant exposes the recipient to additional complications. Nonetheless, cornea, kidney, liver and heart transplantation are established and successful procedures which are of enormous importance and benefit to those who are able to be treated in this way. Five year survival rates vary between 70 per cent and 90 per cent, with the highest rates being achieved for renal transplants, especially from living related donors. Clearly, obtaining organs from living donors is not an option for heart and liver transplants and the falling rate of road traffic deaths has had the consequence of exacerbating the difficulty in obtaining sufficient donor organs to meet the need. Obviously, there are difficult ethical issues involved in selecting those potential recipients who should receive the available organs. People with renal failure are obviously in a better position, because apart from the possibility of receiving an organ from a living, related donor, renal dialysis therapy is able to preserve life indefinitely. However, survival rates are less, quality of life is lower and the cost of the treatment is much greater for chronic renal dialysis than for successful renal transplantation.

Pancreatic transplantation is used in the management of insulin-dependent diabetes mellitus. However, as the risks of treatment with immunosuppressive drugs are greater than those of continued treatment with insulin, its use is limited to insulin-dependent diabetic patients who also require renal transplantation and would therefore be treated with immunosuppressive drugs anyway. In this situation, where subjects are selected who are otherwise relatively healthy, good results can be achieved (about 75 per cent of subjects do not require insulin treatment one year after combined pancreas and kidney transplants).[384] The long-awaited goal of pancreatic islet transplantation (isolation and injection of the tiny clusters of cells in the pancreas which make insulin) as an alternative to the more complicated process of pancreas transplantation remains elusive, with supply of sufficient islets being the limiting factor.

Bone marrow transplantation has allowed much higher doses of chemotherapy in patients with cancer, with improved cure rates in some forms of leukaemia and lymphoma. Best results are obtained with autologous transplantation. In this procedure, the patient's own bone marrow is harvested prior to high dose chemotherapy and reinfused after chemotherapy. The use of peripheral bone marrow derived stem cells harvested from the peripheral circulation has greatly simplified the procedure. Living, related bone marrow transplantation where a good tissue match is obtained is a successful procedure, but unrelated bone marrow transplantation remains a demanding and relatively risky procedure which is performed only in highly specialised centres.

Although it would be considered intuitively that organ-transplantation procedures would be at the very top of the cost-effectiveness or cost-utility ladder, and the first procedures to be dropped in situations of resource constraints, their highly successful outcomes and the high quality of life following successful transplantation make procedures such as kidney, heart, liver and bone marrow transplantation very cost-effective. This is especially so when the alternative costs of prolonged terminal management of kidney, heart or liver failure or cancer by medical means are taken into account. To illustrate the relative cost-effectiveness of transplantation, the average cost per life saved of treatment of mild to moderate hypertension or hypercholesterolaemia by drugs is considerably higher than that of each of the transplant procedures referred to above.

Intensive care

When first introduced, there was considerable controversy about the role and cost-effectiveness of intensive care units, and other types of intensive care such as coronary care units, burns units and specialised units for the management of upper gastrointestinal haemorrhage. In the case of adult intensive care units, in many cases poor selection of cases led to little improvement in outcome, at much greater cost and much greater emotional trauma to the family of the patient. However, greater experience, and resource-driven selectivity for admission to the units have led to a greatly increased survival rate, and cost-effective care. Their particular value lies in the expert nursing care, the availability of highly sophisticated methods of respiratory support, and detailed physiological monitoring combined with specialised medical expertise. The presence of intensive care units combined with advances in diagnostic and surgical techniques has led to markedly improved survival in multiple trauma, and has allowed successful, elective major surgery to be performed in elderly subjects with multiple coexistent medical problems who would never survive such surgery without intensive care support. The introduction of coronary care units together with the multiple improvements in drug therapy derived from the randomised controlled trials referred to at the beginning of this chapter has reduced mortality rates in acute myocardial infarction by at least 50 per cent. The ability to detect and treat previously lethal cardiac arrhythmias has been the major reason for additional benefit of coronary care units, over and above the effects of the pharmacological interventions. Specialised units for the management of gastrointestinal haemorrhage have been demonstrated to lead to a reduction by about one third in the mortality rates associated with this condition.

The role of the neonatal intensive care unit has been somewhat controversial. It used to be extremely uncommon for any infant born prior to 30 weeks of gestation to survive. Now survival is expected, and babies weighing as little as 0.5 kg and born at 24 weeks of gestation can survive. Such infants are more liable to have problems with subsequent intellectual development, throwing an ongoing load on to the health care costs of the community and causing distress in the family. However, the vast majority of surviving, very premature babies managed in neonatal intensive care units, become normal, productive children and adults justifying the costs of such units.

In childhood, the availability of intensive care and specialised management of a variety of conditions previously almost uniformly lethal in childhood, has allowed children with such conditions to survive into adult life. Children with cystic fibrosis and congenital heart conditions provide examples. Our success in maintaining reasonable health in such children into adult life is a success of modern medical management, but simultaneously it throws extra costs on to our health care system.

The introduction of molecular biology into clinical medicine

There is little doubt that the development of the techniques of molecular biology has been the greatest advance in biological science in the last half of the twentieth century. Much of the explosion in medical knowledge in the last two decades has been dependent on the identification of new molecules or the unravelling of complex regulatory pathways using the tools of molecular biology. Understandably, there has been a time-lag between the dramatic advances in our understanding of basic biological mechanisms and their application to clinical medicine, so the clinical impact of techniques dependent on molecular biology has so far not equalled their importance in basic biomedical science. However, the pace of development of knowledge and its application to clinical medicine suggests that many of the advances in medical care over the next two decades will come from the more complete application of the techniques of molecular biology.

First it is necessary to understand the major tools of molecular biology before describing their current applications in clinical medicine. Basically, molecular biology refers to our ability to uncode the genes which determine the structure and function of every living organism, and to manipulate the structure of the genes by a variety of techniques, many of which can be viewed as analogous with the ability to 'cut and paste' words, clauses, sentences and paragraphs using computer technology in word processing. The technology is dependent on the discovery by Watson and Crick in the 1950s that the genetic code for all living matter is determined by the sequence of four simple chemicals linked together in a chain structure, and intertwined with a second chain with a structure complementary to and dependent on the first chain. This double helical structure is known as DNA. All inherited characteristics of all living organisms are determined by the variation in the sequence of these four simple chemicals (called nucleotides). The capacity for huge biological variation is determined by the number of genes involved (about 100 000 in humans) and the enormous number of nucleotides in each gene. Moreover, not only is there variation in the structure of each gene, but the extent to which it is expressed in each cell is determined by a segment of DNA next to the gene known as the promoter. This in turn is regulated by proteins produced by other genes, producing a very complex and sophisticated network based on a very simple underlying structure.

Major progress was made in our ability to unravel and control genetic structure and function in the 1970s. Techniques were developed which allowed detailed genetic sequence to be determined if the structure of a protein was known, and new proteins to be identified by 'pulling out' genes with similar structure to other genes. Elegant techniques for determining the sequence of genes, for modifying their structure and reinserting them in modified forms have been developed. Unravelling the promoter sequences and their regulatory mechanism has allowed the physiological control of gene expression to begin to be understood. A major international effort is underway to map the entire genetic make-up of all the genes carried in the human chromosomes. The exponential growth in our knowledge of human physiology and biochemistry will continue as the secrets of genetic regulation are progressively clarified over the next 20 years.

There have already been significant applications of molecular biology to everyday medicine in developed countries. The most significant applications so far are in the synthesis of biologically active substances previously only obtainable in limited supply from biological sources, the diagnosis of parasitic, bacterial and viral infections, the prenatal or presymptomatic diagnosis of genetic disorders and in vaccine development. Examples of each of these applications will be given, and the potential but still elusive goal of gene therapy will also be discussed.

Until recently, there was a worldwide shortage of insulin, required for the treatment of the millions of insulin-requiring diabetic subjects.

The only source was isolation and purification of insulin from the pancreases of pigs and cattle. The ability to insert the human insulin gene into bacteria, yeast and mammalian tissue culture cell lines turning these cultured cells into 'factories' for human insulin has meant that the supply is now potentially limitless, although expensive purification steps are still required. Moreover, human insulin itself rather than animal insulin is produced and this has the advantage that it does not cause as much antibody formation, producing more predictable activity. Factor VIII, the blood clotting factor deficient in subjects with haemophilia, used to be prepared from concentrates of human blood. This had led to the tragic transmission of the Human Immunodeficiency virus, with the development of AIDS in many unfortunate recipients of human factor VIII concentrate prepared from human blood. Although better testing procedures have made human blood products safer than before, small but significant risks remain. Recombinant DNA technology can now produce totally safe factor VIII, avoiding these risks. Therapy with human growth hormone has been used for several decades to restore normal growth to children with congenital or acquired growth hormone deficiency. Without this therapy these children remain severely growth retarded with poor muscular development. Until 12 years ago, the only available source of the growth hormone was pituitary glands removed from cadavers. Unfortunately, a small number of these glands carried the Creutzfeldt-Jakob virus, and some recipients of human hormone became infected with this rapidly progressive and fatal neurological disease. Human growth hormone prepared by recombinant DNA technology is now widely available (although still very expensive), and is completely safe. Other examples of important therapeutic agents prepared by recombinant DNA technology include the blood cell growth factors (erythropoietin, colony-stimulating factors and thrombopoietin) now widely used (or in the case of thrombopoietin, under clinical trial) in a variety of applications including anaemia or renal failure and to aid recovery of the bone marrow after high dose chemotherapy or aplastic anaemia.

The techniques of molecular biology now allow tiny amounts of genetic material to be amplified by a technique known as the polymerase chain reaction (PCR). This technique had its initial practical application in forensic pathology, where the ability to get a genetic 'fingerprint' from tiny samples of biological material (e.g., blood stains, semen, a single hair, a few skin cells, or cheek cells in saliva) has allowed definitive identification of the individual from which the material derived. The same principle is used in the microbiological diagnosis of disease. Tiny amounts of parasites, bacteria or viruses or of the antibodies elicited by their presence, not detectable by the usual means can be amplified by the PCR so that they become detectable. Modern microbiological laboratories are making increasing use of such methods for routine diagnosis of certain conditions. Apart from increased sensitivity, a considerable saving in time can be involved. For example, the bacterium causing tuberculosis takes several weeks to culture, but the PCR reaction can allow the diagnosis within hours. Moreover, the technique is not dependent on the presence of living microorganisms. A difficulty in the diagnosis of meningitis (infection of the membranes covering the brain and spinal cord) is that the patient has often already received some antibiotics, making it difficult to culture the causative organism. PCR can allow identification of genetic material from the organism, living or dead.

Prenatal and presymptomatic diagnosis of disease is a difficult area because of the ethical issues raised. It is possible to diagnose cystic fibrosis, muscular dystrophy and several other debilitating genetic disorders in the first trimester of pregnancy by obtaining a tiny sample of the placenta or amniotic fluid. Thorough counselling is required, but the parents may well then choose to have a therapeutic abortion. The situation with postnatal but presymptomatic diagnosis of genetic disorders also raises difficult ethical issues. For example, Huntington's disease is inherited as a genetically dominant disorder (on average, one in two of the offspring of an affected individual can be expected to carry the gene). Individuals carrying the genes are normal until middle age (usually the fourth or fifth decade) when they show the first signs of a degenerative neurological disorder characterised by involuntary movements, progressive dementia and premature death. The gene has been identified and it is now possible at any stage of life to identify those destined to develop the condition. This allows informed decisions about whether to have children, financial management and other important life plans, but there can also be devastating and destructive psychological consequences when individuals learn that they (or their relative or spouse) carry the gene. Very skilful and sensitive counselling is required to allow individuals to make appropriate decisions about whether they wish to be tested.

Huntington's disease provides a graphic example of the ethical questions raised, but there is an increasing number of examples of similar dilemmas. It is possible to provide genetic identification of individuals likely to develop a rare type of inherited thyroid and adrenal tumour— potentially fatal, and probably preventable by major surgery in those carrying the gene in childhood. However, the decision to undertake such surgery on a perfectly well child on the basis of a genetic test is a difficult one. Rare, inherited forms of bowel and breast cancer can also be detected in this way.

A variety of techniques to develop vaccines has been used over the years. Increasingly, molecular biology is becoming the most flexible and effective method. Portions of organisms crucial to the infectivity of the organism can be identified and synthesised by recombinant DNA technology and used to generate natural immunity without risk of infections. Such techniques have been used in the highly successful development of hepatitis vaccines and are being used as major approaches in the development of vaccines for malaria and AIDS, two of the huge current challenges.

Gene therapy has been viewed both as the holy grail of recombinant DNA technology and as the greatest threat, with scenarios reminiscent of those in Huxley's *Brave New World* being generated by an exaggerated view of the ability of scientists to manipulate human genetic potential at will. So far, the potential applications and the 'hype' concerning gene therapy have far exceeded the clinical reality.

Gene therapy can comprise either modification of the genetic structure of the germ cell (ovum or sperm) with that modification transmitted to subsequent generations, or modification of the genetic structure of the cells of specific tissues, usually postnatally. Although germ cell genetic manipulation is an extremely valuable tool in basic biological research, it is unlikely that it will ever have a clinical role. This is because there are very few situations where genetic disorders will affect 100 per cent of offspring of a couple. Most genetic disorders are either autosomal dominant (requiring just one abnormal gene from either parent to cause the disease) in which an average of 50 per cent of offspring will be affected, or autosomal recessive (requiring one affected gene from each parent), in which an average of 25 per cent of offspring will be affected. Our ability to provide genetic diagnosis very early in pregnancy and offer therapeutic abortion to mothers carrying affected fetuses provides an effective approach in these disorders, although many have major ethical reservations about this approach. However, those with concerns about the morality of this approach are likely to be just as concerned about the genetic manipulation of the ova of women prior to in vitro fertilisation to avoid transmission of the abnormal gene.

Somatic gene therapy has been the subject of much speculation and research and some clinical trials. The problems of getting sufficient stable and regulatable gene expression to allow production of sufficient protein in the right place at the right time are considerable, but not insurmountable. In conditions such as cystic fibrosis, familial hypercholesterolaemia, muscular dystrophy and a variety of other rarer diseases caused by single gene mutations, it is likely that, over time, methods of applying gene therapy successfully will be achieved. Another potential, but even more difficult, application of gene therapy is to replace the function of damaged or destroyed cells in acquired disorders. Insulin-dependent (type I) diabetes mellitus is an example of such a disorder. In such situations, not only is it necessary to engineer cells expressing the human insulin gene, but additional manipulations are required to allow the insulin release to occur physiologically in response to elevated glucose levels. Other potential applications of gene therapy include the insertion of genes coding for factors which lead to tumour suppression, or inhibit cell proliferation to prevent atherosclerosis.

To summarise, molecular biology has already made major contributions to the prevention and treatment of disease. However, its contribution over the next 20 years is likely to be even more significant. Indeed its potential to alter medical care is difficult to envisage.

A summary of other major advances in sickness care

So numerous have been the advances in almost all fields of sickness care in the last two or three decades that it is impossible to describe or even to list them all. In this section, a very brief mention will be made of some additional examples of such advances.

The technical aspects of surgery have advanced in all fields. Examples include the introduction and outstanding efficacy of coronary artery surgery, carotid artery surgery and the dramatic improvement in the outcome of other forms of vascular and cardiac surgery. Microvascular and reconstructive surgery has allowed limbs to be reattached following trauma and disfiguring congenital deformities to be corrected. Cataract surgery is now a simple, safe and highly effective day procedure. Effective drug treatment for the prevention and treatment of peptic ulceration has been devised, with long-term cure of the disease now possible following identification of the causative organism. New psychotropic therapy for schizophrenia and severe depression has allowed subjects who previously required institutionalisation to live freely and satisfactorily in the community. Many forms of cancer, most notably the majority of cases of leukaemia and lymphoma are now curable by drugs sometimes combined with bone marrow transplantation. High levels of cholesterol and other fats in the blood can be treated effectively with drugs with proven efficacy in preventing recurrence of heart attacks. The outlook for people with diabetes is now dramatically improved, partly because of more convenient and comfortable methods of insulin administration, the development of methods of self blood glucose monitoring and more effective dosage of regimens of insulin, all of which lead to better control and less complications, and partly because of the development of more effective treatments for the eye, kidney and other complications if they do occur. Our ability to treat infections has improved, although this has been parallelled by the development of resistant organisms, and by the emergence of new and deadly viruses including that responsible for AIDS. For the first time, we have antibiotics which are effective against viruses, although this effectiveness is often incomplete and may be associated with toxicity. The effectiveness of treatment of AIDS has improved dramatically in the period since its description just over a decade ago, partly because of suppression of the virus itself using antiviral drugs, and partly because of better prophylaxis against and treatment of the very numerous opportunistic infections which pose the major threat in AIDS. We can be reasonably optimistic that the condition will soon be able to be held in check indefinitely in a high proportion of subjects.

The developed versus the developing world

Most of what has been written in this chapter applies to the developed world and is available to only limited and variable extents in developing countries. In the developing world, neonatal death rates, deaths from diarrhoeal diseases, malaria, bacterial infections, congenital defects and a host of other preventable or treatable diseases continue to be unacceptable, and many, many fold higher than those in the developed world. Many of the new technologies are expensive, and even countries in the developed world are having difficulties meeting the costs through the public purse, leading to a variety of forms of overt, or more often, covert, rationing. In developing countries, much more basic health care is unobtainable by many of the population.

The future

The section on molecular biology has emphasised the potential of the modern scientific approach to increase its impact on sickness care. Major goals which so far have been elusive include prevention or cure for many forms of cancer, AIDS, diabetes mellitus, asthma, rheumatoid arthritis and a host of other chronic illnesses. The ability to prevent or cure Alzheimer's disease, schizophrenia and other psychiatric illness would have a huge impact. However, it should be emphasised that all these past and present advances will not eliminate the need for hospital beds. With more people living to old age, it is likely that an increased prevalence of a variety of degenerative 'wear and tear' conditions such as joint and vascular disease will continue to throw a huge load on our health care system. The extent to which our community is able to obtain access to and to benefit from the huge advances in sickness care may well turn out to be a barometer of the wealth, efficiency and fairness of our society.

REFERENCES

371. Trovato F, Lalu NM. Narrowing sex differentials in life expectancy in the industrialised world—early 1970s to early 1990s. *Social Biology* 1996; 43: 20–37.
372. Novakovic B. United States childhood cancer survival 1973–1987. *Med Ped Oncol* 1994; 23: 480–6.
373. Fabre E, Deaguero RG, Deagustin JL, Tajada M, Repolles S, Sanz A. Perinatal mortality in term and post-term births. *J Perinatal Med* 1996; 24: 163–9.
374. Manson JE, Tosteson H, Ridker PM, et al. The primary prevention of myocardial infarction. *New Engl J Med* 1992; 326: 1406–16.
375. Peltonen M, Asplund K. Age-period-cohort effects on stroke mortality in Sweden 1969–93 and forecasts up to the year 2003. *Stroke* 1996; 27: 1981–5.
376. ISIS-2 (Second International Study of Infarct Survival) Collaborative Group. Randomised trial of intravenous streptokinase, oral aspirin, both, or neither, among 17187 cases of suspected myocardial infarction; ISIS-2. *Lancet* 1988; 2: 349–60.
377. The Scandinavian Simavastin Survival Study Group. Randomised trial of cholesterol lowering in 4444 patients with coronary heart disease; The Scandinavian Simavastin Survival Study (4S). *Lancet* 1994; 344: 1383–9.
378. Singer DE. Randomized trials of warfarin for atrial fibrillation. *New Engl J Med* 1992; 327: 1451–3.
379. Castigliovegertsch M, Johnsen C, Goldhirsch A, et al. The international (Ludwig) breast cancer study trials I–IV—15 years follow up. *Annals of Oncology* 1994; 5: 717–24.
380. Forman WB. The role of chemotherapy and adjuvant therapy in the management of colorectal cancer. *Cancer* 1994; 74: 2151–3.
381. The Diabetes Control and Complications Research Group. The effect of intensive treatment of diabetes on the development and progression of long-term complications in insulin-dependent diabetes mellitus. *New Engl J Med* 1993; 329: 977–86.
382. Sackett D. Cochrane collaboration. *Brit Med J* 1994; 309: 1514–15.
383. Grabowski TJ, Damasis AR. Improving functional imaging techniques—the dream of a single image for a single mental event. *Proc Nat Acad Sci USA* 1996; 93: 14302–3.
384. Sutherland DER, Grussner A, Moudry-Munns K. International Pancreas Transplant Registry Report. *Transplant Proc* 1994; 26: 407–11.

CHAPTER TWELVE

Beyond Medicine: The Wider Determinants of Population and Global Health

ANTHONY MCMICHAEL AND DAVID LEON

Humans, nearly everywhere, are living longer than ever before. What component of this favourable trend is due to modern forms of medical care and their wider-spread availability and what is the result of broader social-environmental influences? This chapter maps the key elements of this relationship, considering those factors that influence health at a global, national and local population level.

International variation in the rate of decline of perinatal and infant death rates over the past three decades illustrates the difficulty in apportioning 'credit' to these different influences.[385] Modern techniques of vaccination, antibiotic therapy, oral rehydration and nutritional supplementation have greatly enhanced infant survival. From the early 1960s infant mortality began declining in southern Europe, while in central Europe (Germany, Austria, Czechoslovakia, and Hungary) appreciable reductions only started a decade later. Outside of Europe it declined more steeply in Canada than in the USA, and more strongly and enduringly in Cuba than in most other Latin American countries. These differences suggest that something more than the acquisition of technical health care facilities has affected the gains over time. The importance of social improvements is suggested by the persistence of low infant mortality rates in Cuba despite its economic difficulties and by the recent upturn in countries, such as Romania and the Dominican Republic, undergoing a loss of social cohesion and stability.

The role of medicine

Differences in medical knowledge, technology and provision are commonly invoked to explain differences in the health status of populations across time and between populations. Today, the substantial proportion of national budgets in developed countries being spent on health

183

care systems leads naturally to the belief that this must translate into improved health and longevity. Meanwhile, among public health practitioners, one often finds the opposite view: that medical practice and the health care system have little influence upon population health.

The work of Thomas McKeown, dating from the middle of this century, stands out as the pioneering contribution to the debate on the contribution of medicine to population health. His central thesis is that the decline of mortality in nineteenth-century Britain was driven by improvements in the standard of living and all things that went with that, especially an improvement in nutrition. Recently, Szreter has argued that McKeown underestimated the importance of the improvements in sanitation and other conscious efforts to improve the public health that occurred in the latter part of the nineteenth century.[386] However, McKeown's general contention that medicine played little role in the mortality decline of the nineteenth century is largely undisputed. Indeed, Guha has recently argued[387] that the timing of the infectious disease mortality decline in relation to specific acts of legislation in the UK, its greater magnitude in women (especially from tuberculosis), and the fact that the decline for many infections was in deaths, i.e., case fatality, rather than in incidence, all point to a substantive protective effect of improved nutrition.

This assessment of a minimal role of medicine in the nineteenth century has coloured perceptions of the reasons for the mortality decline in this century. Often overlooked is the fact that the mortality reductions that have occurred in countries such as Britain since 1900 are far larger than those occurring in the nineteenth century, as shown in Table 12.1.

In the second half of the nineteenth century life expectancy in Britain improved by just over four years, while in the first half of this century it improved by approximately 20 years, largely due to declines in mortality in infancy and childhood. Since the middle of this century the rate of improvement has declined, although it has been of the same order as in the latter part of the nineteenth century. A thought-provoking account of the twentieth century trajectories in life expectancy in a wide range of developed countries is provided by Kinsella.[389] He identifies the widening of the gender gap in life expectancy at birth as one of the dominant features of trends over the past 90 years. In the 15 developed countries that he studied, the gender gap at the turn of this century was typically of the order of two to three years. Today, in most of these countries women outlive men by between five and nine years. This has been mainly due to a reduction in mortality in women at older ages. This divergence between the sexes has occurred along with an overall convergence in life expectancy at birth between countries.

Table 12.1 Improvement in life expectancy at birth in Britain over the past 160 years[388]

Period	1838 –54	1871 –80	1881 –90	1891 –1900	1901 –10	1910 –12	1920 –22	1930 –32	1950 –52	1960 –62	1970 –72	1980 –82	1990 –92
Life expectancy at birth	40	41	44	44	49	52	56	59	66	68	69	71	73

McKeown argued[390] that medical practice and knowledge contributed little to the sharp declines in mortality this century before the 1970s. He emphasised particularly that the major developments in immunisation and treatment of communicable diseases occurred after mortality from these diseases had already fallen dramatically. Instead, he pointed to improvements in diet and environment as the key driving force. A similar conclusion was drawn by McKinlay and McKinlay in their analysis of the mortality decline in the USA since 1900.[391]

This scepticism about the role of medicine has been described by Kunitz as a counter-revolutionary reaction to the over-optimistic view of the benefits presumed to have followed from advances in medical science (particularly antibiotics) in the late 1940s and early 1950s.[392] It may also be seen as a timely questioning of the population health impact of the post-war explosion in health service expenditure. Powles,[393] using British data, and McKinlay and McKinlay,[391] using US data, observed that the enormous increase in expenditure on health since the 1950s coincided precisely with the period in which there was actually an appreciable slowing in the rate of increase in life expectancy. The take-home message from this graphic contrast in trends was that the post-war medical enterprise was not generating the anticipated improvements in population health.

Recent assessments of the contribution of medicine to population health status have been less negative. Mackenbach and Looman,[394] for example, deduced that the post-war introduction of antibiotics had had a major impact upon mortality from communicable diseases in the Netherlands, particularly between ages 10 and 59 years. A computer-modelled simulation of factors affecting the decline in coronary heart disease mortality in the USA during 1980–1990 indicates that just over half of the decline is attributable to reductions in risk factors (primary and secondary prevention) and that 43 per cent is attributable to improvements in treatment of patients with coronary disease.[395] More generally, there has been a growing interest in analysing mortality trends from diseases thought to be at least partly amenable to medical treatment. Charlton and Velez[396] examined trends in mortality from ten such amenable causes—including tuberculosis, cervical cancer,

Hodgkin's disease, cerebrovascular disease and maternal mortality. Death rates from these conditions fell sharply over the three decades from 1950, compared to a much more static picture for other causes of death. More detailed work from The Netherlands[397] concluded that 'the impact of medical care on post-1950 mortality . . . could well have been substantial'. Similar conclusions were reached in an analysis of Finnish amenable mortality 1969–1981.[398] A weakness of these analyses, however, is their assumption that declines in mortality from 'amenable causes' are due to medical treatment rather than to other non-medical influences upon those same diseases.

Bunker and colleagues[399,400] have developed a more direct estimation of the impact of both secondary prevention and treatment on life expectancy today. Using data from the United States, the contribution to life expectancy was estimated separately for 'clinical preventive services', such as screening for hypertension, cervical and colo-rectal cancer and immunisation for a range of communicable diseases, and 'clinical curative services' for conditions including cervical cancer, hypertension, diabetes and trauma. This approach extrapolates directly from what is known about the efficacy of various interventions to their impact on the US population as a whole. While individual components in this inventory generally have small effects measured in weeks or months of life expectancy, when added up these interventions were estimated to account for about five years of life expectancy, with a potential to add another 2 to 2.5 years 'by extending therapies already known to be efficacious'.

When one considers that nearly all of these preventive and curative activities have been introduced in the post-war period—and many just in the past few decades—the size of this total estimated effect is striking in comparison to the overall gain of seven years in life expectancy at birth in the United States between 1950 and 1990. The assumptions made in this analysis by Bunker may be questioned, and other similar analyses need to be carried out by others to see if these conclusions can be replicated. However, this direct approach illustrates how small individual impacts of specific interventions may add together to provide an effect that is relatively substantial compared to the overall gains in life expectancy since the middle of this century.

Recent trends in mortality and morbidity

Life expectancy at birth has risen in all industrialised countries during this century. National trends in life expectancy have been uneven over time and the gains have been greater in women.[389] In most developed countries, recent gains in life expectancy have been greatest above the age of 65. This principally reflects a reduction in heart disease and stroke fatalities.

Meanwhile, what has been the trend in non-fatal disease? In 1977, Gruenberg argued that 'the net effect of successful technological innovations used in disease control has been to raise the prevalence of certain diseases and disabilities by prolonging their average duration . . . the net contribution of our success has actually been to worsen people's health'.[401] To what extent it that a valid assessment today?

Long-term historical data indicate that there has been something of an 'inverse transition', with mortality declines being accompanied by persistence of, or increases in, morbidity.[402] One study in the USA, using a composite measure of mortality and morbidity (the probability of future life-years free of disability), found that although the overall life expectancy had increased over several decades, most of the increase had been in years of disability.[403] Between 1964 and 1985, life expectancy at birth increased by 4.4 and 4.5 years in males and females respectively, but the estimated disability-free life expectancy actually declined by 7.3 and 7.6 years respectively. For persons aged 45 years, the approximately three extra years of life were, in effect, all years of disability. Only older persons, aged 65 years, had gained in disability-free life expectancy. Overall, perhaps the prolonged survival, with disability, of persons with life-threatening illness offsets the reduction of illness incidence in other persons.[404]

These US findings suggest that life-saving medical technology is not necessarily health-preserving technology. But for the population at large, if healthy life expectancy has increased less than total life expectancy this necessarily means that the prevalence of poor health must have increased. However, there are few systematic data on trends in overall morbidity and on the contribution of medical care to its limitation.

Looking to the future it is difficult to estimate to what extent any such future contraction in morbidity will be due to better medical care. There are manifest long-term benefits from contemporary medical interventions for some health disorders, e.g., drug treatment of hypertension, insulin replacement in child-onset diabetes mellitus, bronchodilator treatment for asthmatics, a widening range of vaccinations, surgical treatment of varicose veins and haemorrhoids, hip replacement in elderly persons, and so on. Yet, the incidence of many low-fatality conditions appears to have been rising in Western populations for several decades. These include childhood asthma, non-melanoma skin cancers, eating disorders (especially in young women), obesity, chronic depression, and, in ageing populations, the dementias. Two other categories of health problems also are increasing: the physical and psychological hazards of violence and drug abuse, especially among young adults in inner urban environment, and, second, various types of previously rare or unknown infectious diseases of variable fatality—including HIV/AIDS, several hepatitis viruses, various drug-resistant bacterial infections (including tuberculosis, and many others).

There have been recent attempts to partition life expectancy into its 'active' (disability-free), disabled, and institutionalised components.[405] Indeed, computational approaches have also been developed to take account of individual transitions between these components. Most notable has been the work by the World Bank in developing the disability-adjusted life year (DALY) as a proposed common metric for measuring the duration and quality of less-than-healthy life lived.[406] Using approaches of this kind, it is evident that women in developed countries, who live longer than men, can expect to spend more time in a disabled state. Typically, in such countries, men spend 80–85 percent of their lives free of disability, compared to 75–80 per cent in women.

Non-medical influences on health and mortality

The health of each individual is a composite expression of genetic, social, environmental and personal-behavioural factors, variably modulated by clinical medical interventions. While each of these categories of factor applies at the level of the individual, some have health-influencing properties that can only be understood at the level of groups or populations. For example, while an individual's socioeconomic status (SES) may directly influence his/her personal behaviour and occupation, the steepness of income gradient within a population appears to be an independent determinant of the population's mean level of health.

Factors determining the health status of people thus include their socio-economic status[407-11] and the broader issue of income equity within the society.[412-13] Others argue that social cohesion and health may be related[414-16] and that the Roseto experience[417] provides compelling evidence of the link between social cohesion and health. The next three sections illustrate the importance of several categories of non-medical influence upon health.

East-West European differences in mortality

The collapse of communism in central and eastern Europe and in the former Soviet Union has revealed a startling picture of East-West differences in health. In the early 1990s, it emerged that since the 1960s there had been a widening gap in mortality between the East and West, with life expectancy in the West improving steadily, while that in the

East had reached a plateau or even declined.[418] In 1994, life expectancy at birth in the former communist countries of Central and Eastern Europe (CEE) was 71.3 compared to 77.3 years in the countries of the European Union. The countries of the former Soviet Union, in particular, have undergone a profound crisis in their mortality since the mid 1980s. In Russia, for example, between 1990 and 1994 life expectancy among men fell from 63.8 to 57.6 years, while among women it fell from 74.4 to 71.0 years.

These differences and trends provide a challenge to epidemiologists and public health practitioners. First, there is no intrinsic reason why the populations of the former communist countries should have poorer health than those in the West. Unfortunately, since the early 1990s in these countries, there has been a misdirected tendency (often encouraged by Western advisers) to focus principally upon issues of health service reorganisation and funding—compounding the earlier paradox wherein the ratio of doctors to population in communist countries greatly exceeded that in Western Europe. Much less attention has been given to developing a strategy to reduce the incidence of disease.

Nevertheless, there have been some attempts to synthesise what is known about the East-West health gap.[419-20] These have concluded that environmental pollution is unlikely to play an important part, although in some specific areas there may be appreciable health consequences from degradation of the quality of the environment and toxic effluent from industry. With respect to health care, one analysis has suggested that up to 20 per cent of the difference in overall mortality between CEE countries and West Germany would be eliminated if there were no differences in the levels of mortality from 'amenable causes'. However, as already discussed it is an untested assumption that changes in amenable mortality are necessarily due to differences in medical services. Smoking clearly explains some of the long-term differences in mortality between East and West, especially among men.[421] Dietary factors are also likely to have been important, with one suggestion being that antioxidant micronutrients from vegetables may play an important role.[422] Psychosocial stress has also been advanced as a major explanation,[419] although with little supporting data.

Analyses of the recent mortality crisis in Russia[423-24] indicate that very high levels of alcohol consumption may account for much of the recent sharp downturn in life expectancy. Since 1990 mortality rates have increased not only for accidents, violence and alcohol poisoning, but also for pneumonia, other communicable diseases and circulatory diseases (but not cancer). The marked increases in mortality in middle-age from pneumonia and circulatory diseases could indeed be caused by excessive binge-drinking at levels that are very uncommon in Western Europe. Evidence from other epidemiological studies has suggested that high levels of ethanol intake are associated with death from haemorrhagic stroke, cardiac arrhythmias and pneumonia. Further research is now needed to elucidate the role that alcohol may be playing in the social aetiology of a range of diseases in many countries, not just in Russia.

An adequate explanation for these East-West differences cannot reside in a list of risk factors—whether alcohol, smoking, environmental exposures or psycho-social stress. Via multi-disciplinary research, we now need to learn more from this recent, unusual, European experience about the underlying determinants of these health-influencing behavioural and social patterns.

North-South differences in mortality

In many African, Asian and Latin American countries, the average life expectancy is 20–30 years less than for rich Western countries.[425] Within those countries, it is often much lower for the socially and economically disadvantaged. Infectious diseases remain the main killer, particularly in children below the age of five years.

Much of the health deficit in poor Third World countries reflects the widespread poverty, the adverse social policy consequences of export-oriented economic development, and the environmental adversity that flows from exploitation of natural resources. In today's world-economy, which continues to operate to the disadvantage of poor countries, the exacerbation of land degradation, rural unemployment, food shortages and urban crowding all contribute to health deficits for the rural dispossessed, the underfed and the slum-dweller.

The link between material standard of living and health is illustrated by considering the most basic measure: life expectancy at birth. In the early 1990s, regional life-expectancy figures were: Africa, 55 years; Asia, 64 years; South America, 68 years; USSR and Eastern Europe, 69 years; Western Europe, North America, Australia and New Zealand, 76 years. Nevertheless, the graph of life expectancy against per-person Gross National Product (GNP) contains some surprises. Some countries have much higher life expectancies than their economic indices might predict. Countries with commitments to social justice, and with lesser gradients in income, mass education and primary health care tend to get more health for their per-person wealth. Sri Lanka, where life expectancy is expected to reach 74 years by 2000 (having been 60 years in 1950), Costa Rica, Kerala State (southwest India) and China are four well-recognised examples. Their relatively good health has been attributed to the deliberate strengthening of primary health care systems, to the integration of traditional with modern health care and to progress-ive aspects of social reform and distributive justice.[425]

By contrast, life-expectancy figures in Hungary, Romania and certain of the oil-rich OPEC nations are clearly below their GNP-related expec-tations. In these and some of the more recently industrialised countries, the health deficits relative to national wealth have been primarily due to recent increases in adult mortality, especially cardiovascular disease.

In most Third World countries, a mixed profile of health and disease is now emerging. The persistence of widespread poverty, lack of safe water and sanitation, and urban crowding ensure the continuation of infectious diseases, especially as a source of childhood mortality. The recent spread of HIV and other STDs has added a new and tragic dimension of poor health to many of these poor populations. Rapid increases in extractive and manufacturing industries—often reflecting the largely unregulated spread of transnational companies—cause occupational injuries and diseases.[426-27] Meanwhile, the gains in life expectancy and the increase in urbanisation are transforming the eco-nomy and ecology of Third World populations in ways that substantially increase the prevalence of obesity, hypertension, cigarette smoking, sedentariness and urban traffic. All these are contributing to a rise in chronic non-infectious diseases alongside the persistence of infectious diseases.

A life-course perspective on the origins of disease

Intuition tells us that our health at any particular attained age is the product of our experience and circumstances across the entire course of our life. Freud's views on the importance of events in early life on psychic health in adult life have taken deep root in popular percep-tions about the determinants of adult personality and behaviour. In contrast, the epidemiological model that has dominated much of our thinking about the aetiology of non-communicable disease over recent decades has largely ignored the potential influence of factors operat-ing in pre-adult life. Instead, it has been almost exclusively preoccu-pied with the effect of adult 'lifestyle' and biomedical predictors such as smoking, cholesterol levels and blood pressure.

Recently, this adult-oriented perspective has been challenged by the emerging evidence that circumstances in utero are important determin-ants of a range of non-communicable diseases. David Barker's group in the UK has advanced the generalised notion of fetal 'programming' of adult disease.[428] They have conducted studies showing that, as birth weight declines, blood pressure in childhood and adulthood goes up as does the late-adulthood risk of death from ischaemic heart disease, while being thin at birth (low length:weight ratio) appears to be specifically related to impaired glucose tolerance and non-insulin-dependent diabetes. Strikingly, these effects appear to be continuous across the range of size at birth, and are not restricted to neonates clinically defined as small at birth.

These results have been interpreted by Barker and colleagues to mean that impaired fetal nutrition permanently changes the physiological setting or cell complement of specific organs of the affected individual or in some other way affects susceptibility to later disease.[429] This 'fetal origins' hypothesis has created controversy. Some have welcomed this innovatory shift in view of the aetiology of many adult diseases, while others have been more sceptical (in part because this perspective distracts attention from attempts to persuade the public to alter their adult lifestyle).

Meanwhile, other research groups have replicated the basic findings.[430] Further, the possibility that these neonate-to-later-adulthood associations arise from socio-economic confounding by continuity of socio-economic circumstance from infancy through childhood to young adulthood has now been largely excluded by studies able to take account of these circumstances both at birth and at older ages. It appears, therefore, that the associations between size at birth and risk of later disease are real. In addition to this work on the fetal origins of cardiovascular disease and diabetes, there is some evidence that fetal growth is correlated with the risk of cancer in later life. There is emerging evidence of a link between large size at birth and increased risk of breast cancer in women.[431]

What mechanisms might explain such associations? The proponents of the 'fetal programming' hypothesis maintain that these effects result from variations in the fetal nutritional environment. However, other research indicates that maternal diet during pregnancy has only a minor impact on fetal growth and thus is unlikely to be a major factor. Placental function may well be critical, being the active conduit through which all nutrients reach the fetus. With present knowledge, however, we cannot preclude the possibility that some of the observed associations are due to genetic factors that may influence both fetal size and adult disease risk. For example, given the importance of insulin for both fetal growth and diabetes, a genetic factor that influences either insulin production or its action could plausibly explain the link between thinness at birth and later-life non-insulin-dependent diabetes.

From an historical perspective, this recent interest in the fetal origins of adult disease may not be quite as novel as is sometimes perceived.[432] In the first four decades of this century, good childhood circumstances and nutrition were believed to be central to ensuring adult health. The emphasis in the pre-war period, however, was very much on nutrition in childhood in contrast to the focus on nutrition in utero that characterises the current interest in the pre-adult origins of adult disease.

Constructing a framework in which these serial, potentially interacting, influences at different points in the life course may combine to determine adult disease risk presents an important challenge.

Conclusions

Recent gains in life expectancy in Western populations have not been matched by gains in healthy life expectancy. Indeed, as populations age and as infectious diseases have been overshadowed by chronic non-infectious diseases, the prevalence of overall morbidity may be increasing. Increasingly, we are encountering the unavoidable reality of a prolonged adulthood that entails the risk of considerably more chronic disability and disease than occurs in other animal species, most of whom do not survive beyond middle adulthood.

Meanwhile, we are making further gains in understanding and improving human health. Infant mortality has fallen rapidly in most countries as vaccination, sanitation, family planning and nutrition have improved. Many adult-age risk factors for non-infectious diseases have been identified—although achieving changes in personal health-endangering behaviour continues to prove difficult. There are new ideas about how stresses during fetal development can 'program' the human organism's biology and thus influence susceptibility to the diseases of later adulthood.

The profile of health and disease is never static. The quickening pace of technological change and of long-distance human migration in recent centuries has amplified the mismatch between human biology and ambient environment that influences various disease risks. Patterns of infectious diseases are changing on a broad front. Aspects of health, safety and well-being are declining in many of today's large cities. Food production resources and fresh water supplies may yet become inadequate for many in a world population that will almost double by 2050. The global impact of human economic activity on Earth's atmosphere, biodiversity and other large-scale natural systems now casts an unprecedentedly long shadow over the health prospects of future generations. Have we, in part, been improving population health by a non-sustainable consumption of natural capital?

Good population health should be a central objective and a recognised key indicator of social and economic policy. Our history shows us that, while advances in medical care will continue to defer the time of death, alleviate much suffering, and cure some illnesses, it is the shifting ecology of human community life—its social relations and its compatibility with sustainable ecosystems and environmental amenities —that sets the boundaries of population health.

REFERENCES

385. La Vecchia C, Parazzini F, Levi F. Perinatal and infant mortality: a worldwide issue. *Eur J Pub Hlth* 1996; 6: 157–8.
386. Szreter S. The importance of social intervention in Britain's mortality decline 1850–1914: a re-interpretation of the role of public health. *Social History of Medicine* 1988; 1: 1–37.
387. Guha S. The importance of social interventions in England's mortality decline: the evidence reviewed. *Social History of Medicine* 1994; 7: 89–113.
388. Office of Population Censuses and Surveys. *Mortality Statistics 1992*, England and Wales, DHI no 27, London, HMSO, 1994, Table 14.
389. Kinsella KG. Changes in life expectancy 1900–1990. *Am J Clin Nutr* 1992; 55: 196S–1202S.
390. McKeown T. *The role of medicine: dream, mirage or nemesis*. The Nuffield Provincial Hospitals Trust, 1976.
391. McKinlay JB, McKinlay SM. The questionable contribution of medical measures to the decline of mortality in the United States in the twentieth century. *Millbank Mem Fund Q* 1977; 55: 405–28.
392. Kunitz, SJ. The personal physician and the decline of mortality. In: Schofield R, Reher D, Bideau A (eds). *The decline of mortality in Europe*. Oxford: OUP, 1991; 248–62.
393. Powles J. On the limitations of modern medicine. *Science, Medicine and Man* 1973; 1: 1–30.
394. Mackenbach JP, Looman CW. Secular trends of infectious disease mortality in The Netherlands, 1911–1978: quantitative estimates of changes coinciding with the introduction of antibiotics. *Int J Epidemiol* 1988; 17: 618–24.
395. Hunink MGM, Goldman L, Tosteson ANA, et al. The recent decline in mortality from coronary heart disease, 1980–1990. *JAMA* 1997; 277: 535–42.
396. Charlton JR, Velez R. Some international comparisons of mortality amenable to medical intervention. *Brit Med J Clin Res Ed* 1986; 292: 295–301.
397. Mackenbach JP, Looman CW, Kunst AE, Habbema JD, van der Maas PJ. Post-1950 mortality trends and medical care: gains in life expectancy due to declines in mortality from conditions amenable to medical intervention in The Netherlands. *Soc Sci Med* 1988; 27: 889–94.
398. Poikolainen K, Eskola J. The effect of health services on mortality: decline in death rates from amenable and non-amenable causes in Finland, 1969–81. *Lancet* 1986; 1: 199–202.
399. Bunker JP, Frazier HS, Mosteller F. Improving health: measuring effects of medical care. *Millbank Mem Fund Q* 1994; 72: 225–58.
400. Bunker JP, Frazier HS, Mosteller F. The role of medical care in determining health: creating an inventory of benefits. In: Amick BC, Levine S, Tarlov AR, Walsh DC (eds). *Society and health*. Oxford: Oxford University Press, 1995, pp305–41.
401. Gruenberg EM. The failures of success. *Millbank Mem Fund Q* 1977; 3: 24.
402. Riley JC. Long term morbidity and mortality trends: inverse transition. In: Caldwell JC, Findley SE, Caldwell P (eds). *What we know about health transition: the cultural, social, and behavioural determinants of health*, vol 1. Canberra: Australian National University, 1990, pp165–88.

403. McKinlay JB, McKinlay SM, Beaglehole R. A review of the evidence concerning the impact of medical measures on recent mortality and morbidity in the United States. *Int J Hlth Serv* 1989; 19: 181–208.
404. Poterba JN, Summers LH. Public policy implications of declining old-age mortality. In: Burtless G (ed). *Work, health and income among the elderly.* Washington DC: Brookings Institute, 1987.
405. Suzman R, Harris T, Hadley E, Weinbruck R. *The robust oldest old: optimistic perspectives for increasing healthy life expectancy in the oldest old.* New York: Oxford University Press, 1991.
406. Murray CJL, Lopez AD (eds). *Global comparative assessments in the health sector. Disease burden, expenditures and intervention packages.* Geneva: WHO, 1994.
407. Davey Smith G, Bartley M, Blane D. The Black report on socioeconomic inequalities in health: 10 years on. *Brit Med J* 1990; 301: 373–7.
408. Whitehead M. *Inequalities in health. The health divide.* Harmondsworth: Penguin Books, 1990.
409. Blane D, Brunner E, Wilkinson R. *Health and social organisation.* London: Routledge, 1996.
410. Amick BC, Levine S, Tarlov AR, Walsh DC. *Society and health.* Oxford: Oxford University Press, 1995.
411. Davey Smith G, Leon DA, Shipley MJ, Rose G. Socio-economic differentials in cancer among men. *Int J Epidemiol* 1996, 1991; 20: 339–45.
412. Wilkinson RG. *Unhealthy societies. The afflictions of inequality.* London: Routledge, 1996.
413. Wilkinson RG. *Health inequalities: relative or absolute material standards? Brit Med J* 1997; 314: 591–5. Wilkinson 1997.
414. Putnam RD, Leonardi R, Nanetti RY. *Making democracy work: civic traditions in modern Italy.* Princeton, NJ: Princeton University Press, 1993.
415. House JS, Landis KR, Umberson D. Social relationships and health. *Science* 1988; 241: 540–5.
416. Mosk C. *Making health work. Human growth in modern Japan.* Berkeley, CA: California University Press, 1996.
417. Wolf S, Bruhn JG. The power of clan: a 25-year prospective study of Roseto, Pennsylvania, 1993. New Brunswick, NJ: Transaction Publishers, 1993.
418. Feachem R. Health decline in Eastern Europe. *Nature* 1994; 367: 313–4.
419. Bobak M, Marmot MG. East-West mortality divide and its potential explanations: proposed research agenda. *Brit Med J* 1996; 312: 421–5.
420. Hertzman C, Kelly S, Bobak M (eds). *East-West life expectancy gap in Europe: Environmental and non-environmental determinants.* London, Kluwer, Academic Publishers, 1996.
421. Peto R, Lopez AD, Boreham J, Thun M, Heath C. Mortality from tobacco in developed countries: indirect estimation from national vital statistics. *Lancet* 1992; 339: 1268–78.
422. Ginter E. High cardiovascular mortality in postcommunist countries: participation of oxidative stress? *Internat J Vit Nutr Res* 1996; 66: 183–9.
423. Ryan M. Alcoholism and rising mortality in the Russian Federation. *Brit Med J* 1995; 310: 646–8.
424. Shkolnikov VM, Nemtsov A. The anti-alcohol campaign and variations in Russian mortality. In: Bobadilla J-L, Costello C (eds). *Mortality and adult health priorities in the new independent states.* Washington: National Academy of Sciences, 1996.
425. World Bank. *World Development Report 1993. Investing in health.* Oxford: Oxford University Press, 1993.
426. McMichael AJ, Woodward AJ, van Leeuwen RE. The impact of energy use in industrialised countries upon global population health. *Medicine and Global Survival* 1994; 1: 23–32.

427. Pearce N, Traditional epidemiology, modern epidemiology, and public health. *Am J Pub Health* 1996; 86: 678–83.
428. Barker DJP. Fetal origins of coronary heart disease. *Brit Med J* 1995; 311: 171–4.
429. Lucas A. Programming by early nutrition in man. In: *The childhood environment and adult disease*. Ciba Foundation Symposium 156. Chichester: Wiley, 1991, 38–50.
430. Leon DA, Ben-Shlomo Y. Pre-adult influences on cardiovascular disease and cancer. In: Kuh D, Ben-Shlomo Y (eds). *Life course influences on adult disease.* Oxford: Oxford University Press, 1997.
431. Michels KB, Trichopoulos D, Robins JM, et al. Birthweight as a risk factor for breast cancer. *Lancet* 1996; 348: 1542–6.
432. Davey Smith G, Kuh D. Does early nutrition affect later health? In: Smith DF (ed). *Nutrition in Britain: science, scientists and politics in twentieth century Britain.* New York: Routledge 1996, 214–37.

PART FOUR

DILEMMAS IN
MEDICINE

CHAPTER THIRTEEN

Current Distortions

PETER BAUME

Introduction

Much of the improvement in average longevity in Western countries during the twentieth century has come from application of public health measures, from the development of antibiotics, and from immunisation (see Figure 13.1). Many of the other interventions of disease-oriented medical practitioners have had more to do with the comfort and relief of individuals than they have had to do with the health of whole societies.[433,434,435] It has been estimated that only 10 per cent of the mortality from ten leading causes of death in the United States is related to inadequate health care while 50 per cent of the premature mortality was thought to be related to unhealthy behaviour and lifestyle.[436] Nevertheless, many disease-oriented practitioners believe that their efforts have achieved most of the manifest improvements during the last 100 years. Medical practitioners have certainly responded to the needs, often significant and urgent, of sick people, but their contribution to the health of the whole society is less certain. These matters are discussed further in other chapters.

The maximum quantity of life (that is, the time that the longest lived persons survive) has not increased[437] and there may be a limit to human existence determined in part by intrinsic qualities of the cells which make up the human body. No-one lives longer than about 110 years and all people over the age of 95 live with some significant disability. Figure 13.2 puts finite human life into context,[438] while observing that the development of artificial intelligence will cause new and different major changes and challenges. Nevertheless, colleagues continue to work to overcome one disease after another, considering little or not at all the lives which people will have to lead should the diseases they study be mastered. Since death is universal, every success leaves people susceptible to death from some other cause—as any one cause disappears, another will increase. So the rising incidence of deaths from cancer has, as one cause, the decreasing incidence of deaths from other causes.

Background

The medical advances of this century have not been achieved without associated costs. Some medical practitioners have forgotten how to relate to the people they serve, to their frailty, to their troubles, to their suffering, to their fears, to their humanity. Medicine has become more sophisticated in its understanding of disease, but less personal in its relation to people. It is harder and harder to find a modern practitioner interested in patients as people. Many citizens are bitter about the failure of their own medical attendants to communicate empathetically or effectively or equally (that is, as one person talking to another) at times which are the most significant and most emotionally charged in their lives. Some medical publications, recognising the problem, have set out detailed accounts of empathy and of some of the techniques which practitioners might use to relate better to people in practice.[439]

Figure 13.1 Tuberculosis, Australia—age adjusted mortality rates per 100 000 population per year, 1860–1988

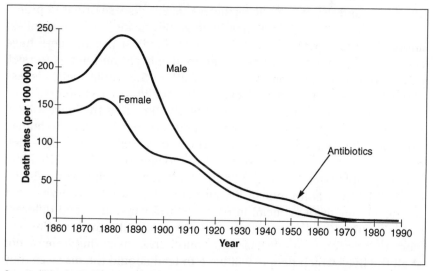

Sources (1) Lancaster, HO, *Tuberculosis Mortality in Australia, 1908 to 1945*. Medical Journal of Australia, 1950, p655; (2) Australian Bureau of Statistics, *Causes of Death: Australia*, Cat. No 3303.0, Australian Bureau of Statistics, Canberra, 1972–90; (3) Commonwealth Bureau of Census and Statistics, *Causes of Death*. Bulletins 1–7. Commonwealth Bureau of Census and Statistics, Canberra, 1962–72.

Reproduced with permission from Lawson, JS. Public health Australia: an introduction. Sydney: McGraw-Hill, 1991.

Financial distortions

More and more practitioners are tailoring what they do for patients, and how long they spend, to economic signals like repayments, subsidy, co-payments, and bulk-billing arrangements rather than to the needs of people for care and attention. Most payment systems reimburse patients by item of service and, only where practitioners receive payment for a preventive activity (like immunisation or the performing of a Pap smear), is it possible to justify activity to maintain health. In a piece-work system, some Australian primary care practitioners claim that they are forced to offer an average of six minutes for standard consultations (one minute more than a 'short' consultation) if they are to remain economically viable. Because it is sometimes not possible to respond to patients in such a short time, many consultations are inadequate and truncated. Although provisions exist for higher payments for longer consultations, it is economically more advantageous, in a piece-work system, for practitioners to conduct more shorter consultations than it is to conduct a smaller number of longer consultations.

Some problems

There are serious distortions in the present systems of care which operate to the disadvantage of people. The purposes for which hospitals and medical practices are organised are sometimes related as much to the perceptions, needs and agendas of care providers, or of systems of payment, or of the rules of insurers, or of central budget planners, as they are to the needs of care users. Cynical private hospital planners sometimes say that, if a choice is to be made, it is more important to have adequate parking for the practitioners who will use and refer patients to the facility than it is to have adequate hotel services for those who will be patients. Conventional providers (medical practitioners, nurses, therapists) simply do not believe complaints from patients that the providers themselves are a cause of unhappiness for many, believing instead that unhappiness is the result of disease processes, or of the outcome of disease, or of psychological factors within people, or else is the result of ignorance and misunderstanding of medical science on the part of citizens. Those factors are often, but not always, the cause of patient distress. If practitioners understood that they are often part of the problem, they would have to think about changing—and some are too driven by circumstances, and are unwilling anyhow, to change.

Present hospital and medical systems are organised in ways that leave citizens desperate and alienated.[440] To walk along the corridors of many busy hospitals is to see insiders who are comfortable and the people they care for who are mostly uncomfortable. Insiders are often in uniforms, have an air of authority about them, sometimes carry 'badges of office' such as stethoscopes, and are frequently busy and pre-occupied. The people they care for wear ordinary clothes or pyjamas or hospital gowns, seldom smile, look lost, are sometimes visibly ill, frequently try to catch the eye or talk to any care provider who has time to share, and appear to be what they are—the less powerful partners in a desperate game. So not only are hospitals unsafe places to be in as a consequence of widespread iatrogenic disease,[441] they are unfriendly and alienating to many people, their hotel services (for example, food services[442]) are poor—and no-one seems able to fix these matters.

Many users of care are interesting and important and powerful people in their own rights. Powerful or otherwise, many users have important lessons to teach medical practitioners—but they generally are not allowed to take any role but that of the passive grateful patient into hospital with them. No-one seems interested in the other lives that these people have, in their capacities, or in their skills, or in their personalities.

Little[443] has summarised with eloquence the adverse experiences of famous medical practitioners who themselves have suffered within the system when ill, and has then gone on to say that the moving personal stories produced little or no lasting change, so strong and accepted is the reductionist, biomedical paradigm and the restricted behaviours to which it leads.

The hospital system does not always deliver care which is kind, or even efficient in the communication sense.

Another problem relates to high technology, high-cost medicine. This is able increasingly to deliver new things for sick people but usually only at high cost of money or other resources. Increasingly decisions are being made about how much of the new technology should be supported through public funds. The resolution of questions like this involves considerations of several kinds of equity and opportunity cost, and the whole polity plays too little part in making these decisions at present.

Purposes

Central to present distortions is a misconception of what are the purposes of medicine. The principal purpose should be the care of people with problems. For too many practitioners, it has become instead the subsidiary purpose of the management of diseases which are attached only co-incidentally to suffering people. The distinction is important.

People are 'untidy'. They are a nuisance. They do not fit neatly into pigeonholes. They often describe symptoms in flowery or non-classical terms. They do not understand and often misuse terms (words like 'shock' or 'system') with specific meanings for medical practitioners. Not only that, people might elect for a course of considered 'non-intervention'[444]—even to the extent of not gaining a 'complete' diagnosis —if allowed to make decisions about themselves for themselves.

Disease, on the other hand, is impersonal. It is tidy and the textbook descriptions are clear—if seldom seen. When dealing with disease one can play down or even ignore the suffering, the deaths, the loss, the grief, the loneliness of individuals. One can concentrate on group statistics rather than on personal outcomes. This is not possible when one concentrates on individual people, on their dislocation, on their unhappiness, on their desires, on their understanding, on their needs for support and interest, and nurturing, and love, and care.

What medicine has done increasingly well is to deal with disease, so that many of the killer diseases of yesterday can be dealt with effectively now. One has only to think of most infectious diseases, of most childhood malignancies, of most lymphomas, of many cases of ischaemic heart disease. But, since people are all mortal, the control of one fatal illness leaves people to die of another, an awkward fact that too few medical scientists confront or consider, even while they do deliver a longer, more comfortable better quality life to many people.

A century of science

Thanks to medical science this has been the century of scientific advances in medicine, when we use different belief systems and do things routinely that were unthought of, and impossible, 100 years ago. Followers of Thomas Kuhn[445] will acknowledge that today's paradigms, which fit current data and knowledge, will probably be overtaken in time by new paradigms better able to explain new observations. Those who are not Kuhnians may believe that present knowledge is satisfactory and that while observations will be added, gaps in knowledge filled in, current frameworks will not be challenged. If history is any guide such beliefs are childish and romantic.

Power maintenance

All healers are powerful figures and many of the activities of some medical people are directed towards maintaining that powerful position.

Figure 13.2 Human survival over time
(Human life span has increased on average over time as economic conditions have improved. In ancient Rome the average lifetime was 22 years, in developed countries around 1900 it was 50, and now in the US it stands at 75. Still, these curves share the same maximum. Even if we found cures for every plague, our bodies would probably wear out after roughly 115 years.)

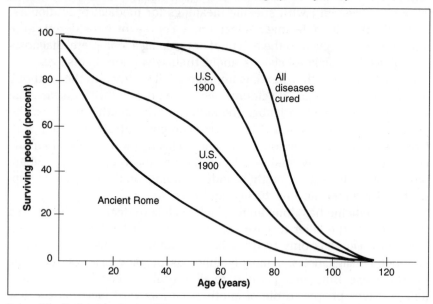

Source: *Scientific American*, October 1994.
Reproduced with permission.

This is so especially in relation to questions of income or influence and is so almost irrespective of the 'evidence' available on any significant matter. For example, there is Australian evidence pointing to great regional inequalities in the rate at which particular operations are done,[446] and one has to suspect that at least some of the differences are related to income maintenance[447] rather than to the presence of disease differentials between geographical areas. If indeed there are real regional differences in the incidence of disease requiring surgery then this would be of great interest to many people—but current belief is that the differences reside in the carers, not the patients.

Practitioners and people

Many citizens feel, some strongly, that their individuality is undervalued in the 'medical' system which predominates today. In some instances people feel that their individuality has been lost completely, that they are of interest solely because of the diseases they have, and that considerations of disease detection and treatment come too often ahead of considerations of them as people. In fact, they feel that any intrusion of personal, individual matters by them into the medical transaction is likely to be treated with annoyance or disdain. Such interventions might even be regarded by some practitioners as a 'waste of time'. In spite of improvements, too many patients believe still that they must be silent and patient, passive and grateful, to earn any commendation from their carers.

A person with newly-detected glaucoma took some questions to her eye doctor only to be told: 'I ask the questions around here'. A surgeon told a group of medical students that no woman with a lump in her breast was in a fit emotional state to make a decision for herself. Had both not happened in the mid-1990s, each might have been regarded as an apocryphal story from another age—but both did occur, and recently and in apparently well-trained Australian practitioners.

It is desirable that practitioners should possess, as part of their armory of skills, expertise in communication and sensitivity towards the people with whom they come into contact. This should include a capacity for active listening, an ability to perform precise reflective listening, and an ability to feel (and to show) empathy and sympathy towards patients. These skills are taught today in some undergraduate medical courses. The skills should be taught in all courses for all carers and should be valued more than they are in the large hospitals in which many carers are trained. Today, sadly, many of our students have their sensitive and substantial communication skills 'knocked out of them' in the large hospitals where capacities in sensitive communication are, too often, not valued highly. Those who have not done so should read *The House of God*[448] for an iconoclastic view of what teaching hospitals can be like at their worst.

What the medical model does well—superbly—is to detect and treat illness. The medical model makes it easy for the most modern science to be brought to bear for the benefit of individuals with identified diseases. What the medical model does less well is help people with illnesses that cannot be cured, and what it does least well is deal with the problems of people whose symptoms and distress do not conform to the textbook descriptions of any disease.

Health today

Much daily activity undertaken by people is actually harmful to health. For example, it is widely known that cigarette smoking harms health and yet thousands of young people, especially young women, encouraged by cigarette companies, take up smoking each year. It is known that excessive speed is a cause of many traffic crashes and yet many cars are driven at excessive and unsafe speeds. It is known that alcoholic excess is bad for health and yet many people drink alcohol to excess. It is known that promiscuity encourages the spread of sexually transmitted disease and yet many people engage in predatory and mindless sexual pursuit. It is known that regular aerobic exercise promotes health and yet many people undertake no regular exercise at all.

A societal myth is that medical interventions 'save lives'—when everyone dies and what medical care does is add valuable quality and years to finite lives. This is more than an academic point—those medical practitioners who believe that they are involved in saving lives will continue to misdirect their professional and research activity in the short as well as in the long term. A public that colludes with this view will embrace the hope that lives are saved as part of humankind's unceasing longing for immortality.[449]

The Cartesian view of medical science would lead inevitably to a race of long-lived people—and this is not what many people find attractive or desirable. It would lead inevitably to reduced births if the population of the earth was to remain within sustainable limits. Cartesian thinking is discussed in Chapter Six in this book.

During the twentieth century, medical scientists have sought to study more and more diseases with a view to controlling them. What has been lacking is some associated recognition within medicine of universal mortality, a recognition which places advances in disease management within a context of finite human life and eventual death.[450] One might ask what purpose is there in a 'war against heart disease' (to select just one of the Cartesian slogans) if mortal people are then left to die of something else. It is the failure of the medical profession to answer these questions to the satisfaction of a wider public that has been its greatest failure of the twentieth century. Put crudely, the profession has become irrelevant to much of what has occurred to human beings who do not share its obsessional fascination with disease and who live complicated and difficult lives. Leadership has passed often to those who will try to answer some of the questions that organised medicine ignores and who will recognise and deal with human need as well as with disease.

The needs of people

What do humans want? Most of us want a satisfying life leading to a gentle or a sudden death; but this many of us cannot have.

When human beings are suffering or dying (and that will be all of us) they want someone to care for them.[451] If living is difficult, or stressful, people want someone to share their problems and troubles. If a practitioner has to seek expert input on some details of illness, people will accept that provided they know that the practitioner cares and that he/she will stand by them. It is the capacity to listen, to share, to understand, to hear, to care, to respond, to explain patiently in simple words and concepts, that makes people feel secure and valued. So the work of groups like the Tavistock Clinic associated with the Balints[452,452a] is important, adding skills that can be used by any practitioner.

People want to feel that they are important, that they are unique, that they matter to the practitioner, and that their problems (rather than their diseases) are understood and accepted by the practitioner. They want to know that they, rather than their disease, will be looked after.

Too often this is just what they do not receive. They are told sometimes by practitioners that 'there is nothing wrong' when this response means too often that the practitioner can find no organic illness within his/her specialty area. But the response means something quite different to the patient. The person would not have come to the practitioner in the first place without some distress, and the answer given above is only the negative part of what is required. What the patient hears from the response 'there is nothing wrong', unless they have come for reassurance only, is that they are malingering, that they are without value, that their suffering is insignificant, and that they are wasting the time of the practitioner.

It is no wonder, in such circumstances, that so many responsible people turn to alternative practitioners who listen to them, who give sensible general advice, and who concentrate on well-being rather than on disease.

People with chronic diseases present a different reason for seeing practitioners. They may be suffering from a separate second condition not related to their chronic illness, in which case they should be handled with sympathy and understanding like any other patient. But if they come with some complaint related to their existing illness, a judgment will have to be made about whether there is any underlying, unspoken question they have about the chronic disease itself. They may need extra care and reassurance about the new manifestation, about how it relates to the chronic illness, whether the new manifestation represents a threat to their continued existence, and about how the management of the latest episode fits naturally with the longer-term management of the problem.

People with a chronic illness may need symptom relief rather than cure. They may be more interested in coping, in maintaining their independence and their comfort than they are in cure. In fact, many people will accept a diagnosis of a chronic illness if they can remain comfortable, if their autonomy is protected to the maximum extent, if efforts are made to allow them to remain independent, if a program is developed with them to allow them to cope with disability, and if their symptoms are controlled.

People reaching the end of life need care too. Too often senior practitioners avoid seeing those who are dying, or else offer them perfunctory visits with platitudes instead of real communication. People read 'signals' well and the perfunctory visits and platitudes are understood by patients—even if the message people receive is not felicitous. If everyone dies, practitioners should be specially skilled at dealing with dying people, should be comfortable with dying people, should have time to spend, and should build up excellent communications with such people. And the more senior the practitioner, the more skill in this area should he or she be able to demonstrate. Since people need 'validation' to feel that they can speak openly, failure to encourage communication will often result in important messages being retained by patients and hidden from practitioners—sometimes for reasons which relate to the comfort of the practitioner rather than to the comfort of the patient. So some patients die lonely and isolated when this is neither desirable nor necessary.

Medicine needs a balance between science and humanity. Today the pendulum has swung too far towards science and away from the caring skills of medicine.

It is scientists and medical practitioners today who should ask what consequences are likely to flow from the continual advance of medical science if it is unmatched by a commitment to the ancient art of medicine. It is the teachers and the medical faculties who must ensure, more than they do today, that medical students are introduced to ancient arts of caring as well as to modern bioscience.

Perhaps the response by teaching faculties in this area will be one way by which they will be judged over the next quarter century.

REFERENCES

433. Marmot MG, Zwi AB. Measuring the burden of illness in general populations. In: White KL, Connelly JE. *The medical school's mission and the population's health*. New York: Springer-Verlag, 1992.
434. Lawson JS. *Public health Australia: an introduction*. Sydney: McGraw-Hill, 1991.
435. Harper, AC., Holman CD'A, Dawes, VP, Snow J, quoted in Harper AC, Holman CD'A, Dawes VP. *The health of populations: an introduction*. Edinburgh: Churchill Livingstone, 1994, p49.
436. Centre for Disease Control, Atlanta, quoted in Australian Institute of Health and Welfare. *Australia's Health 1994*. Canberra: AGPS, 1994, p2.
437. Comfort A. The biology of senescence. Quoted in Harper AC, Holman CD'A, Dawes VP. *The health of populations: an introduction*, ibid, p18.

438. Minsky M. Will robots inherit the earth? *Scientific American*, October 1994; p88.
439. Niselle P. Empathy: another tool in the bag. *Australian Doctor*, 17 May 1966, p54.
440. Mendelsohn RS. *Confessions of a medical heretic.* Chicago: Contemporary Books, 1979, ch 4, p67.
441. Court C. Britain tries to cut the rate of hospital acquired infection. *Brit Med J*, 1996, 312: 660.
442. Sweet M. Hospital food 'a health hazard'. *Sydney Morning Herald*, 31 May 1996.
443. Little, JM. *Humane medicine.* Cambridge: Cambridge University Press, 1995, p5.
444. Fowler, D., *A case for non-intervention*, Brit Med J, 1995, 311: 1691.
445. Kuhn TS. The structure of scientific revolutions. *International encyclopedia of unified science, foundation of the unity of science*, vol 2, no 2. Chicago: University of Chicago Press, 1970.
446. Baume P. *A cutting edge: Australia's surgical workforce.* Canberra: AGPS, 1994: refs 13, 14, 15, 16, 17.
447. Mendelsohn RS. *Confessions of a medical heretic,* ibid, p12, p50.
448. Shem S. *The house of God.* London: Black Swan, 1985.
449. Saul JR. *Voltaire's bastards: the dictatorship of reason in the West.* New York: Vintage Books, 1992, ch 15, p347.
450. See for example Cawte J. Aboriginal medicine. In: Joske R, Segal W (eds). *Ways of healing.* Ringwood, Vic: Penguin Books Australia, 1987, p69.
451. Elias N. *The loneliness of the dying.* Translated by Jephcott E. Oxford: Blackwell, 1985.
452. Balint M. *The doctor, his patient and the illness.* London: Pitman Medical, 1957.
452a. Elder A, Samuel O (eds). *'While I'm here, doctor': a study of the doctor-patient relationship.* London: Tavistock, 1987.

CHAPTER FOURTEEN

Death or Immortality

R OBERT J. M AXWELL

Death and context

Throughout human history, until about 50 years ago, death was part of everyday experience. It still is in some parts of the world; but not for the prosperous in the wealthier countries. For us, death has become separated and to a degree shut away, the province of professionals in hospitals and residential institutions.

Death is at times admirably dealt with. The hospice movement in particular, has made an outstanding contribution to the control of pain without unnecessary loss of mental alertness, recognising the need to talk and listen to the dying person and their family, and emphasising that death is a spiritual event as well as a physical one.[453] But sadly we often do not come close to this standard.

The purpose of this Chapter is first to set out some fallacies that get in the way of appropriate responses to death, then to discuss some dilemmas in modern medical practice, and finally to suggest some propositions that might help us. Let us begin, however, with some real cases since that will focus the mind and help prevent the discussion from becoming too abstract. In the following example the death of an elderly lady is described by her nephew, a physician:

My 93-year-old great aunt lived in Cheltenham. She had diabetes. She fell over and fractured her hip which was pinned. Three months later, and after she had been partly rehabilitated and was once more back with my rather frail mother, she suffered a mild stroke. She was then admitted to hospital where it was found that one of her legs was gangrenous from atherosclerosis and diabetes and required amputation. I learnt this on a Friday evening and I went to the hospital, arriving around 11pm. I met the orthopaedic registrar, who confirmed that they had decided to carry out the operation the following morning. I suggested that it was not necessary as she was dying, but he said they thought it was desirable to make it easier for her nursing. I pointed out that she also had Cheyne Stokes respiration; from where we were standing near her bed it sounded as though she had pneumonia. He then said they had already put her on a third generation cephalosporin antibiotic intravenously to prevent infection. It became totally bizarre, with me asking them for permission to stop my aunt's antibiotics, which eventually I did, signing the prescription form. Nonetheless, they operated the following morning, removing her leg. She was declared dead at midday.

This case illustrates the temptation to treat aggressively even where it is inappropriate and inhumane. Because intervention is possible, it seems difficult for physicians and surgeons not to intervene. Sometimes a good recovery and a grateful patient will confirm that the aggressive approach was right. At other times it will become clear that the approach was wrong—that someone who was ready for death has been subjected to additional suffering and indignity to no good effect, at considerable cost. A patient described in a publication[454] illustrates this point:

Miss Hazel Welch was a 92-year-old woman with severe peritonitis from a ruptured peptic ulcer, arthritis and atherosclerosis. She told the surgeon that she had been on this planet 'quite long enough young man' and did not wish to go on. Nevertheless, she was in the end persuaded by the surgeon to have the operation. 'I'll do it', she said, 'but only because I trust you.' Though she survived the surgery, she told the surgeon that she had been through too much and that she did not trust him any more. The only good to come out of it was the surgeon's recognition (as he wrote) that he had been guilty of distorting the evidence in persuading her, and the worst sort of paternalism. Two weeks after her discharge from hospital, back to residential care, she died from a massive stroke.

The next case is another where the technological imperative to treat appears to have gained the upper hand over what the patient wanted. Here a physician describes the death of his godfather:

My godfather, who was in his seventies, was a Catholic priest who had trained as a lawyer and practised as a barrister before taking orders. I was very close to him as a boy and, in his latter days I was, in effect, his closest relative. After his retirement he was looked after by a group of religious sisters in a house in London. His health was poor and he was in chronic heart failure. A hospital general physician whom I trusted had seen him and explained that it was due to atherosclerosis and there was really nothing by way of treatment that would be effective. He had very limited exercise tolerance. He then had a mild stroke from which he made some recovery. He also had an inguinal hernia, his prostate was giving him trouble and he had arthritis in his hip which, in other circumstances, might have led to hip replacement. He understood the position perfectly.

He developed an acute chest pain one night, was seen by the GP relief service and transferred into the nearby teaching hospital. I spoke to the Senior House Officer on the geriatric ward where he had been admitted and they agreed to discharge him back to the nursing sisters. A few weeks later he had a serious heart attack. Unfortunately, once more the emergency GP service was called; presumably they had no knowledge of his previous history. He was transferred into the same hospital as before and on this occasion they admitted him to the coronary care ward. I went there to be greeted by the Sister in charge of the ward with what she regarded as good news, namely that he had an arrest, but they had managed to restart him. It was obvious that they had no knowledge of his previous care, either in the hospital concerned or beforehand. When I found him he was in pulmonary oedema, semi-conscious and distressed. He was on an isosorbide drip, but had not been given any pain relief. Twenty-four hours later his condition had not improved and I spoke to his consultant. I explained my godfather's life history and we agreed that heroic measures were not indicated. We agreed that he could be given morphia to relieve his distress from pulmonary oedema. In effect, however, I had then to go to the ward and insist it was given as they were not keen to comply with this policy. They maintained him on his isosorbide drip, but fortunately he lapsed into coma. Only then, after an interval of 48 hours, did they remove him to a side room and accept that he was dying.

After two days of Cheyne Stokes respiration and coma, the most extraordinary thing happened. He suddenly grabbed my arm while I was sitting at the bedside, sat up in bed, and said very clearly to me: 'Charles, something has gone wrong with the chronology of this.' I assured him I was doing my best to sort it out. He thanked me, fell back on his pillows and was once more unconscious. This, as I recall, was on the Thursday evening, and he died on the Saturday morning. The last week of his life was a denial of how he had lived the rest of his life and of his spiritual ambitions. Goodness knows what it cost the National Health Service.

On reflection, what went wrong was the failure to communicate within general practice. His NHS records must have contained the letter from the hospital physician, setting out his view of my godfather's overall health and his GP ought to have been there to organise his care at the end. The lesson I have learned from this is the need to break down the barriers between primary and secondary care. They may have served us well in the past, but in my view they are no longer appropriate today, certainly not in the inner city.

The last case is a happier one where the clinical staff wholly satisfied my informant, a sophisticated and sympathetic observer, about the care given to her mother. The crucial factors seem to have been, first, the care taken to keep the family informed; second, the willingness to listen and to go no further in terms of rescue than those who knew and loved the patient judged to be appropriate; third, the imaginative compassion with which care was given to both patient and relatives. In the following a daughter describes her mother's death:

Given a free choice we would all choose to die quietly and without ill health as our passport out of this world. Most of us would choose also to die in our own homes, with those we love near us. However, for many of us, the reality increasingly is that, as we live beyond our allotted three score years and ten, we will suffer a measure of decline before our death and may die in some form of care, be it a nursing home or hospital, with uniformed staff and paraphernalia of clinical activity around us.

In the case I describe, the death of an elderly person on an acute and busy surgical ward, the professional care given was wrapped in a garment of intense affection—for a gentle old lady of 80 years, known to none of the staff, save for a few brief hours when she was admitted semi-conscious. For another 10 days she was cared for and protected, largely unaware of the world around her or of the voices which soothed her and the hands which held her own in moments of quiet.

My mother was admitted to an acute surgical ward in a busy general hospital in a state of collapse, lapsing in and out of consciousness. She had been increasingly frail, both physically and mentally, for several months. This was not her first admission, although it was the first to the particular ward. A frightened and diminutive old lady, with few resources of her own, except a remarkable reluctance to relinquish her tenuous hold on life, her baggage included a distressed 82-year-old husband and two daughters. The Sister rang me on my mother's admission and, given her condition, suggested that I should travel from London to the South Coast hospital to which she had been admitted. This was to happen three times over the next two weeks before I ceased travelling home and was accommodated at the hospital. On the second day I spent some time with the Senior Registrar who explained in detail, without prevarication, that my mother was suffering from peritonitis, that antibiotics were being given to handle the infection, but an operation was necessary to establish the exact cause of the problem and probably to save her life. The choice to go ahead was mine. Since I had already spoken to my sister, I made it clear that we believed an operation was an unnecessary extension of her struggle. I also observed that she seemed unlikely to survive it. The Senior Registrar agreed and we moved on to discuss how my mother would be cared for. In the ten days that followed I saw a doctor daily and received a telephone call at work from the Consultant asking if his team was giving mother all the care I would wish for. While it became increasingly clear that she would not get better, nor indeed leave the hospital, the staff continued to behave as if she would recover. Other patients came, had their operations and went home.

The nurses turned my mother three-hourly, although because they knew that lying on her left side caused her discomfort, she was never left long on that side. They knew that my father was afraid about her death: if my sister or I were not there, one of them would keep an eye on both old people. If in the ward at mealtimes, my father was always fed. The day before my mother died was my father's birthday. I mentioned it to a nurse in passing, because it was clear that my mother was near the end and I was concerned at the effect on him of her dying on his birthday. When we arrived that morning, a birthday card, signed by all day and night staff, was waiting for him.

Accommodation was made available for my sister and me to stay with my mother and three days before her death she was moved to a side room. It was not unusual for me to walk into the room to find a nurse sitting, holding her hand and talking to her, using her first name. On the last night Sister came in and said quite simply: 'You have been here for 36 hours. You have said goodbye. I think you should go.' At 8.00 o'clock the following morning she telephoned me to say that mother had died just after midnight—she had seen out my father's birthday.

What can we learn from this brief glimpse at the death of one old lady? That:

- Personal care is possible within a busy, clinical and apparently impersonal environment.
- Professionalism and care go hand-in-hand, but they are not the same.
- Care is better given where staff know one another and have worked together over time.
- Care has a price for the staff and it needs relatives who also care, to share the process.
- You cannot pay for what my mother received.

Six modern fallacies

We have been led by our inexperience of dying and our unwillingness to accept its inevitability, and by the power of modern medicine, to a number of contemporary fallacies about death:

1. That death is unnatural. The opposite is the truth. A plant grows, flowers and dies. An animal does the same, albeit to a different time clock. Why should we be any different? There are many religious beliefs about immortality but they tell us more about the hopes and fears of human beings than about objective reality. If there is an immortal life, it is something very different from life here.

The truth is that death is natural. There is a time to be born and a time to die.[455] Were it not so, the world would be intolerable. We lose sight of that reality at our peril.

2. That death constitutes a medical failure. In the cases described above, the most common single fallacy is the assumption that death is a failure. There are many instances where this is true, especially in the case of premature deaths. But, as the Bible has it, 'all flesh is grass'.[456] We can escape particular deaths not Death itself. An essential feature of our maturity is acceptance of the inevitability of our own end. The same is true for physicians and nurses, both for themselves and for their patients. Medically untimely and unnecessary deaths must be fought. Not so, timely death.

Men must endure,
Their going hence, even as their coming hither:
Ripeness is all.[457]

Because death is inevitable and natural, medicine must recognise a duty to see us as peacefully as possible out of the world, just as it has a duty to see us safely into it. If, as in Cases 1 to 3 above, medicine (with the best of intentions) contributes to the pain and indignity of our passing, then it fails.

3. That disease, rather than the whole person, is the appropriate focus for medical skill. Medical progress has depended on specialisation. While there remains an important place for the generalist, as general practitioner or family physician, the body of medical knowledge is now too great for any individual to be expert in more than a part of it. It follows that anyone who is seriously ill is likely to need the help of specialists in the condition(s) concerned. These specialists will be selected on the grounds of their technical expertise, not by whether they happen to know the individual patient previously. This concentration on disease or specialty as the basis for referral has obvious advantages, but it tends to reinforce the metaphor of medical care as a struggle to gain the upper hand against (say) cancer, heart disease or stroke, rather than the care of each patient as an unique individual who has their own life to lead and, some day, their own death to die. The more, however, that the patient suffers from multiple conditions, the less close is likely to be the identification with any one person or team. As my third case illustrates, communication is crucial between the primary care physician, who should know the individual as a person, and the specialist team. All too often, as in the case quoted, this communication fails. The metaphor of treatment as a military campaign then takes over, with the patient relegated to the role of battle field.

4. That death is primarily a technical or specialist matter best left to experts. The roots of this fallacy probably lie less with medicine than with a society influenced by fear of death and, for most, by unfamiliarity with it. In Britain most deaths now take place in an institution of some kind, whether it is a residential or nursing home, a hospice or a hospital. Those who work in such institutions encounter death frequently. Those of us who do not, meet it at first hand relatively seldom. To hear that someone has died is not the same as to be with them when they die. Because of the taboos around death, it is only too easy to go along with this separation of death from life, accepting that it is best hidden and that the experts will cope. But this is not good enough. It helps the majority to avoid a painful but fundamental part of life. It puts upon a minority—nurses, doctors, care staff, often relatively unsupported—a heavy load of coping with what is often a traumatic and distressing experience. Death can be peaceful, but by no means always. Finally, and worst of all, it can too often mean that people face their own death surrounded by strangers.

In recent times nothing has done so much to counteract the dehumanisation of death as has the hospice movement. However the lessons from it need to permeate other institutions and home care programs. Marvellous places as hospices are, most deaths will take place elsewhere. Their approach and expertise are too precious to be confined to hospices as inpatient centres, and must spread out much more widely. The growth of home-based hospice care is therefore most welcome. The influence of hospices on hospital practice still has a long way to go.

5. That death is best not talked about. Again the roots of this fallacy lie less with medicine than with society, though the segregation and medicalisation of death reinforce the conspiracy of silence. How often do most of us discuss death? Yet the issues are profound.

In preparatory work for this chapter I visited one of the leading medical libraries in London. The librarian had nothing under the classifications 'death' and 'dying', but a lot on diseases causing death.

I suspect that most nurses and doctors have had some traumatic experiences of death that they will not forget, particularly early in their careers when they were least well prepared. How much discussion about death have the young typically had during their professional education? To what extent are they aware of religious, cultural, philosophical and literary approaches to understanding the mystery of death?

6. That any doctor can ever properly say 'there is nothing more I can do.' This links back to the second and third fallacies, that death is a medical failure, and that the appropriate focus of medical skill is the disease. The patient is not the battleground, but the principal in this particular drama and the place of medicine and nursing is there, to the last breath and beyond, for medicine is not only about cure, but also about care and comfort. In fatal illness there will often be pain to alleviate, fears to allay and peace to make. Nobody should die feeling abandoned or that professionals are too busy to give them time. Of the cases I described earlier, the last demonstrates how important emotional support is to both patient and relatives. As the writer concludes: 'You cannot pay for what my mother received.'

Some contemporary dilemmas about medical care and death

While death has tended to move out of everyday experience into the shadows, modern medicine has also raised new dilemmas at the margins between life and death. For example, life support prolongs life, but does not necessarily restore independence and meaningful personality. In what situations should life support be given, and under what circumstances should it be withdrawn?

This is a classic 'wicked problem' in the sense that it has no 'correct' solution, unlike a technical puzzle which has a single right answer and is therefore 'tame'. Wicked problems will not lie down. Also, people can disagree fiercely about the right course of action, on grounds of principle. Abortion illustrates this. Some will argue that the decision to abort should lie solely with the mother: that until the child is born it is part of her body, without separate rights. Others will argue, with equal but opposite conviction, either that all life is sacred and abortion is therefore almost always wrong, or that the fetus has (at some stage of development) some rights, independent of its mother.

At the extremes, these views are quite simply irreconcilable, based on conflicting definitions of right. Often however, there will be some middle ground on difficult ethical dilemmas, where people can agree a way forward despite important differences of opinion among them.

These are not theoretical questions. They lead directly to decisions and actions that shape life and death. They are like other dilemmas such as when not to resuscitate, rationing decisions for treatments that prolong or transform life, assisted suicide, voluntary euthanasia. Readers will add other examples. Such dilemmas do not so much raise questions about technical skills as about what sort of people, what sort of society, we are.

Ethics has a contribution to make to tackling such dilemmas as these, not in prescribing answers, but in providing frameworks for clarifying principles and a tradition of discussing dilemmas and differences. Some such articulation of principles can be profoundly helpful, for example the principles of autonomy and justice. By the first of these, the patient's right to decide takes precedence, subject to the law, their mental competence and the impact on others (for example, because NHS resources are limited). The best contemporary exposition of the principle of justice is by Rawls.[458] He suggests, for example, the idea that justice for a society is best developed as though behind a veil of ignorance, that one should examine arrangements, policies and procedures without knowing what position in that society you yourself will hold, nor whether you stand to gain or lose by the rules you put in place.

The law has a contribution also. In some fields (e.g., rationing, consent to treatment, voluntary euthanasia) the law is shifting. While professional ethics can challenge the law, medicine has in the end to work within the law, since it is the only framework we have for determining society's definition of what is just.

Four propositions

Let us end this chapter with some specific suggestions.

1. Each of us needs, in our own way, during the course of our life, to come to terms with the inevitability of ageing and death, including our own death. In part this duty is personal and private. Nobody can do it for us. But it also calls for a collective determination not to shut death out of our lives, nor to romanticise it.[459] In schools, in families, on television, we need a much more mature understanding of what ageing and death are actually like, and of some of the issues they raise.

2. Death and dying should have an important place in medical and nursing education at the undergraduate level as well as the postgraduate. While the focus should include the pathology of ageing and death, it should also embrace the ways in which men and women have faced them in different cultures, historical contexts and religions. Literature and philosophy (along with cases) are likely to be more help than standard medical textbooks. The aim is to begin to understand what death has meant to others, and to lay the foundations of each individual's own values and beliefs.

3. Every doctor and nurse should accept that talking and listening to patients, families and friends about death is a fundamental part of their role and responsibilities. Of course, some patients do not want to talk about death, and their choice must be respected. Often though, people do want the chance to have the subject out in the open, yet find it hard to broach it, and virtually impossible if the health professionals are too busy or too embarrassed to help.

4. Senior doctors and nurses should take special care to support juniors in these roles, both by example and by discussing anything that worries them. Too frequently, young clinicians have had a traumatic experience of feeling inadequate in relation to a patient's death. They deserve help. All too often also, some of the worst tasks are delegated to juniors because their seniors do not want to do them. As a general principle, the main responsibility for confronting difficult issues around bad news and death should lie with the leader of the clinical team, while the rest of the team should be involved in these discussions.

The distinctive features of the last of the cases described at the beginning of this chapter have little to do with spending more money. Indeed, good care at death will sometimes cost less, because it is cautious about heroic efforts at rescue. What are needed are compassion, imagination, good two-way communication and an acceptance of the naturalness and inevitability of death.

REFERENCES

453. Saunders C, Summers DH, Teller N (eds). *Hospice: the living idea.* London: Edward Arnold, 1981.
454. Nuland SB. *How we die.* New York: Alfred A Knopf, 1994, pp250–4.
455. Ecclesiastes, 3: 1. See for example Cohen JM, Cohen MJ *The Penguin dictionary of quotations.* London: Penguin Books, 1960, p41.
456. The First Epistle General of Peter, I, 24.
457. Shakespeare W. *King Lear,* Act V, Scene 2, 9.
458. Rawls J. *A theory of justice.* Oxford: Oxford University Press, 1972.
459. Callahan D. *Setting limits.* New York: Simon & Schuster, 1987.

CHAPTER FIFTEEN

The 'Disease model' Challenged

DEBORAH SALTMAN

Introduction

This chapter explores the current disease model and postulates that it no longer provides an universal framework for contemporary health care. Because the disease model is limited by the medical nature of the problems it describes, it does not encompass all the broader issues of health and illness which are important to consumers.

Diseases and symptoms

Modern practitioners concentrate on the notion of disease. Symptoms remain an important entrée into this disease framework. Symptoms, from the doctor's point of view, provide the reason for interaction between providers and consumers. For clinicians, symptoms are still the beginning. Constellations of symptoms still direct doctors on the disease pathway. However, in the usual practice of medicine, this pathway is unidirectional. It leads doctors to disease. The patient is no longer part of the process, other than the disease carrier. Patients' reasons for seeking help are often lost or subsumed in this process.[460] The symptoms revealed in a consultation may never be dealt with directly, if at all. As a result, patients are often left dissatisfied with the interaction.[461] Their symptoms are downplayed or not relieved too frequently and often are replaced by a diagnosis that is at best unhelpful or at worst frightening.

In contrast, alternative and complementary practitioners have embraced symptom models.[462,463] Validation of symptoms is an essential component of an alternative consultation. In fact, the constellation of symptoms may be enhanced in the questioning by an alternative practitioner. Terms not currently used by conventional medicine or patients may be postulated such as 'dullness, oiliness and sliminess'.

Alternative practitioners have learnt far earlier than medical people that focussing on patient concerns leads to a more successful interaction. Satisfaction and empowerment are linked. Patients feel more in control when their concerns are validated.

Recently the disease model has also disappointed clinicians.[464] There is a widening gap between disease and treatment. The disease explosion has led to a large increase in the number of diseases known, but without an equivalent increase in the number of treatments. It may be possible that a disease can be named but not treated or cured—a situation unsatisfactory for both patient and doctor.

In the case of chronic diseases or continuing problems, a lot of treatment is still possible. However where symptoms persist and cure is generally recognised as unattainable, something must substitute for the cure. The consultation process itself, between patient and doctor or series of consultations, then assumes greater importance. The therapeutic component of this consultation is well recognised. For example, in psychiatry, the therapeutic role of a series of consultations has been validated.[465]

The question of what is an appropriate outcome is also not clear from either provider or patient perspective. Outcomes need to be determined collaboratively between all players. However, not until patients' concerns are addressed can this be adequate. To this end, symptoms must be taken seriously.

Functionality is also an important outcome. Patients present themselves because there is some disruption in their lives which they want at best removed, at worst minimised. The rest of this chapter explores the relationship between functionality and health outcome.

Medical scientists claim disease

I can get no remedy against this consumption of the purse: borrowing only lingers and lingers it out, but the disease is incurable.[466]

So said Sir John Falstaff on behalf of his king. It was a battle weary and broke Henry IV who was depicted by Shakespeare in the play of the same name. The 100 years' war with France over, the last British territory on the European mainland was in full flight. Ultimately, Calais would fall and with it the end to England's claims.

For Henry IV, war was an incurable disease. He held no illusions. Both the words 'war' and 'disease' could only lead to suffering. That Shakespeare should choose a medical analogy for war is not surprising. Even in Elizabethan England, 'disease' had a bad name. For centuries to come, disease would be identified with problems and disaster. The 100 Years' War was lost as were the battles with many diseases.

In the early twentieth century, both terms were viewed more sympathetically. World War I was 'the war to end all wars'. However, the realities and the aftermath of war made a positive view of war short-lived. Clearly, whatever the aetiology, war was personally and socially devastating and financially crippling. During this century, war has declined as a positive cultural icon. Wars still continue, but rarely are they now seen as a solution to any problem.

Disease on the other hand has become more palatable. The advent of good public health measures has helped this process. Some diseases can now be cured and even eradicated. The reputation of the World Health Organization, for example, was based on its capacity to co-ordinate the eradication of smallpox.[467,468] Where diseases could not be cured, there was still the promise that adequate treatments would be available. For example diabetes, asthma and hypertension could be treated and monitored. Unlike war, not all diseases ended in death. People were living longer, but carrying incurable diseases.

This scenario is particularly relevant for the elderly. Unfortunately for our now ageing population, cures are becoming less commonplace. Many cancers, viral illnesses and chronic conditions cannot be cured. Whilst everyone talks and searches for 'the cure to end all cures', the prospects are not good. The number of diseases without definitive cures is increasing daily.

When diagnosis of disease is not connected to a cure, patients are left with unsatisfied expectations. It is of little comfort to the patient that the term 'diagnosis', at best, describes a disease. In fact, diagnosing a disease that cannot be cured is of little benefit to anyone besides the diagnostician.

There is also an increasing number of instances where cures are available but the resultant problems from the treatment may be worse than the disease in the first place. The example of impotence after trans-urethral prostatectomy springs to mind.[469] When weighed up by male patients, the benefit of an unhesistant urinary stream is quite often less desirable than a post-resection impotence or urine leakage.[470] In fact, not even the spectre of untreated prostatic cancer can convince a vocal, but small, group of male patients to forego sexual potency and undergo the surgery.

Of course, for clinicians, aetiology or cause of disease has always been more significant than its name or impact on the patient.[471] Treatment and patient satisfaction were later objectives.

The naming and recording of disease was essentially driven by scientific discovery. As the twentieth century progressed and microscopes became bigger, they were able to view smaller and smaller objects. With this scientific advance our microscopic knowledge of disease has increased. This increasing knowledge has led to increased complexity not clarity.[472]

Medical nosology has continued to grow and accommodate the descriptions of the findings. However, this sequence of events is not just due to the technological improvements in diagnostic processes but also it is driven by other forces.

Reproducibility and transportability of scientific discovery is one of these imperatives. An empiric finding is little more than superstition until it has occurred a respectable number of times. The current fad of evidenced-based medicine is a direct result of this research 'bean counting'. Also, a recognised system of coding and nosology are essential for the translation of local findings into global concepts.

What is in a name?

Internationally, the global issues surrounding the naming of diseases has been enhanced by the involvement of the World Health Organization. The World Health Organization's medical road map, the International Classification of Diseases (ICD) is now in its tenth edition (ICD 10).[473]

The huge task of producing a universal nosology is so complex that it requires the efforts of a specialised group of non-clinical health professionals. Thus the process of developing and revising this classification system is quite slow. It is also health provider focussed.

ICD 9 was first published in 1975. It contained a total of 7600 codes covering clinical conditions and health status. In the 18 years it took to produce ICD 10, 14 000 categories were included—an 84 per cent increase, almost a doubling of numbers of categories.

It is not surprising, therefore, that advances in clinical knowledge and terminology surpass the capabilities of any classification system almost as soon as it is produced. Where the dissonance between what is available and what is necessary is great, often transportability and generalisability are sacrificed. One example is ICD 9CM. Clinicians in the United States recognised the deficiencies in ICD 9 and published ICD 9CM (the clinical modification of ICD 9) in 1978. ICD 9CM is currently the coding system of choice of clinicians.

In coding, the process of naming diseases has been essentially additive. There has been an overall increase in codes.[474] It was not until 1996 that subtraction occurred. It was recognised that some codes were able to be deleted or collapsed into other codes. This process is best described using ICD 9CM. The following figure traces the changes in the number of codes in ICD 9CM over the past few years. The tracking is achieved by backward mapping of codes. That is, each year's new codes are assigned to a previous year's code. Figure 15.1 shows the number of new codes assigned for the years 1992, 1993, 1995, 1996 using 1992 as the baseline.

Figure 15.1 ICD 9CM code analysis

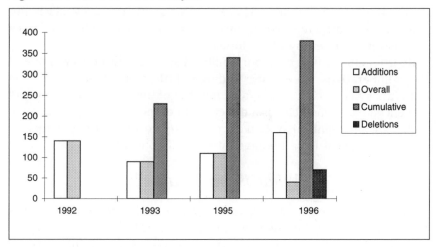

Overall, the number of additions far outstrip the number of deletions, even in 1996 when deletions were first recorded.

Treatment response

The rise in the number of diseases would lend hope for a medical system on the right track if the number of diseases was matched by the
number of treatments available. Unfortunately this is not the case. The
treatment response to the exponential growth in new diseases has not
been as rapid or widespread. The number of new procedures listed in
ICD 9CM in the years 1992, 1993, 1995 and 1996 are shown in Figure 15.2.

The generally low procedure index shows that an increase in new
diseases is not always accompanied by a new range of treatments.
Also, where treatment is available, the treatment response in Western
medicine is often non-specific.

The potential for a classification system which had both provider
and consumer applicability has never been explored. It follows that
the further separation of patient from disease is enhanced by this
process.

Symptoms, side-effects and consumers

The treatment of breast cancer has not been related to diagnostic
advances. Initially the treatment of breast cancer was surgical.[475]

Figure 15.2 New procedures listed in ICD 9CM

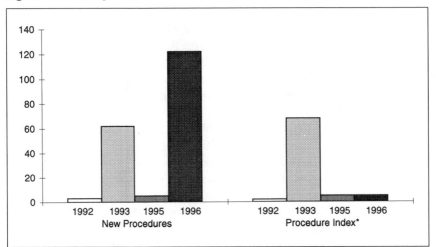

* Procedure Index is the ratio of new procedures to new diagnoses, expressed as a proportion of the total.

Mastectomy was the surgery of choice despite the knowledge that breast cancer was a discrete multi-focal disease. The optimal surgical treatment for breast cancer initially was total removal of the breast, including the underlying pectoral muscles and lymph glands in the axilla.

The surgery was very deforming. Not only were women left without a breast, but also the removal of lymph glands in the axilla resulted in poor drainage of fluid from that arm. Swollen, tender arms were common and almost impossible to treat.

Clearly, the surgeons used their skills to ensure the majority removal of the tumour. Extending a woman's life was the ultimate objective. The ensuing major disfigurement was not viewed by the profession as reason for altering treatment. The prospect of bodily disfigurement was minimised by the surgeons. A cancer successfully removed was the measure of success, despite the lack of scientific evidence that such mutilating treatment was necessary. Despite such radical treatment, the mortality rates for women who had breast cancer did not improve.[467] Treatment and side-effects were not integrated with diagnosis. Surgeons operated from a purely individual and interventional perspective. The voice of women consumers was to change this situation. Initially these treatments occurred in the absence of informed debate from women. Women were offered no reasonable choice. They were trapped between the choice of following the suggestions of their (predominantly male) surgeons and death.

The entry of the epidemiologists (population medicine specialists) into the breast cancer debate signalled a decisive change in the relationship between diagnosis, description and treatment. Doctors, usually more interested in smallpox and malaria than breast cancer were, like the women consumers, questioning the appropriateness of treatment. From within the medical ranks, the autocratic model of dealing with women was challenged on a non-gynaecological issue.

Epidemiologists all over the world were exposing the failure of surgeons to deal adequately with breast cancer. Questioning of the traditional surgical model of treatment of breast cancer became widespread within the profession. Surgeons, who had until this point managed breast cancer as a disease (once cut out, able to be forgotten), were invited to reassess their management.[475]

The medical profession struggled with the relationship between intervention and outcome within the medical model, urged on by data and by the voice of consumers. Clearly, if the outcome and treatment could not be directly related to cause and diagnosis, other issues were important. A group of surgeons in Milan listening to the voices of women and the non-surgical medical community devised a less invasive procedure for the surgical management of breast cancer. In 1990 it was shown conclusively that small scale surgery, with minimal disfigurement was as effective as radical mastectomy.[468]

The example of breast cancer surgery shows that women's concerns, which were largely symptom related, were important in effecting a change in medical activity. The replacement of radical mastectomy with more conservative surgery can be seen as a victory not only for the women's movement, but also for the recognition of the importance of symptoms.

The recognition of side-effects or the validity of symptoms is not uniform. Some clincans accept the available evidence relating to outcomes, while others do not. Whilst the mutilating effects of radical surgery have been minimised, the extension of treatment modalities without involvement of women consumers has continued. For example, radiotherapy and/or chemotherapy (drugs) are considered essential, non disfiguring adjuncts to breast saving surgery by clinicians.

Disease with many names

Advances in Western medicine, clinical knowledge and professionalisation of the naming process are the main drivers of the worldwide increase in diagnostic and therapeutic terminology. However, an understanding of disease and treatment is not limited by the lack of scientific knowledge alone, cultural and language issues also contribute.

The language of medicine is English. ICD 9CM and all the ICDs have been produced initially in the English language. When translations into other languages occur, the cultural bias in the disease classification becomes evident.[476] Certain diseases well described in non-English speaking cultures are not represented. For example, spasmophilia, a French condition affecting the liver does not appear in the classification system. Similarly, 'hertzinsufficenz', a German cardiac condition, has no translation.[477] In China, neurasthenia is viewed quite differently from its perception in English-speaking countries.[478]

Despite the quest for consistency across languages, culture, hubris and local usage also determine naming rights. This is particularly evident where medical science is not sufficiently advanced to provide a credible basis for a terminology. At these times, culture and mythology are strengthened.

The naming of new infectious diseases is one such area. Epidemics often spread faster than the medical knowledge about them. They are emotive and cannot be confined to the electron microscope or agar plate. The public often knows more through the media than the medical profession give credit for. However, the medical agenda is driven by the pursuit of knowledge and understanding of disease, rather than the need to inform the 'non-agar' media. In an epidemic, defining the spread is more important than finding the cause. The naming of the epidemic by the media usually reflects this fact. For example, the Ebola virus sent a clear message to the worried multitudes that the disease was confined to an obscure part of Africa.

The naming of an epidemic by public conferral of a title and not medical investigation also can reflect the level of community anxiety about the severity of the disease. The case of Mad Cow disease illustrates this point. In cows, the condition is named after a deprecating description of the altered appearance and behaviour of the animal. The response of the medical profession once again is to negate and perhaps sterilise the population's emotion by sanitising and reclaiming the name of the disease. The disease in humans is Creutzfeldt-Jakob disease, not 'mad human disease'.[479,480]

Similarly, the AIDS virus, initially associated with gay men, underwent a transmogrification into the supposedly more technically correct human immunodeficiency virus. A close examination of this term reveals that it is as value laden and as inappropriate for the community as its predecessor. The reader's mind could easily slip into the belief that anyone with human immunodeficiency virus was missing something more than T-cells. The missing cells are a result, not the true cause, of the viral illness. In fact, the immunodeficiency profile of cells is not exclusive to infection by the HIV.

The new 'diseases'

The descriptive power of public health at large and health promotion initiatives within communities have also had profound effects on the definitions of disease. Understanding the demography of the population has become as important as, or even more important than, the diagnostic category.

As we age, we are more likely to become sicker and die. Thus age correlates well with illness and mortality. Gender is also a prominent determinant of health and disease. Women live longer than men. Often age and gender can compound the sickness. For example, the problem ages for men are adolescence, when the suicide risk is highest and until middle age when men fall into the 'black hole'.[481,482] That is, they do not undertake preventive and health-promoting activities, nor visit their doctor for advice on these issues.[483] Similarly, there are ages in which women are sicker, comparatively, for example during their reproductive years.[484] Age and sex can tell us quite a lot of information about the community. Information from patients can add much more.

Forget the patient: symptom denial in Western medicine

The focus on scientific discovery and disease has maximised the impact of the analytic and quantitative components of medicine. The descriptive processes, whether they are macroscopic, microscopic or election microscopic, have contributed significantly to the development of modern medical knowledge. Initially, the process of description was accompanied by a series of medical actions which improved health. The discovery of the mechanism of action of bacteria led to antibacterial agents. The description of relationship between water and disease led to improved sanitation. Unfortunately, in the last 50 years, this process of scientific discovery has not been so closely linked to health outcomes.

This process is evidenced by the fact that pathophysiology, or the description at a microscopic level of the disease process, has far exceeded the level of sophistication of symptom identification. At the same time the input of patients in the process of their own health care has been minimised. Symptoms belong to patients and are often expressed in their terms. Consequently they are relatively non-specific. This vagueness of individual symptoms has led to their decreasing use as diagnostic instruments in medicine. Patients and their problems are largely sidelined, or in extreme cases, considered 'difficult'.[485]

At best, discussion of symptoms in a medical consultation has become part of the courtesy banter between doctor and patient. This situation is more true for consulting physicians than general practitioners.[486] Often a symptom is viewed as an abstract commentary on health status at the commencement of a consultation. The following transcript of the first two lines of general practice consultations highlight the role of a general symptom in providing a prelude to exploring the diagnostic physical signs.

Doctor: How are you today?

Patient: I'm well Doc, I suppose, but I've got a bit of a backache.

In this interaction the patient has immediately focussed on a disease specific symptom relating to a particular part of the body. The patient may have been prompted to do so by previous experiences with medical practitioners or because they seek an anatomical explanation. For whatever reason, the original question 'How are you?' which related to global issues concerning the patient may never be answered.

Sometimes the early consultation symptom chat can be a proxy for exploring emotional symptoms as the following first two lines illustrate.

Doctor: How can I help you today?

Patient: Ah well, I'm not *feeling* the best.

Without any symptom specificity this beginning may not lead to any further exploration of the patient's reason for the visit. 'Not feeling the best' does not lead to an organ or diagnosis.

The non-specific nature of symptoms can mean that an individual symptom can be attributed to several diseases. In such cases symptoms may be downplayed by the clinician. For example, the symptom 'abdominal pain' tells a diagnostician very little about the aetiology of the disease at a cellular level. The problem could be anything from bowel cancer to appendicitis. Similarly, constellations of symptoms have no greater disease specificity. For example, the combination of abdominal pain, altered bowel motions and nausea does not increase the specificity of a diagnosis.

Symptom recognition and alternative and complementary therapies

The response of less orthodox medicine to the symptom-diagnosis dilemma is interesting. Holisitic medicine purports to focus on the whole person.[487] Many alternative and complementary therapies historically have based their healing activities on symptom identification.

Western herbal medicine, for example, seeks to treat the person, not the condition. Emotional and environmental issues for each patient are incorporated into the overall description of the patient. Mind and body symptoms are connected.

In the Ayurvedic System of medicine, the symptoms are broadly related to body forces. Largely related to the caste system in India and therefore racial in origin, the Ayurvedic System nevertheless highlights the potential range of symptomatology available for description. Table 15.1 below describes the range of attributes and abnormal symptoms for three major human body forces.

Table 15.1 Human body forces and attributes in Ayurvedic medicine[488]

Attributes	Abnormal functions
Bayu dryness, lightness, clearness, coolness, motion, formlessness	twitching, tremors, falling out, displacement, extension, enlargement, bursting of limbs, cheerlessness, joy, thirst
Pitta heat, keenness, lightness, slight oiliness	burning, warmth, suppuration, sweat
Kafa whiteness, coldness, heaviness, oiliness sweetness, firmness, sliminess, softness	dullness, heaviness, oiliness, paralysis, impure secretions, lightness, sweetness in mouth

Clearly, one of the successes of current alternative therapies is their responsiveness to patients' needs not diseases. Many consumers cite the fact that alternative practitioners acknowledge and deal with their symptoms as a necessary part of a satisfactory outcome.

Outcome focus

Outcomes are now very important in health care. The health outcome movement has gained credence around the world as a valid driver of health care systems. Identification of appropriate outcomes goes some of the way to replacing the disease and treatment nexus. Where treatment is not achievable, other outcomes may be used as indicators of a successful health intervention. Patient satisfaction with the health service and alleviation of symptoms are two consumer-based outcome measures.

Measuring outcomes is not easy, in fact no measurement in health care is easy.[489,490] Traditionally, mortality has been used as a reliable marker of outcome.[491] Death, apparently, is the easiest to measure.

In some countries this is not the case. For example, of the estimated 50 million deaths occurring in the world each year, medical certification of cause of death is obtained in less than one quarter.[492] Resistance to recording causes of death may be more than just technical. Mortality data only provides retrospective information about existing health care. Mortality data only records an endpoint, without any description of the pathway of health care prior to the event. Even morbidity, whilst a living measure, only records a level of health status that occurs at one particular point in time.

The measurement of health care costs appears to be a more current and easily derived outcome indicator.[493] Cost is rapidly becoming the extension of the disease model, in that it seeks to define the economic parameters of disease. The economic rationalist approach firmly links outcome to economics. Costs, like disease labelling, cannot explain the cause of the problems, nor do they acknowledge nor remedy them. Such a process denies both the patient and the health care provider their say. It is little wonder that consumers at large cannot be drawn into supporting cost-cutting exercises in health care.[494]

Economic reductionism or reducing health care funding by analysing smaller and smaller costing units has been achieved through the use of disease nomenclature. Casemix is an example of this process. In casemix, diagnosis and outcome are united by hospital accounting. Widely used as a diagnosis-based mechanism for estimating and funding expenditure per patient in hospital, casemix is one example where accountants, administrators and medical coders have been victorious over doctors in the battle for control of the hospitals. It is a fight from which consumers have been largely excluded and patients' feelings ignored.

In fact, casemix has become the new link to diagnosis. Casemix has turned diagnosis into an outcome measure. Casemixers have used the tenuous links between diagnosis and countable measures of outcome, for example, length of stay in hospital and repeat surgery, to forge a new causal role and meaning for an increasing array of diseases.[495]

In some circumstances, this link is entirely appropriate. For example, casemix works best when the diagnosis is surgical and the treatment is operative. Pain shifting from the umbilical region to the right iliac fossa + temperature + tenderness in the pouch of douglas = acute appendicitis = appendicectomy. The equation, barring mishaps, is simple.

Casemix descriptions and funding arrangements can only benefit institutions which favour the well-defined or low-risk cases. For this reason, casemix has been most effective in achieving the outcomes of cost containment and user responsiveness in health maintenance organisations, where the populations are highly selected and usually fairly healthy. This selective process is focussed on the institution. As such it is unacceptable in the public sector where unhindered access, empowerment of patients and equity of care should be important. In such settings, casemix descriptions and ensuing funding cannot be correlated with consumer outcome measures.

Most complex, multiple diagnoses, chronic conditions, and long-stay conditions do not lend themselves to simple equations. This observation is particularly salient for the elderly where casemix has been shown to be no better than functional assessment in analysing patient stays in hospital.[496,497]

Patients seek care when their functioning is diminished in some way or has the potential to be diminished if some intervention action is not taken. Surely, the goals of any treatment should be to restore optimal functioning. Yet, doctors do not routinely measure functioning in their consultations. As patients grow older, they accumulate more problems. The continuing nature of many of these problems results in patients carrying multiple health agendas.

Judging functionality and severity are routine informal occurrences in any consultation. Unfortunately without measurements over time we cannot tell how well we are addressing these issues.

Partnership and outcome: the consultation

The outcome of effecting change in patients' health status can be achieved through the medical consultation. Doctors use the consultation to effect changes. Acting as a catalyst, in the traditional consultation the doctor remains essentially unaltered by the process. The emergency consultation where the patient is unconscious is one example of this style of medicine. Other examples include the consultations where the problem/s are easily defined and treatments clear-cut both in delivery and outcome, for example, prescribing for bacterial infections. A patient has a bacterial condition and the doctor facilitates the cure by prescribing antibiotic medication. In this model of interaction, there are very few challenges to the diagnosis-treatment pathway. This model is essentially biomedical, and is shown diagrammatically in Figure 15.3.

Figure 15.3 Biomedical model

	Catalyst	Desired Outcome
Patient$_{time\ 1}$	Doctor	Patient$_{time\ 2}$

But in the majority of consultations the problems may be from any or all of the domains present in health care—biological, psychological or sociological. In these consultations sickness and adversity form a bonding relationship between a doctor and a patient. The goals of management also become collaborative.[498] In this sharing relationship, doctors are also changed. The change in the doctor during the consultation is usually viewed by the patient as a beneficial side-effect.[499] The doctor is seen as understanding, caring or effective. In some countries this style of consultation, for example the checkup, is the most frequent reason for encounter with a general practitioner (9 per cent of all reasons for consultations).[500]

Such a collaborative framework allows both patient and general practitioner more autonomy in the consultation. Shared goals can be developed. Goal setting is best described in a consultation for a chronic illness. With longstanding knowledge of the progress of similar conditions and a working relationship with the patient, a management plan can be tailor-made to both individuals. This model of the consultation is often described as the biopsychosocial model and is reflected in Figure 15.4.

Figure 15.4 Biopsychosocial model

	Catalyst	Desired Outcome
	Consultation	
$Patient_{time\ 1}$		$Patient_{time\ 2}$
$Doctor_{time\ 1}$		$Doctor_{time\ 2}$

In a long-term patient-doctor commitment it is difficult not only to describe the beginnings of this relationship, but also to define what roles doctor and patient should have and what keeps it going. In this continuing relationship the outcome of an individual consultation may not be very significant. Also, traditional indicators of a successful consultation, such as cure or patient satisfaction, may not be helpful. The consultation must be viewed as a variable in itself which is subject to changes over time. This model can be described as the continuity of care model and is shown in the following figure.

Figure 15.5 Continuing or chronic model

	Catalyst	Desired Outcome
	Time	
$Patient_{time\ 1}$	$Patient_{time\ 2,\ 3,\ 4}$	$Consultation_{time\ 1}$
$Doctor_{time\ 1}$	$Doctor_{time\ 2,\ 3,\ 4}$	$Consultation_{time\ 2,\ 3,\ 4}$

In the management of arthritis the disease is accompanied by a constellation of symptoms and the treatments are at best, non-specific and not aimed at the cause. Often the situation occurs where there are no clear-cut definitions or outcomes. In such situations both doctors and patients must learn to deal with uncertainty.

In this new consultation both patient and doctor must share responsibility for owning knowledge not only about disease and treatment but also symptomatology. The doctor must use their knowledge base in disease and treatment to help the patient expand theirs. The patient must use their expertise in symptomatology. Both participants may not have time in an individual consultation but may have time over a series of consultations in which to establish a working arrangement. The continuity element is particularly relevant in psychiatric or psychological consultations.[501]

Often patients have cogent or compelling reasons for seeing their doctors. The timing of the consultation is a reflection of the urgency of these reasons. The 'reason' for seeing the doctor is often a new problem (70 per cent of encounters), however nearly half the problems described in the consultations are old ones.[502]

Conclusion

There is debate about the suitability of the disease model as a continuing framework for health care. Within these polemics, there are many signs that indicate that patients' needs are not met. Historically, the medical profession has been able to shift this focus by discovery. Scientific innovation, usually signifying a paradigm shift in thinking, has come to the rescue of medicine.

In recent times, few of these innovations have heralded sustainable change. Rather critics have been silenced and patients awed by the sheer power of a handful of major therapeutic discoveries. For example, medical advances such as pasteurisation and penicillin have occurred in a time of medical medievalism philosophically. Unfortunately, since the discovery of penicillin, little has occurred to support the view that medical science will conquer all.

Economics and medicine have forged new links. With accurate disease data, it is argued by the economic rationalists that appropriate decisions about treatments and services for communities and societies can be made.[503] The promise has remained unfulfilled. These disciplines have yet to reconcile the competing needs of individuals with those of communities.[504,505] It is also questionable whether the current methodology available to researchers in these areas is robust enough to look at longitudinal issues which are the growing concern of health care.

In this context, some long-term consequences of medical intervention and health care provision have come into question. For patients the only legitimate vehicle remains the consultation and exploration of symptomatology. Despite its best efforts, medicine is in the Dark Ages again. Today patients are scared by science not superstition, however, the effect is the same. A cure or a sign from a deity is awaited.

REFERENCES

460. Weiss S, Wengert P, Martinez E, Sewall W, Kopp E. Patient satisfaction with decision making for breast cancer therapy. *Ann Surg Oncol* 1996; 3: 285–9.
461. Schwartz L, Overton D. The management of patient complaints and dissatisfaction. *Emerg Med Clinics of North America*, 1992, 10: 557–72.
462. Bayley C. Homeopathy. *J Med Philos* 1993; 18: 129–45.
463. Lynn J. Using complementary therapies. Reflexology. *Prof Nurse* 1996; 11: 321–2.
464. Saltman D. *With a little help: choosing and assessing mental health therapists.* Sydney: Choice Books, 1996, pp89–92.
465. Saltman D. *With a little help: choosing and assessing mental health therapists.* ibid, p46.
466. Shakespeare William. *Henry IV*, Part II, Act 1, Scene 3, line 237.
467. Greenough P. Intimidation, coercion and resistance in the final stages of the South Asian smallpox eradication campaign. *Social Science Medicine* 1995; 41: 633–45.
468. Hopkins D, Ruiz-Tiben E. Surveillance for dracunculiasis, 1981–1991. *MMWR CDC Surveill Summ* 1992; 41: 1–13.
469. Polascik TJ, Walsh PC. Radical retropubic prostatectomy: the influence of accessory pudendal arteries on the recovery of sexual function. *J Urol* 1995; 145 (1): 150–2.
470. Fowler FJ, Barry MJ, Lu-Yao G, Wasson J, Roman A, Wennberg J. Effect of radical prostatectomy for prostate cancer on patient quality of life: results from a Medicare survey. *Urology* 1995; 45 (6): 1007–13.
471. Bolton J. Medical practice and an anthropological bias. *Social Science Medicine* 1995; 40 (12): 1655–61.
472. Harris HW, Schaffner KF. Molecular genetics, reductionism, and disease concepts in psychiatry. *J of Medicine and Philosophy* 1992; 17 (2): 127–53.
473. *International statistical classification of diseases and related health problems*, 10th edition. Geneva: World Health Organization, 1992.
474. Official Mapping ICD9CM Codes. National Coding Centre, University of Sydney, 1996.
475. Veronisi U, Costa A. Conservative surgery in breast cancer. In: Suartini E, Bevilacqua G, Conte PF, Surbone A (eds). *Breast cancer: from biology to therapy.* Annals of the New York Academy of Sciences, 1993, vol 698: 212.
476. Pelicier Y. Les Concepts d'asthenie et de fatigue. *Encephale* 1994; 3: 541–4.
477. Payer Lynn. *Medicine and culture.* New York: Penguin Books, 1989.
478. Lee S, Wong KC. Rethinking neurasthenia: the illness concepts of stenjing shuairuo among Chinese undergraduates in Hong Kong. *Cult Med Psychiatry* 1995; 19 (1): 91–111.
479. Marwick C. Views of reason for mad cow disease vary widely. *JAMA* 1996; 276 (6): 438–40.

480. Collins S, Masters CL. Iatrogenic and zoonotic Creutzfeldt-Jakob disease: the Australian perspective. *Med J Aust* 1996; 164 (10): 598–602.
481. Diekstra RF, Garnefski N. On the nature, magnitude, and causality of suicidal behaviors: an international perspective. *Suicide and Life-Threatening Behaviour* 1995; 25 (1): 36–57.
482. Saunders L, Ntoane C, Wilson T. Why don't patients return for anithypertensive treatment in Soweto? *South Africa Med J* 1983; 64 (6): 208–10.
483. Brett K, Madans J. *Long-term survival after coronary heart disease. Comparisons between men and women in a national sample. Annual Epidemiology* 1995; 5 (1): 25–32.
484. Waslien C, Stewart L. Nutrition of the Asian adolescent girl. *Asia Pacific Journal of Public Health* 1994; 7 (1): 31–3.
485. Sharpe M, Mayou R, Seagroatt V, et al. Why do doctors find some patients difficult to help? *Quarterly Journal of Medicine* 1994; 87 (3): 187–93.
486. Williams P, Peet G. Differences in the value of clinical information: referring physicians versus consulting specialists. *J Am Board Fam Pract* 1994; 7 (4): 292–302.
487. Ward B. Holistic medicine. *Australian Family Physician* 1995; 24 (5): 761–2, 765.
488. Kaviraji Nagendra Nath Sen Gupta. *The Ayurvedic system of medicine.* New Delhi: Logos Press, 1919.
489. Avis M, Bond M, Arthur A. Satisfying solutions? A review of some unresolved issues in the measurement of patient satisfaction. *Journal of Advanced Nursing* 1995; 22 (2): 316–22.
490. Murphy R. Work reengineering: the benefits and the barriers, an analytical review. *Journal Soc Health System* 1995; 5 (1): 73–84.
491. Bradbury R, Golec J, Stearns F, Steen P. Inter-hospital mortality and morbidity variation in Pennsylvania. *Journal Soc Health System* 1993; 4 (1): 48–67.
492. Murray CJL, Lopez AD. Evidenced-based health policy—lessons from the global burden of disease study. *Science* 1996; 274: 740–3.
493. Rich M, Beckham V, Wittenberg C, Leven C, Freedland K, Carney RA. Multidisciplinary intervention to prevent the readmission of elderly patients with congestive heart failure. *New Engl J Med* 1995; 333 (18): 1190–5.
494. Knickman J, Hughes R, Taylor H, Binns K, Lyons M. Tracking consumers' reactions to the changing health care system: early indicators. *Health Aff Millwood* 1996; 15 (2): 21–32.
495. Ansari M, Collopy B. The risk of an unplanned return to the operating room in Australian hospitals. *Aust NZ J Surgery* 1996; 66 (1): 10–13.
496. Carpenter G, Main A, Turner G. Casemix for the elderly inpatient: Resource Utilization Groups (RUGs) validation project. Casemix for the Elderly Inpatient Working Group. *Age & Ageing* 1995; 21 (1): 5–13.
497. Soderlund N. Product definition for health care contracting: an overview of approaches to measuring hospital output with reference to the UK internal market. *Journal of Epidemiology and Community Health* 1994; 48 (3): 224–31.
498. Frederikson L. Exploring information-exchange in consultation: the patients' view of performance and outcomes. *Patient Educ Couns* 1995; 25 (3): 237–46.
499. Winefield H, Murrell T, Clifford J. Process and outcomes in general practice consultations: problems in defining high quality care. *Social Science Medicine* 1995; 41 (7): 969–75.
500. Bridges-Webb C, Britt H, Miles DA, Neary S, Charles J, Traynor V. Morbidity and treatment in general practice in Australia 1990–1991. *Med J Aust* 1992; 157: s1–s56.
501. Crossley D, Myers M, Wilkinson G. Assessment of psychological care in general practice. *Brit Med J* 1992; 305: 1333–6.
502. Bridges-Webb C, Britt H, Miles DA, et al. Morbidity and treatment in general practice in Australia 1990–1991, ibid.

503. McPherson K. The Cochrane Lecture. The best and the enemy of the good: randomised controlled trials, uncertainty, and assessing the role of patient choice in medical decision making. *Journal of Epidemiology and Community Health* 1994; 48 (1): 6–15.
504. Witte D. Measuring outcomes: why now? *Clin Chem* 1995; 41 (5): 775–80.
505. O'Connor A. Validation of a decisional conflict scale. *Med Decision Making* 1995; 15 (1): 25–30.

CHAPTER SIXTEEN

Better Health

STEPHEN LEEDER

The Better Health Commission

In 1985, Dr Neal Blewett, Federal Minister for Health, convened a group that he named the Better Health Commission, and I was a member of it.[506] We'd had health commissions before—many of them—but not a *better* health commission. It provoked a derisive response from those whose fortunes depended upon their membership of the health industry—had Blewett completely lost the plot? And as for establishing a health commission comprised of individuals drawn from the media, sport, trade unions and academia—surely this was lunacy writ large.

In fact, I look back on the time I spent with the Better Health Commission as one of my most enjoyable and creative professional interludes. The Commission's report was entitled *Looking Forward to Better Health*,[506] and proposed how we might gain more health by establishing goals and targets and a strategic direction in three exemplary areas—heart disease, nutrition and trauma. These examples were chosen for their intrinsic health importance and because each, in some way, showed that to achieve better health, the health professions could not expect to 'go it alone'.

In the case of injury, unless preventive changes are mandated and implemented in industry, on our roads and in our schools, we will stagnate with a fixed level of untreatable, and yet potentially preventable, disasters however clever we become at rescue, triage and intensive care. Changes in our national diet require intersectoral action—by the producers of our food, those wholesaling it and retailing it.[507] Such efforts will likely achieve more than would any number of diet sheets put in letterboxes or doctors' surgeries by foundations for pure living and more health benefits than those obtained from the $200 million we spend each year on cholesterol-lowering drugs.[508] Likewise with heart disease: improvements in the medical and surgical care of coronary disease account for between one third and one half of the encouraging 60 per cent decline in the death rate in Australia since the mid 1960s.[509] Much of the rest of the downturn reflects changing lifestyles—more exercising, people eating better and smoking less.[510]

By the choice of these three target areas we hoped to demonstrate that the pathway to achieving better health—of living better as a nation—lay outside as much as within the health care system. Had we chosen other goal and target areas—the impact of unemployment, housing, the physical and built environments come to mind—again factors beyond those of the health system would have featured. If politics is too important a topic to be left to politicians, then better health is too broad, too deep a matter to be left entirely to therapists.

If the thesis that underpinned the efforts of the Better Health Commission is correct—and virtually all public health professionals would argue from the evidential base of their discipline that it is—then to achieve better health, to live better from a health perspective, will require a close examination of the motivation and intention of the broader community. And when this examination is begun, it becomes apparent that health is but one among several phenomena, including education, that depends heavily upon the values and priorities of society. Put at its simplest, if there is no special worth placed upon health beyond what an individual can buy for themselves, then community efforts—essential, by public health reckoning, to move beyond good health to better health—wither. Moreover, if there is no social capital— that store of community goodwill which leads a community to be altruistic, caring and concerned with equity—then you can kiss goodbye to the idea of achieving better community health. For instance, if a community has such low levels of social capital that parents of young children consider the very small risks of immunising their child to be unacceptable, the levels of immunity within the whole group of similarly aged children fall, making them all much more susceptible to an epidemic (which we know would not be an epidemic had the levels of immunity in the group been higher). Put this way, if a community does not nurture, support and value altruism, then ultimately individual levels of health suffer and the achievement of better health becomes an impossible dream.

As I have said, the Better Health Commission was generally regarded unenthusiastically by the health establishment. Indeed, as preventivists we were some of the first in Australia to map the barriers to prevention from a social health perspective for the nation as a whole. In our ventures, the lessons we learned were that:

- doctors and other health professionals need to develop a more energetic approach to advocacy on behalf of the knowledge they possess that might direct society toward a healthier future;
- funding for health promotion should be in line with funding for other health care—on the basis of cost and outcome and determined by prevailing community values but generally more than the trivial proportion currently allocated to it;
- mechanisms should be developed to work more synchronously with other sectors such as transport and education whose impact on health is every bit as important as the health sector;
- we must draw upon, protect and enhance our reserves of social capital—which I believe exist in the form of a metaphorical soil deposit —to achieve better health outcomes.

Prevention for better health

I have a health economist colleague who is very sceptical about prevention and health promotion. I spoke to him about Australia's success in controlling tobacco. 'When was the evidence about smoking hazards known?' he asked me. 'It was known to doctors 30 years ago,' I replied. 'And what is the smoking prevalence among men now?' he prodded. 'About 30 per cent,' I said. 'And you call that a success!' he said, amazed. 'What would you call a failure?'

I don't often disagree with this health economist, but given the politics and history of tobacco, we have done well, and better than many countries. People such as Nigel Gray in Victoria and Simon Chapman in New South Wales stand out as exemplars in the pursuit of health gains and life-saving through smoking reduction, especially given the heavy artillery brought against them by the tobacco industry.

Nevertheless, smoking stands as a national folly, as Barbara Tuchman calls those historical phenomena that occur when societies, heading for a stone wall, put their foot ever harder on the accelerator instead of the brake, pushing, pushing until final impact and destruction.[511] The steadfast support by government for the tobacco industry through subsidies indicate the height of the barrier we face when trying to achieve prevention. Terry Dwyer in Hobart has shown that younger Tasmanian women have made a historic crossing: they now have a greater likelihood of dying of cancer of the lung than do men.[512]

Who can provide a leadership role? The health professional community should quit its silent comfort and be heard more often on these matters, assuming a much higher profile in regard to advocacy for safety, and the removal of destructive and health damaging elements in our environment.

The medical profession has never been backward in its advocacy for the protection of its commercial base which trades under the name of the doctor-patient relationship. We can be powerful advocates when we wish to be. Crusades that have more to do with health outcomes rather than medical incomes are rare. Brendan Nelson, past president of the Australian Medical Association, took on some of these social issues, including Aboriginal health, and we need a cast of a thousand behind him.

Instead, we have often medicated prevention, but without applying all the medical insight and power at our disposal. We have reduced prevention to the prescription of drugs—for cholesterol, for blood pressure—trusting in these chemicals to treat high-risk people. But we have done less than we might to support population health initiatives which require action outside the health care system.

The medical profession is contemporary society's carrier of profoundly powerful knowledge about health and disease. Strategies for political action based on this knowledge should involve doctors prepared to move out of the surgery or the hospital ward, to achieve the breakthroughs that Australia deserves. And nowhere is the need so obvious or so urgent as in the area of Aboriginal health where a suspension of medical commonsense and public health management clarity and purpose has occurred over many years.

If doctors and health professionals took the lead, I believe the community would come in behind them. Too often we assume the community is ignorant about health whereas we find in western Sydney, for example, that people are strongly motivated toward health but their environment holds them back. I admire the work of the Victorian Health Promotion Foundation—contributions have been made through it to prevention by many doctors and other health professionals, and in a breadth of health issues it has engaged the Victorian community. Once the community appreciates its own efficacy in tackling preventive issues, the climate changes. Too often we have viewed the community as the passive recipient of our advice and not as a group from whom preventive action and choices should derive. Making health rather than tobacco the sponsor of sport, as was done first in Victoria and then in other states, may not only reduce tobacco sales but also enable the community to associate prevention with something positive, in this case sport. That will flow on to its attitude toward other opportunities for prevention and increase our stores of social capital.

Health promotion funding

Estimates vary as to the amount going into disease prevention, but it is probably at best 10 per cent of all health and welfare expenditures, and may be as low as 2 per cent. Yet death and irreversible brain damage from trauma, sudden cardiac death, a substantial component of coronary artery disease and stroke, some suicides, cervical cancer, the lifestyle-associated disorders of minority communities such as Australian Aborigines, are all within reach of energetic prevention programs (providing these are well-conceived and adequately financed), and, most importantly, each is largely out of the reach of medical and surgical care.

If prevention is as cost-effective as commonly used treatments for heart disease, as health economist Rob Carter from Monash University[513] has shown for example, it may ethically be preferable for society to prevent the problem than to wait until it presents as a medical crisis. An opportunity exists for aligning investment and action with social goals by consultation with the community to gain information about what people might expect for additional investment in various preventive programs. Of course, no perturbation to our lifestyle is ethically or morally free: reducing opportunities to do oneself harm are taken by some to be infringements of civil liberties. And so they are. The issue really is one of comparison of cost and consequence, balancing individual rights within a setting of community values, and engaging an informed community in consultation. I believe this can best be done within the same framework as a discussion about the provision of health services where choices are posed based on evidence of cost and likely consequence of alternative strategies.

Social capital

Such exchange of information between community and professional assures a relationship of trust. Much has been written in recent years about trust within the social setting, and an interesting term has been given currency by the Harvard professor Robert Putnam.[514] The term is 'social capital'. He was not the first to use it and certainly will not be the last. It is a slippery term but it has been used to excellent effect in jolting us into realisation that a preoccupation with the $ variety of capital is altogether impoverishing—that $ is treasure that 'moth and rust doth corrupt'.[515] Trust, altruism, generosity and participation are energies that must be invested to be preserved, and they strengthen our social defences against the depredation of greed, individualism, isolationism, racism and an inwardness born of social poverty. The word 'capital' may stir homo economicus, caught in mesmeric economic trances, in a way that no other word would do. It has an arresting and exciting resonance that provokes people who might never otherwise think once, let alone twice, about the importance of investing in social interaction and trust, and if this is all it did it would be more valuable than diamonds.

Putnam's definition of social capital is this—'. . . features of social organisation such as networks, norms and social trust that facilitate co-ordination and co-operation for mutual benefit'.[516]

Putnam identifies an interesting aspect of discussions about social capital. He refers in conversation to his amazement that the debate has been 'orthogonal' to the political spectrum extending from the right to the left. 'Orthogonal' is not a word that my spellcheck thesaurus recognises, but it means essentially that the spread of opinion about the validity of the idea of social capital is not such that lefties believe in it and conservatives don't. Support comes from across the political spectrum—antagonists come from both the left and the right, too. This is a standard feature of post-modern society, at least from my experience in public health, where coalitions of interest are very transient. Campaigners against fluoride in the water may be (or may not be) the same people who campaign against immunisation. So orthogonality is a familiar phenomenon to public health.

What Putnam fears is that people may take the term and use it for ultimately socially perverse purposes. While social capital appears to be built up by participation in social life, campaigners on the right can use the idea as an excuse to send women back to the kitchen in bare feet; as a nostalgic claim for the old ways of doing things—accumulating social capital for the family by their devoted contribution to reproduction and child-care at home. Others have expressed concern that the World Bank appears to have taken the idea of social capital to its heart and may be using it to distort the terms and conditions for investment required of developing countries. Furthermore, conservative governments may invoke it in an argument to return the care of chronic patients to families, as they assume more responsibility for looking after their own ill.

Thus some negative aspects of the term 'social capital' are associated with its economic essence, and there is a risk that it will be used by exploitative politicians and bureaucrats to push individuals into assuming more responsibilities, such as the care of the aged and infirm at home, with a view to saving taxes. There is another problem, associated with the derivative function of capital—to be productive—which suggests that the purpose of society and all individuals in it is always to produce. That worries those who fear that ageist attitudes towards the unproductive elderly will find support, albeit through distortion, from the messages proclaimed by the advocates of social capital, or be used as a nasty weapon of exclusion against the disabled, elderly or mentally ill. Social capital, and implied notions of productivity, run all the risks of utilitarianism in the name of which all sorts of evils have been visited on minorities, including the very ill, throughout history.

So the term 'social capital' has some serious drawbacks. Putnam pleads that people using the term begin to approach it empirically, by which he means that much more measurement should be done on the relation between social capital and other desirable social goals and qualities. Intuitively we may believe that a community that has a fair working knowledge of its members and fosters mutual support will be a happier and healthier place to live in than one where anonymity and lack of trust beyond the front door are key features. But we cannot be sure. High trust communities, says Putnam, have choral societies, by which he means that people get together for purposes other than industry and commerce to celebrate their living together in the same time and place, and having harmony in their relationships. But what is the relation between choirs and better health?

Putnam's expression of his ideas in the USA has led to an outpouring of empathy, some of it nostalgic for a lost age, but some of it more basic in terms of the American traditions of openness and trust. He writes:

> There is rising unhappiness about the performance of major social institutions, including (but not limited to) the institutions of representative democracy. At least in the USA, there is reason to suspect that some fundamental social and cultural preconditions for effective democracy may have been eroded in recent decades, as a result of the gradual, but widespread, process of civil disengagement.

By civil disengagement he means spending more time meditating alone, watching TV, waxing your car, sitting on a computerised exercise bike at home and counting down the calories, instead of belonging to a church, a car club, or athletics club—opting out of society in favour of anonymity and doing things on your own or within a very nuclear group.

In Australia the idea of social capital was given an immense boost by Eva Cox's thoroughly engaging and altogether splendid 1995 Boyer Lectures for the ABC entitled 'A Truly Civil Society'.[517] Cox explains Putnam's thesis as implying that:

> high levels of social capital bring co-operation and norms which may be called civic virtues. These virtues in turn are the basis of truly civil societies . . . if we trust others as we trust ourselves, prosperity and economic growth follow.[517]

Cox has progressed the exegesis of the term 'social capital' brilliantly, locating it in the world of human encounters, politics, disadvantage and advocacy in a way that I find exciting. She draws a helpful distinction between social capital and other forms of capital such as financial and physical capital which 'can be used to produce wealth, as can human capital and our individual skills'. But only social capital is a measure of process, a measure of our satisfaction with the way we interact. Positive social capital ensures a high level of social trust while social capital deficits create distrust. The assumption is that when we experience positive experiences with a wide range of other people, we begin to trust, and akin to investment in a bank, we begin to accumulate this trust. We become willing to transfer the trust to strangers and be generally optimistic that others will act positively towards us.

This is not the only source of social decay. For example, big business can cause social devastation—through exploitation and the troubled towns they leave behind as they downsize or move offshore—and of course war, above all the nuclear variety, can obliterate everything—not just humans and the societies in which they live. But the benign arm of government, where health and welfare reside—the very expression of government by the people for the people—that's different. One of the strongest claims to legitimacy available to liberal-democratic states is their association in people's minds with security, with assistance in times of trouble and a generally benign social purpose. This trust may be misguided in some respects, but it is taken to be the norm where the goals of government are supposed to be about the protection of our lives, our liberty, and our well-being. When this is added to the relationship with the health professionals we consult—when we go to a public hospital for instance—we have a very strong brew: trust is all important! A public hospital is, in a sense, a potent symbol and keystone of the liberal-democratic state.

I believe that unless agencies, such as the health service, reward the investment of communities in them of altruism and care, and respect the activities that reinforce these values and avoid behaviours that erode them, then we are in very deep trouble indeed. I suggest that a health service that erodes humanistic values is an immensely destructive force.

Resources and health care

In health service provision whenever draconian policies are brought in which are devoid of community sensitivity and free of the encumbrance of community consultation social soil erosion is threatened. I subscribe fully to the view that most (bar the really highest tech) hospital and community support services should be distributed so that they are easily accessible to people where they live. For this to occur the population needs to be grouped into areas or regions of reasonable size (say 300 000–500 000 people) in urban settings, and public health resources need to be made available accordingly on a formula that relates recurrent investment to the size, age and need of the population in each region. This is not hard to calculate, and many public health services, both in Australia and other countries (notably New Zealand and the UK) are tending this way. New South Wales has had a formula for progressively more equitable annual allocation of its $3 or $4 billion recurrent (not capital) public health dollars for its several health areas for over a decade, endorsed by political parties of both persuasions. Steady progress has been made to reallocate resources accordingly, although not as quickly as some hoped for.

The achievement of equitable resource allocation for public hospitals and affiliated community services is now made somewhat easier by virtue of change in the most basic notion of what a hospital is and does. Hospitals are no longer halls of neatly made up beds which people occupy in their infirmity for weeks at a time. Instead, they have become more of an organisational base and emergency care centre, with fewer horizontal and more vertical users. Hospitals are becoming less permanent, more modular and flexible, and resources to support them also are now more portable. Keyhole surgery has transformed such diabolical operations as removal of the gall bladder into a two-day wonder and now there are prospects of thoracoscopic surgery extending routinely to coronary artery grafting. The management of aortic aneurism has been transformed by new approaches from inside rather than outside that vital abdominal blood vessel. Heart attack patients who once spent weeks in hospital are now out in days. Most cancer care is now managed as an outpatient procedure, people coming to hospital only for the initial diagnosis and care of complications and on occasions for palliative support late in their illness. The idea that St Mother's should always remain there as an immortal, unchanging icon, is losing its charm and more importantly its conviction as a reflection of medical and surgical reality. Hospitals, one way or another, are already on the move.

That said, it is possible to screw up the shift of resources, especially the shift of hospital resources, to growth communities in a big way. Unless the meaning of a hospital is understood from the community's point of view, social soil erosion can take a devastating grip.

Closing a hospital is a very big deal: there is often a heavy community investment in it—raffles to buy equipment, births and deaths, and pain and repair associated with it in the community's mind—and it is usually embedded deeply in the social soil from which its nourishment comes, based on commitment, generosity and care of society, even if supplied via the tortuous channels of Medicare and taxes. Hospitals, even the modular, treat-you-on-your-feet variety, are often the focus of a lot of community participation. In my own hospital in Westmead, which sits on what was once a favourite community trotting track in the west of Sydney, humming quietly, akin to *Battlestar Galactica* on standby, volunteers from surrounding neighbourhoods help bamboozled people to find their way around its labyrinth of wards and corridors. Fêtes and women's support groups and Rotary and a host of other agencies provide support. Local industry contributes to research funding. Police bands used to play in one of the courtyards regularly at lunchtime. Hospital staff (and there are 3000 of them to chose from) form choirs (R Putnam, please note) to sing carols at Christmas in the vast entrance. The hospital revue brings out delicious talent from the same staff who daily fulfil all the functions of keeping the hospital running. Our hospitals fulfil multiple social purposes, among them being employment. Attend to these other functions and hospitals can be moved; ignore them, close a hospital, and wait for the bang.

So we have a paradox: for the sake of justice resources may have to move; for the sake of the host community this must be done with extraordinary sensitivity (never mind the vested interests of professionals which often cloud the issue) or social soil is lost.

A particularly bad example, where social soil was eroded in tanker loads, occurred in New South Wales with the proposals announced on 21 June 1996 to close St Vincent's Hospital and simultaneously to move its staff and principal functions to the St George Hospital at Kogarah, about 20 kilometres south but in the suburban heartland of Sydney. St Vincent's has a proud history and longstanding religious basis for its provision of services to its community, but the survival of the hospital depends upon a significant redefinition of its catchment area. The community it once served has changed radically and as large inner city hospitals have discovered worldwide, they are offering a service to patients who have moved. The hospital has recognised this transition and has been looking to see what could best be done with its capacity, contemplating at one stage a move to Liverpool, further south-west, but this was not regarded positively by the local community because of the religious overlay.

St George Hospital, which I can recall attending as a lad of five to have a blood test to rule out rheumatic fever, also has its proud history and the religious affiliations if they can be so called, to the local community. Concurrently moves to shift other resources from other hospitals, together with a $100 million overall health budget cut, were mandated from the inner sanctum of the health minister's office without further consultation and proclaimed as edicts with the due sounding of brass from atop the city wall.

The public outcry was instantaneous and interesting. It had little to do with any objection to the basic principle of equity, the principle which seeks to arrange health care services in such a way that equal need has equal access to equal care. I have no doubt that the principle of equity was one (alongside cost-cutting to pay back debts incurred during an odd campaign to reduce waiting lists for elective surgery by one half in the year before) which inspired the offending proclamations, given the Minister's unequivocal personal commitment to equity. Rather, most of the decibels had to do with the process by which the moves were being engineered. It is as though a community understands intuitively when it is being shoved by big bulldozer blades and immediately reacts to protect itself and its social assets.

Not to receive the signal of yes for equity, no for non-consultative proclamation, could lead to the false conclusion that no-one in New South Wales is willing to contemplate ever giving up anything on behalf of anyone else. That would be a disastrous outcome, akin to shooting the messenger when he/she delivers the Mastercard monthly account.

Conclusion

Beyond the business of providing sickness care, which consumes more than 90 per cent of the $35 billion we spend on 'health' in Australia each year, there is the small matter of health promotion and prevention through the organised efforts of society directed toward achieving better health. Although the amount of $ capital consumed in this pursuit is relatively small, Australia has a proud record of achievement, not least in the last two decades. During that time an exemplary approach to the control of HIV/AIDS infection was mounted from the Federal Health Minister's (Neal Blewett's) office in Canberra—exemplary in the sense that participation was a key principle, involving the gay community especially right from the start. Others have written extensively about the opposite approach taken in the USA where the Gipper (President Reagan), for all his folksy popularity, never did get to grips with AIDS, leaving it to the states worst affected, such as California and New York, to battle through with makeshift arrangements and financially crippling burdens. What was missing was an appreciation of the necessity to deposit social soil, to increase social capital if that metaphor is more pleasing, from which the community response to this disaster could be supported.

Even if one is committed, as many of our politicians these days are by virtue of prevailing fashion if for no other observably sensible reason, to moving from a communal market garden to a reformed model where we all grow (by choice) our own lettuces once more, through complex privatisation and voucher-based systems, social soil is still necessary. Waste it with provoked cynicism, squander it by ripping things out and leaving the ground bare, and there is nothing to support further life.

The path to better health is by engendering community values that transcend selfishness and greed. Reform that ignores the fact that society depends upon an organic life support and that you can't rip down social structures that grow in it with impunity, adds to the environmental burden, and erodes social soil. This diminishes our capacity to support initiatives aimed at achieving better health. These indiscretions are readily avoidable. They require insight and sensitivity to be applied—just like leaving trees in vital places and keeping your sheep out of some paddocks for some of the year allows the soil to recover and rejuvenate.

Can we discern and learn? I am confident we can. I know we must.

REFERENCES

506. Better Health Commission. *Looking forward to better health, report of the Better Health Commission.* Canberra: AGPS, 1986.
507. O'Dea K, Traianedes K, Chisholm K, Leyden H, Sinclair AJ. Cholesterol lowering effect of a low fat diet containing lean beef is reversed by the addition of beef fat. *Amer J Clin Nut* 1990; 52: 491–4.
508. Barratt A, Irwig L. Is cholesterol testing/treatment really beneficial? *Med J Aust* 1993; 159, 10: 644–7.
509. Barrat A, and Irwig L. ibid.
510. Wise M, Graham-Clarke P. *Cardiovascular health in Australia: a review of current activities and future directions.* Department of Human Services and Health and AGPS, Canberra, 1994.
511. Tuchman BW. *The march of folly: from Troy to Vietnam.* New York: Random House, 1984.
512. Dwyer T, Blizzard L, Shugg D, Hill D, Ansari MZ. Higher lung cancer rates in young women than young men: Tasmania, 1983 to 1992. *Cancer Causes and Control* 1994; 5, 4: 351–8.
513. Carter R. In: *Pathways to better health: national health strategy health issues, paper no 7.* Canberra: Treble Press, 1993.
514. Putnam R. Bowling alone: America's declining social capital. *Journal of Democracy,* 1995; 6, 1: 65–78.
515. *New Testament,* St Matthew, 6: 19.
516. Putnam R. Bowling alone: America's declining social capital. *Journal of Democracy,* 1995; 6, 1: 68.
517. Cox EA. *A truly civil society.* The Boyer Lectures, ABC, Sydney, 1995.

CHAPTER SEVENTEEN

How Much Should We Spend on Health Services?

JEFF RICHARDSON

Introduction

Providers of health care generally dislike the idea of restrictions upon the services they offer their patients. Professional training encourages the collection of the maximum possible information before diagnosis and aggressive treatment with the most recent and often the most expensive therapies. Concern for patient's well-being and personal and financial considerations usually reinforce the dislike of restrictions. Patients similarly expect unrestrained access to health services. For some time the prevailing attitude has been that health care is a right; that when sickness occurs there is a fairly well defined and appropriate therapy which should be universally available.

These attitudes have been challenged in the last decade. Many now accept, albeit reluctantly, that without fairly vigorous measures to control spending the health sector will face an even greater crisis than at present. The common argument runs somewhat as follows:

> Health care spending is rising too rapidly. Its growth is fuelled by an ageing population, by the existence of universal health insurance and by the introduction of new and expensive technologies. In the first three post-war decades the rate of economic growth was sufficiently high to support this trend. But with the slowing of GDP growth in the 1980s and 1990s the economy cannot sustain the continued inflation of medical costs. In particular, the tax burden has become so great that the Government cannot continue to underwrite the expansion of the health sector at its historical rate. The population cannot continue to receive unrestricted access to all possible medical care. It is therefore inevitable that explicit rationing will eventually be introduced and if this rationing is not sufficiently severe then governments will be forced to hand back responsibility for health spending to the private sector.

The theme of this chapter is that there is some truth in the diagnosis but that the aetiology of the problem is far more complex than implied

by the simple view above. It is certainly true that health services con-
sume an enormous share of the GDP and that they may continue to
expand rapidly. For this reason it is also likely that we will adopt some
form of explicit rationing. Indeed, it is argued later that such rationing
is ethically desirable. However, it is agued that there is no inevitability
about the level or source of health funding and that these decisions
are largely matters of social choice; that they are not driven by some
economic or technological imperative.

The chief difficulty in making a decision regarding the appropriate
level of health spending arises from the imperfect information available and from the imperfect analytical tools for making the decision. In
this respect economics makes a valuable contribution but it does not
(and cannot alone) resolve a number of the ethical issues that underlie
the decision. In particular there is no fully satisfactory method for placing a dollar value on a human life, although a judgment must inevitably
be made if limitations are to be placed upon life-extending services.
Similarly, judgments must be made about the appropriate distribution
of health benefits. Despite these difficulties there is a fairly clear agenda
for reform. In the short run health service efficiency must be improved.
This is a prerequisite to any sensible decision about how many resources
we should finally spend on health services.

Current and future spending

While it is generally recognised that the health sector is big, very few
people appreciate its true magnitude. This is shown in Figure 17.1[518]
by comparison with Australian GDP expenditures in other sectors. The
figure reveals that the health sector is as large as agriculture and mining
combined and over 50 per cent the size of the entire manufacturing
sector. By 1994/1995 health consumed \$(1994) 38.5 billion.[519] At the
underlying growth rate the burden on an average family of four in 2000
AD will be about \$(1994) 10 185.

While the distribution of the expenditure is highly skewed the figure
indicates the average sacrifice that will be made to permit the use of
medical services.

As two thirds of the spending is financed by government, it is also
true that the health sector imposes a heavy tax burden and that changes
in the level of government support have a significant impact upon the
budget. This is illustrated in the passage below.

> To give some perspective to the fiscal implications of changes in health
> policy, consider the following arithmetical figuring. Over the five years
> to June 1976 the ratio of health expenditure to GDP increased from
> 5.8 per cent to 7.8 per cent and the Commonwealth's share of the
> bill rose from 28.5 per cent to 48.0 per cent. If the Commonwealth's

Figure 17.1 The relative size of the health and other sectors: 1974–1995

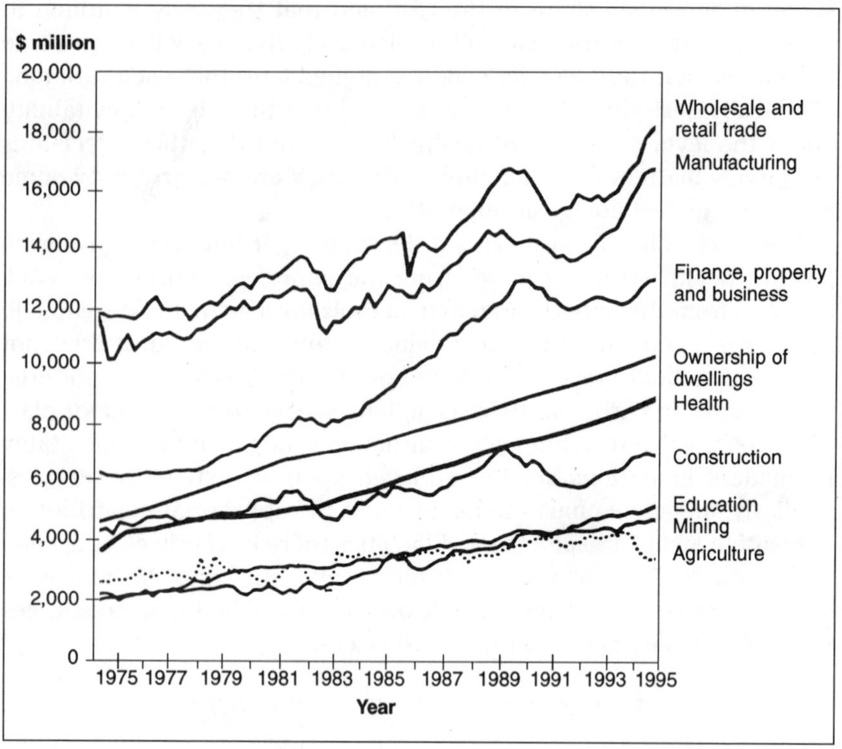

Source AIHW: *Australia's Health* p123.

percentage share of total health expenditure had remained at the 1970 level, its 'revenue savings' from the reduced contribution to the total health expenditure of 1976 would have been almost sufficient to finance a doubling of the Commonwealth's outlays on education or defence; alternatively, Commonwealth social security and welfare payments could have been increased by 30 per cent, or personal income taxation reduced by one-quarter.[520]

The period discussed in this quotation was atypical as it included the introduction of Medibank 1, Australia's first compulsory health insurance scheme which extended health insurance to the 15 per cent of the population previously uncovered. Nevertheless it indicates the magnitude of the budgetary savings that could be achieved by a full or partial reversal of the government share. It also indicates the problem facing a tax-minimising government if health expenditures grow more rapidly than the GDP and general revenue.

Australia is not alone in spending so much on health care. The international comparisons shown in Table 17.1 indicate that the percentage of the GDP devoted to health care in Australia is fairly typical for a

Table 17.1 Health expenditure as a percent of GDP in the OECD[521]

	1960	1970	1975	1980	1990	1994
Australia	4.9	5.7	7.5	7.3	8.3	8.5
Austria	4.4	5.4	7.3	7.9	8.4	9.7
Belgium	3.4	4.1	5.9	6.6	7.6	8.2
Canada	5.5	7.1	7.3	7.3	9.2	9.8
Czech Republic	—	—	—	—	5.3	7.6
Denmark	3.6	6.1	6.5	6.8	6.5	6.6
Finland	3.9	5.7	6.4	6.5	8	8.3
France	4.2	5.8	7	7.6	8.9	9.7
Germany	4.8	5.9	8.1	8.4	8.3	9.5
Greece	2.4	3.4	3.4	3.6	4.3	5.2
Hungary	—	—	—	—	6.6	7
Iceland	3.3	5	5.8	6.2	7.9	8.1
Ireland	3.8	5.3	7.6	8.7	6.7	7.9
Italy	3.6	5.1	6.2	6.9	8.1	8.3
Japan	—	4.4	5.5	6.4	6	6.9
Luxembourg	—	3.7	5.1	6.2	6.2	5.8
Mexico	—	—	—	—	—	5.3
Netherlands	3.8	5.9	7.5	7.9	8.4	8.8
New Zealand	4.3	5.2	6.7	7.2	7.4	7.5
Norway	3	4.6	6.1	6.1	6.9	7.3
Portugal	—	2.8	5.6	5.8	6.6	7.6
Spain	1.5	3.7	4.9	5.7	6.9	7.3
Sweden	4.7	7.1	7.9	9.4	8.6	7.7
Switzerland	3.3	5.2	7	7.3	8.4	9.6
Turkey	—	2.4	2.7	3.3	2.9	4.2
United Kingdom	3.9	4.5	5.5	5.6	6	6.9
United States	5.2	7.2	8.2	9.1	12.7	14.3

Source OECD data file.

Western nation. Indeed, if health expenditure is (statistically) 'predicted' it is almost exactly what would be expected for a country with its GDP.[522] When the data from Table 17.1 are plotted in Figure 17.2, two interesting facts are highlighted.

First, and most obviously, expenditure in the USA significantly exceeds expenditure in any other country. In 1995 its per capita spending was 74.9 per cent greater than in Canada which has the world's second most expensive system. This supports the nearly universal belief that a more free market approach to health insurance and health care delivery is inflationary. The atypical US pattern became most evident in the 1980s, the decade in which a concerted attempt was made to reduce spending through the use of market competition.

The second interesting observation is that, with the exception of the USA, the growth in the relative share of the health sector was brought under control in the mid 1970s with Australia being one of the first countries to achieve control. In most cases, including Australia, this was achieved by the imposition of (fairly indiscriminate) budget caps applied, in particular, to hospital spending. Budget caps were not generally applied in the USA. It is increasingly questioned whether this

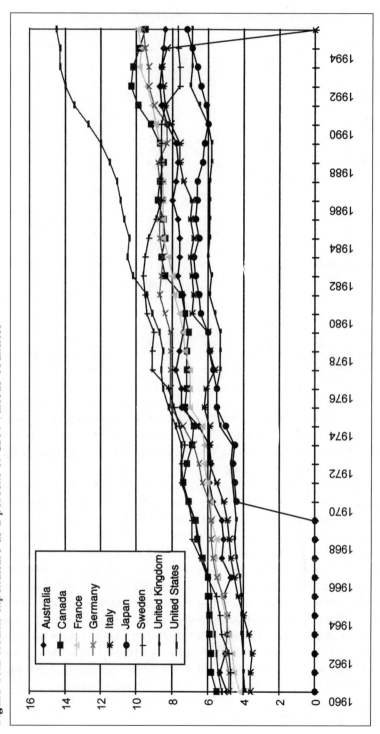

Figure 17.2 Health expenditure as a percent of GDP: Various countries

Figure 17.3 US health expenditure as a percent of GDP 1965–2030

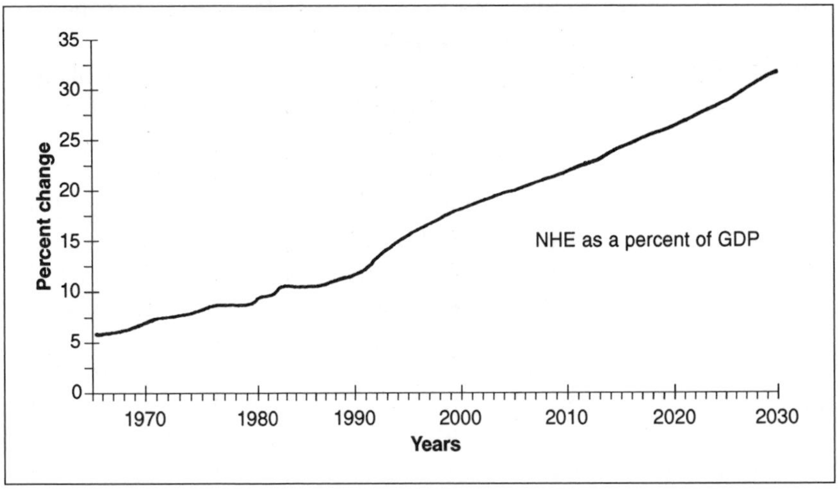

Source Health Care Financing Administration, Office of the Actuary: Data from the Office of National Health Statistics.

mechanism of cost control can continue. It is likely that the initial and relatively easy economies that could be achieved in the hospital sector have been exhausted and that further economies will be far more difficult to achieve.

An important question in the present context is whether health expenditures will continue to grow at their present or at a greater rate. The capacity to spend has already been illustrated. US per capita outlays are already 133 per cent greater than in Australia and there is no technical reason why Australians could not spend this much, i.e., more than double their current outlays. There is also no reason to suppose that US expenditure has reached its limit. Various attempts have been made to predict future US health costs. One projection, made by the US Health Care Financing Agency is reproduced in Figure 17.3.

Based upon the assumption that the current excess spending in the health sector continues at its historical rate, it is estimated that by the year 2030 the USA could be devoting 26.1 per cent of its GDP to health care; that is, allowing for economic growth, more than double its current spending. By contrast, the National Commission of Audit (1996) has suggested that Australian health spending may reach 12.5 per cent in the next 50 years. At least part of this difference could be attributed to the role of excess medical inflation in the USA; that is, the increase in the apparent unit price* above the general inflation rate. Between

---

* This calculation is problematical as it is difficult to define a homogeneous unit of health care and thereby separate pure inflationary effects.

1975 and 1994 the excess in the USA and Australia were 46.6 per cent and 5.7 per cent respectively, suggesting, prima facie, a relative increase in the incomes of US health care providers.[522a]

The more important issue is whether such trends are really likely to emerge. Prediction is, of course, hazardous and especially when it is about the future! However, a sensible judgment may be based upon an examination of the historical reasons for the growth of the health sector and an assessment of whether or not these causal factors are likely to continue. The chief explanatory factors have been considered by a number of authors (for example Newhouse,[523] Weisbrod,[524] Fuchs,[525] and Abel Smith[526]) and the relative importance of different explanatory factors is fairly clear.

Surprisingly the chief economic variables do not play a very important role. Even in the USA where out of pocket costs faced by consumers have fallen fairly significantly with the extension of medical insurance, the authors of the definitive RAND experiment into the effects of medical co-payments calculated that only about 10 per cent of the increase in US costs between 1950 and 1984 could be attributed to the extension of medical insurance.[527] In Australia, Richardson[528] estimated that reduced co-payments could account for a maximum of 6 per cent of the growth in medical costs. Similarly, rising expenditure cannot be attributed to the direct effect of income upon the demand for services as the direct effect of income upon expenditure is known to be small. This is pariculary true when consumers face small co-payments as in the case for hospital and medical expenditure. In the absence of significant user charges there is no reason why personal income should affect a person's demand for services and none of the studies carried out to date have suggested that direct income effects are of particular importance. However, the close association observed between per capita GDP and national health expenditures suggests an important indirect income effect. It is clear that the pressure for increased expenditures generated elsewhere can be accommodated more easily as GDP rises, although the precise mechanism by which this occurs has never been clearly articulated.

Equally surprisingly, the effects of ageing per se do not appear to have been particularly important historically and projections suggest that they will remain of marginal significance. For example Abel Smith[526] reports that over a 20 year period in the UK the changing demographic profile could only account for an 8 per cent increase in service use. In France and the Netherlands ageing only led to a 0.3 per cent per annum growth in service costs. Richardson[529] estimated that in the decade to 1986 the changing age/sex structure of the population explained between 3 per cent and 6 per cent of the actual change in Australian service use—very similar to the growth in France and the Netherlands. The future impact of demographic change per se is also likely to be under-whelming. By 2030 the percent of Australians over the age of 65 will be only slightly greater than the percentage in Germany, the UK, Austria and Sweden in 1980, and yet these countries absorbed the impact of ageing upon health expenditures without devoting an exceptional share of the GDP to health care. More generally, the impact of ageing has been exaggerated and the effects of future changes in the age structure in Western countries will be no greater than the impact already experienced and accommodated in the last 50 years.[530]

By elimination, the chief explanation for rising health costs appears to be associated with the supply and not the demand side of the health sector.[526,531–33] In particular, changes in medical technology are increasingly regarded as the main factor fuelling expenditure growth although this is accommodated by the increasing supply of medical practitioners, supplier-induced demand and the permissive role played by rising GDP. While it is difficult to predict the impact of future technology the consensus appears to be that for the immediate future it is likely to be cost increasing and particularly when it is associated with more sophisticated and costly diagnostic procedures and with the introduction of therapies for previously untreatable conditions.

However, it should not be assumed that technology is inevitably cost-increasing. New procedures have dramatically reduced the average length of hospital stay (although it is not clear how much this is attributable to quicker, cheaper treatments and how much to quicker and more expensive interventions). As Fuchs[525] notes, the most significant technological change in the late 1940s and 1950s was the introduction of antibiotic drugs which sharply reduced the length and cost of hospitalisation.

Why do we limit resources?

Observing the level and growth of medical expenditures does not explain why we should wish to limit what to many is a self-evidently desirable use of our resources and, in the case of potentially life-saving expenditures, a morally necessary activity. Adoption of this view would imply that future rationing of health services should be resisted. A possible rejoinder to this conclusion is that health services are already rationed both by their exclusion from the National Health Service or by their limited supply. The extreme variability in the rate at which services are provided to different populations implies that there is an enormous amount of care that could still be provided and that current service levels have more to do with a somewhat arbitrary set of historical decisions than with the maximum benefit that could be obtained with existing technology.

This rejoinder would imply the desirability of an immediate increase in our present health budget as well as an acceptance of future growth: and there is no technological reason why this should not occur. In principle we could double our expenditure and double it again. The US HCFA projections cited earlier did not imply a declining standard of living as health expenditures rose to 26 per cent of the GDP. Rather, almost all of the benefits of general productivity growth in the US economy would be absorbed by the health sector. Even if health sector growth implied a lower material standard of living elsewhere this does not imply its impossibility or even its undesirability if the medical expenditures were providing benefits to people that exceed the benefits from spending on fast food, television, travel, etc. In short, there is no well defined technological or economic limit to the share of the GDP that could be spent of health care. The final level is a matter of social choice.

Similarly, it is entirely a matter of social choice whether health services are financed collectively through taxation or through some private mechanism. The claim that governments cannot or will soon be unable to afford the cost of a health service but that the private sector can, is simply untrue or, at best, a convenient myth to obscure some other objective (possibly the political objective of reducing taxation) which reflects (or promotes) an unwillingness by the healthy/wealthy to transfer resources to the unhealthy/poor. This is particularly true for countries such as Australia where the government share of the health budget is lower than in most comparable countries (at 68 per cent it was the fifth lowest in the OECD in 1994 after the USA, Portugal, Turkey and Austria) and where taxation as a percentage of the GDP is the fifth lowest in the OECD after Mexico, Turkey, the USA and Japan.[534] More generally there is no known relationship between the overall level of taxation and the performance or growth of the economy.[535] This implies that the decision concerning government or private financing in the foreseeable future is not subject to some economic imperative but should reflect social attitudes towards collective versus individual responsibility for the financing of health care.

However, social choice will inevitably result in a level of service delivery that is less than is necessary to maximise health and this implies some form of rationing. The reason for this, as emphasised by economists, is that an activity is only desirable when the benefits from the activity exceed the 'cost'. Conceptually, 'cost' does not refer here to dollar expenditures but to the 'opportunity cost' which is the value of benefits or opportunities foregone by carrying out the activity. The economist's dictum that benefits should exceed cost may therefore be translated as the rule that the desirability of benefits associated with an activity should exceed the benefits foregone.

Within this framework there are at least three reasons why health care expenditures should be limited. Each is based upon the theme that people should spend where they obtain the greatest benefits and this may not always be from health care services. First, people do not only want maximum possible health. They also want a good quality of life and this depends upon expenditures outside the health sector. The compromise between health and non-health related expenditures implies less medical care than is technically possible. Secondly, to the extent to which people seek health improvement, this will not always be achieved by expenditure on formal health care. As emphasised by Evans and Stoddart[536] health is now known to have far more to do with social position, the environment and nutrition than with health services, and the best path to better health will often involve spending in these sectors. Thirdly, and related to this, there is considerable uncertainty about the benefits of many of the procedures that are currently delivered. The effectiveness of most procedures have not been demonstrated. In one survey of Dutch physicians the estimated number of proven procedures varied from 20 per cent to 40 per cent of those covered by the social health insurance scheme.[537] One OECD study reported that 80 per cent of medical procedures and two thirds of medical goods have never been evaluated.[522] On occasions the eventual evaluation of existing technologies has revealed an overall harmful impact.[526]

In addition, proven services may often be used inappropriately. Abel Smith reports estimates of 30–60 per cent of services in some countries being unnecessary (although Abel Smith considers that the figure is probably exaggerated). Finally there is growing evidence of the iatrogenic effects of many interventions. For example, the recent 'Quality in Australian Health Care Study' reported the results of detailed analyses of the medical records of 14 179 patients admitted to 28 selected Australian hospitals.[538] Extrapolation of the results implied that medical errors of omission or commission add about 420 000 additional admissions per annum to Australian hospitals and result in about 50 000 permanent disabilities and 18 000 deaths.

This uncertainty about the benefits of many services at the 'micro' level is reflected in a corresponding uncertainty about the benefits at the 'macro' or population level. The limited evidence available here suggests that these could easily be overstated. For example, Bunker et al[539] examined the cumulative impact of all demonstrably effective clinical preventive and curative services and concluded that in the twentieth century these have added roughly five years to life expectancy. McKinley et al[540] present evidence that most of the increase in life expectancy that has occurred over several decades has been years of disability.

Finally and most provocatively, Cochrane et al[541] found a systematic perverse and positive relationship between age specific mortality and the doctor supply between developed countries after standardising for other relative variables. A similar result was found in Australia by Richardson and Richardson[542] in an analysis which explicitly sought to disentangle the direction of causation in the association. (This study is currently being replicated.) A more recent cross national study of total mortality by Kim and Moody[543] using a different statistical model did not replicate Cochrane's results. However it did not find a statistically significant relationship between doctor supply and declining mortality.

In sum, while no one seriously doubts the beneficial effects of medical care *overall* there is a serious question about the benefits from *further increasing* expenditures except when this is on new and demonstrably effective care. Benefits are uncertain; costs—foregone benefits—are certain and significant. There is therefore a legitimate basis for restricting resources and for rationing when it appears that the overall benefits from expenditures are greater outside than inside the health sector.

While accepting this conclusion it is still possible to maintain that there should be no limit on the amount spent when life itself can be saved. The basis of this argument is that 'you can't put a dollar value on life' or (as in the case of some religions) that life has 'infinite' value. The implication of accepting this view would be far reaching. It would imply that any therapy or diagnostic test with even a finite probability of extending life should be carried out (and in preference to medical care which increased the quality of life). However small the probability, the repetition of such interventions with a sufficiently large number of patients will eventually result in the saving of lives. The case for unlimited expenditures would be re-established albeit for a different set of interventions.

This argument may be analysed as two separate questions: (1) as an empirical observation, does life per se always take precedence over the quality of life and, (2) as an ethical proposition, should this occur? The answer to the first question is unambiguously 'No'. It is clear that neither individuals nor society treat life as having infinite value, i.e., always taking precedence over the quality of life. The evidence for this is obvious when a broad view is taken of the range of activities that can preserve and prolong life. Individuals do not minimise the personal risk

of death. They voluntarily undertake a range of life-threatening behaviours in full knowledge of the risk. The individual does not, of course,
face the certainty of death. However when society permits its members
to undertake these activities it is accepting the inevitability of increased
mortality. The existence of cars, electricity, life threatening industries,
dangerous sports, smoking, the consumption of fatty foods, etc, etc all
ensure premature death.

We do not even minimise the risks associated with these activities.
And the reason for this is also obvious. The benefits of each of these
activities exceeds their costs. That is, the resulting improvement in the
quality of life is valued more highly than the small number of deaths that
occur. Life is, in effect, treated as having a finite value that is traded
off against the quality of life.

It is, of course, still possible to argue that life *should* take precedence
over the quality of life. However while the abstract principle may obtain
some support it is likely that this would evaporate once the practical
consequences were understood. A society incorporating the principle
would be condemned to a relentless quest to reduce death. No effort
would be too great. This would imply the crippling of industry as we
now know it as much of this involves a finite—if negligible—risk of
death to its work force. The residual output from our emasculated
economy would be largely devoted to risk reduction. All resources not
needed for preserving life directly would be devoted to the achievement of a risk free environment. Freedom of choice would need to be
significantly curtailed in case individuals recklessly chose risky activities. For all these reasons our quality of life would be dramatically
reduced.

This scenario is, of course, ludicrous. It simply demonstrates by
reductio ad absurdum that the absolute precedence of life over the
quality of life is unsustainable as an ethical principle. The true question
is how to determine the acceptable trade-off between life and quality
of life and how to quantify this trade-off.

How should we decide how much to spend?

By definition medical expenditure is equal to the price times the quantity of the services provided. Price is identically equal to the provider's
gross income. The identity may therefore be restated as 'expenditure
is equal to the provider income per service times services received per
patient'. This highlights two decisions which must be taken. First, what
income should providers receive? And, secondly, how many services
should patients receive? The decisions are not unrelated. As providers'

incomes rise the cost to the remainder of the population increases and the ideal level of health and health services will fall.

The issue of appropriate provider incomes is complex, unresolved and beyond the scope of this chapter. It is worth noting, however, that governments have been concerned with reducing unit medical prices and, by implication, medical incomes. Governments, at least, have recognised the trade-off between real medical incomes and service availability.

In principle, the second decision concerning the number of services should be made by the application of the economic rule that all services should expand to the point where the additional (marginal) benefit is equal to the marginal cost. Application of this principle is, however, difficult and for this reason a variety of other approaches to prioritisation and resource allocation have been proposed such as 'goals and targets'. To the extent that their methods deviate from the economic prescription it follows, as a matter of logic, that they will result in less health for any given cost. For example, suppose that the unit of benefit was the life year and that the application of the alternative methodology resulted in the adoption of two interventions where the marginal costs of obtaining a life year were $2000 and $10 000 respectively. Scaling down the second intervention would lead to the loss of one life year; but the reallocation of the $10 000 to the first intervention would gain five life years. According to economic principles, all else being equal, this reallocation should continue until it was no longer possible to obtain life years more cheaply from the first intervention. Alternative approaches to resource allocation typically do not employ this logic and often fail to consider costs and benefits at the margin or even fail to consider costs at all.

Economists have developed three basic techniques to assist with the implementation of the general rule. These techniques are described in most text books of health economics[544] and are summarised in Table 17.2. The defining characteristic of the first technique, cost benefit analysis (CBA), is that benefits must be measured in dollars. Because of the difficulty in converting the value of human life into dollars, economists have attempted to side step this issue through the use of cost effective analysis (CEA). This allows the comparison of any interventions where there is a single and common unit of benefit. This, of course, is a serious disadvantage as it is often necessary to compare quite different outcomes and interventions which affect both the quantity and quality of life. Consequently, cost utility analysis (CUA) was developed in which the unit of benefit, the quality adjusted life year (QALY), combines both of these dimensions of outcome. The techniques for doing this are still relatively new and controversial.[545] However CUA represents an explicit recognition of the importance of the

Table 17.2 Three types of economic evaluation

Alternative economic analyses for health and health care evaluation		
Type of Analysis	*Benefits (outcomes) Included*	*Defining Characteristics*
1 Cost benefit analysis	Only outcomes which can be valued in $ are included. Often excludes 'intangibles'.	Benefits measured in dollars. Only one project needs to be considered. Selection Criteria: Benefits exceed costs (no budget constraint).
2 Cost effectiveness analysis	Only one 'dimension' of outcome is relevant, e.g., lives, life years; cases detected.	More than one project must be considered: projects are ranked. Different 'levels' of the outcome are obtained in different projects. Selection Criteria: Minimise cost/unit output.
2(a) Cost minimisation	Relevant outcomes identical.	More than one project must be considered: projects are ranked. No assessment of the 'value' of outcome. Selection Criteria: Minimise cost.
3 Cost utility analysis	Outcome is multidimensional. Quality of life is quantitatively important.	Quality of life is combined with life years. Life years are weighted to obtain 'quality adjusted life years' (QALYs). Projects are 'ranked'. Selection Criteria: Minimum cost/QALY.

quality of life and the inevitability of judging its relative importance when health outcome is compared with cost.

A common characteristic of all of these techniques is that they are applicable at the 'micro' level; that is, they are designed to determine whether particular small scale interventions are or are not desirable. To assist with the global allocation of resources the results of individual evaluations must be combined in some broad framework. The most direct approach is the one adopted in the famous (or infamous) Oregon experiment.[546,547] In Oregon the public was involved in an exercise in which broad service categories were defined according to ethical principles and these categories ranked according to the value placed upon these principles. Strict CUA was only applied within each category. Simplifying somewhat, all of the possible services which could be offered to the Oregon Medicaid population were ranked according to their cost per QALY. Services with the lowest ratio were to be selected progressively until the Medicaid budget was exhausted. The underlying value judgment in Oregon was that as the budget contracted it was desirable to eliminate less cost effective services rather than to restrict population eligibility to participate in the scheme.

The chief difficulty with this approach is the magnitude of the evaluation task. The Oregon experiment was based upon research that was arguably inadequate. Costings were rough, quality of life values were doubtful and cost to QALY ratios were obtained for very broad intervention categories which did not distinguish marginal from intra-marginal services. Despite this, the Oregon experiment remains an impressive model for one approach to global prioritisation within the health sector. Despite measurement error, each of the steps required for correct decision making was subject to explicit investigation and the overall analytical framework had the potential to maximise health from a given budget. The scheme was never implemented as it was deemed to violate US anti-discrimination legislation. The logic of this strange decision is discussed by Kaplan.[548] An emasculated scheme was subsequently accepted which did not include costs or the quality of life in the prioritisation process.

An alternative framework has been suggested and trialled by Segal and Richardson[549,550] in which more comprehensive evaluations are conducted within a disease category but, initially, only for those interventions where there is a serious possibility of expansion or contraction. Global efficiency is envisaged as being achieved iteratively by the progressive elimination of the least cost-effective and the progressive expansion of the most cost-effective services.

While these techniques may make an important contribution to achieving efficiency in the health sector—maximising health per unit of cost—they fall short of determining the appropriate level of overall expenditure in two important respects. First, the techniques purport to place a value or relative value on health benefits. They do not assist with the measurement of benefits in natural units; that is, they require information about the impact of health services upon the quantity and quality of life. This must be obtained from the medical literature and, as indicated above, the majority of health services have not been clinically evaluated, or evaluated in a way that is a suitable basis for economic evaluation.

Secondly, CEA and CUA and both of the broader frameworks discussed above only rank projects. They cannot unambiguously indicate whether or not a service should be provided. In the short run this is all that is required. There is overwhelming evidence of allocative inefficiency in the health sector and, as in the Segal-Richardson frame-work, the greatest health gains may be obtained initially by reallocat-ing resources to where the greatest health benefits can be obtained.

Of course, even in the short run, the application of CEA or CUA implies a dollar value of life. If, for example, we do not provide services when the cost per life year gained exceeds \$50 000, then this is the implied value of a life year. The point here is that in the 'short run' when the health budget is relatively fixed, significant health gains can be obtained without any explicit recognition or endorsement of this figure.

Eventually, however, a comparison must be made between benefits inside and outside the health sector. This implies a common unit of measurement with which to make the comparison and, as most bene-fits outside the health sector cannot sensibly be measured in QALYs this implies that the value of QALYs, life years and lives must be meas-ured in dollars.

Some benefits are directly comparable. Road and public safety meas-ures for example, save lives and improve the quality of life. Expend-itures on sanitation and nutrition may even have a greater impact on health than some disease-directed health services. However, the major benefits outside the health sector arise from the consumption of non health-related activities, that is, goods and services, and it is these benefits that are hard to convert into QALYs.

If this could be satisfactorily achieved then cost benefit analysis could be used for the economic evaluation of all health projects and, in principle the frameworks discussed above could determine, not simply the appropriate ranking of projects, but whether or not bene-fits exceeded costs. The iterative application of CBA could eventually determine the appropriate level of health expenditures; that is, the level where marginal expenditures were just producing the same value within the health sector as they could produce elsewhere. (Program evaluation is usually carried out on the assumption that the price of resources will not vary because of the projects. This assumption could be violated if a large scale reallocation of resources occurred as a result of CBA and explicit prioritisation. This is an additional reason for preferring an iterative approach to reform in which changing prices were employed in later analyses.)

The value of life

Various attempts have been made to measure the dollar value of life. These, of course, require a precise quantifiable criterion of value and two have been suggested. The first is the 'human capital' criterion. In the 'material welfare tradition' of Marshall and Pigou this treats the 'value' of the human life as being external from the individual[551] and 'value' is equated with the present value of future earnings (as with capital generally). The approach, pioneered by Mushkin[552] and Rice[553,554] has been widely used because of its simplicity. Calculating the value of human life only requires information on future earnings and these may be estimated from the age specific earnings of similar groups of individuals in the workforce.

Despite this, the approach is generally recognised as being theoretically unsound for at least two reasons. First, by equating 'value' with earnings it discriminates against those with low earnings; women, various ethnic and low income groups and the unemployed. By this criterion the retired have no value and projects which only saved their lives would be worthless. Secondly, it is clear that individuals are valued for more than their output. There is an intrinsic value of a person's life to their families, friends and to society which must be measured and quantified. At best, the human capital approach measures the contribution of an individual to the (measured) GDP and this is a sub-set of the factors that determine the value of a human life.

The second criterion is that 'value' is what people are willing to pay (WTP). Influential economists such as Mishan[555] have argued that despite its practical difficulties this is the theoretically correct approach as it is the criterion used more generally in the economy. The argument reveals a surprising but widespread misunderstanding of the role of social values amongst economists. While it is true that willingness to pay is the generally used and generally accepted criterion of value in much of the economy, this does not imply that it is, or should be, accepted as the correct criteria in every context. It is, nevertheless, a serious contender as a criterion of value.

The chief practical difficulty with this approach is that there is no market for life *per se* in which we can observe the price of life. Some have suggested that the WTP can be inferred from court decisions involving compensation for the loss of life, or from government (i.e., collective) decisions regarding projects involving the gain or loss of life. Such an approach is clearly circular. Such decisions cannot be used to infer a value of life that is then used to assist with such decisions. It is also common for court determinations to be based upon lost earnings (human capital) which is not equivalent to a willingness to pay. The more common solution is to observe the WTP, not for life, but for an increased probability of life or, conversely, to observe the compensation paid when there is an increased risk of death. If, for example, an individual is prepared to accept $200 for a 1 in 10 000 risk of death then it is inferred that the value of life is $200 \times 10\,000$ or \$2 million. Typically, the value of the compensation is 'observed' statistically. Wage rates in a variety of high risk industries are observed, the relationship between increasing risk and compensation is estimated and from this the implicit value of life is calculated.

This second approach has produced a wide variety of estimates. For example, in his review Viscousi[556] found values for a single life as low as \$US 0.6 million and as high as \$US 16.2 million (1990 dollars). A more serious difficulty is that the process of extrapolation from the risk of death to the value of life relies upon the famous axiom of von Newman and Morgernstern that choices under risk are not altered by 'linear transformation' i.e., it is possible to carry out the type of multiplication described here. However there is evidence that this axiom is both theoretically and empirically invalid. For a review of the theoretical and empirical evidence see Richardson[557] and Schoemaker[558] respectively.

In principle, a third approach to the quantification of the value of life could be to ask people directly what they, or society generally would or should be prepared to pay in different circumstances. If it were clear that the answer to the question could affect the amount that would, potentially, be spent upon the individual then this modified willingness to pay alternative would also incorporate the principles of Rawlsian justice. In practice, such an approach would be enormously difficult and does not appear to have been attempted to date. The relationship between stated and true preferences is problematical and it is not clear whether, in the case of human life, people have preferences which could be easily converted into dollars. At best the approach would require that decision makers be fully informed of the context and consequences of the decision and possibly involved in discussion of the issues.

Despite these reservations, stated preferences are increasingly used as the basis for decisions. In the environmental literature stated preference techniques (contingent valuation) have been used to assess the value of the compensation payable because of environmental damage. In the most famous case, the 1989 Alaskan oil spill from the US super tanker *Exon Valdez*, the controversy resulted in court action. To help resolve the issue, the US National Oceanic Atmospheric Administration (NOAA)[559] commissioned a panel chaired by two Nobel laureates in economics, Kenneth Arrow and Robert Solow, to review the evidence and theory relating to the validity of contingent valuation methods. Their report concluded that, if conducted carefully and subject to the various methodological safeguards discussed in the report, the methods were capable of correctly measuring preferences and placing a valid dollar value upon intangible benefits.[559]

Equity and values

Most of the methods discussed above assume a simple form of consequentialist utilitarianism. First, benefits are determined by health outcomes, the quantity and quality of life; and, in the tradition of preference utilitarianism, the value of these outcomes is determined by the strength of people's preferences. It is possible to obtain a willingness to pay valuation or even a time trade off score for scenarios which include process as well as outcome. In practice this is seldom done.

Second, there has been an implicit and simplifying assumption that there is a single value of each outcome (albeit an average of many individuals' values) which can and should be employed in economic evaluation. It is as if there were a single purchaser of health services who had placed the same value on health outcome no matter who received it. Neither of these assumptions is tenable.

There is compelling evidence that people have a very strong preference, not only for the maximisation of health outcomes, but also for an equitable distribution of health benefits. For example, Table 17.3 summarises the results of an Australian study designed to test the commitment to maximising life years, QALYs and health more generally when this implies less equity.

Table 17.3 Equity vs maximum health: Summary results

Distribution of benefits: Summary of results			
Issues	*Option**	*% Choosing each option*	*Maximisation option*
Age/life gain	Favour young	17.6	*
	Against very old	40.5	
	Equal priority	41.9	
Age/QoL gain	Favour young	21.5	*
	Against very old	2.9	
	Equal priority	75.6	
Newborn	Favour young	44.2	*
	Against very old	1.2	
	Equal priority	54.7	
Potential gain	Favour most helped	52.8	*
	Equal priority	47.2	
Children	Favour parents	33.4	
	Equal priority	66.6	
Smokers	Favour non-smokers	59.5	*
	Equal priority	40.5	
Cost/number treated	Favour least costly	18.6	*
	Equal priority	81.4	
* Summary of fuller statement of option.			

Source Nord E, Richardson J, Street A, Kuhse H, Singer D (1995).

From the second last column it can be seen that the health maximising option is not usually selected. The last result is particularly striking. The 551 survey respondents rejected the principle that, all else being equal, the least costly option should be adopted because this would permit more patients to be treated. Subsequent and more intensive questioning of a sub-set of the sample did not alter this opinion.[560] Other results from the same survey suggest that, all else being equal, there is a preference for more equally shared benefits;[561] that is, a smaller number of health years may be preferred when they are shared amongst a larger number of recipients.

The failure to take account of the distribution of benefits in economies is often justified by the argument that, in principle, benefits (money) may be redistributed after the event to compensate those who lose from an activity. This is often not possible in health care as health benefits cannot be traded or, even in principle, redistributed to those who lose.

More generally, it is not known exactly what ethical principles people wish to incorporate in the overall health sector and what price they are prepared to pay for these principles. A small number of economists has commenced investigation of these issues.[562,563] But to date these explorations have not proceeded very far. They have been concerned with the appropriate importance weights that should be given to different benefits in a micro-evaluation program. There has been no conceptual means suggested for determining how the value of equity should influence the decision regarding the overall level of health expenditure.

The second simplifying assumption is equally untenable. Various values exist depending upon who is asked and the perspective they are asked to adopt. Patient values are different from those of the general population and it is possible to argue that either group should be the appropriate judge of the value of public programs. Values differ when individuals are asked to trade-off the quantity and quality of life for others and for themselves.[564] Most obviously, if a willingness to pay criterion of a value is adopted, individuals will generally be willing to pay more for a health benefit that they receive personally than for a benefit received by an anonymous third party. The failure to distinguish these two sets of values is particularly obvious in the WTP literature where it is assumed that the WTP of an individual or the amount the individual is prepared to accept as compensation for personal risk is the appropriate basis for calculating the value of others i.e., the individual's valuation of themselves is not distinguished from the amount they would or should pay to assist an anonymous beneficiary.

The latter point is particularly important and highlights a potential conflict with the strong preference for egalitarianism noted above.

Health services in all Western countries have had a very large collectivist element in their financing and organisation, with European governments generally undertaking 75–85 per cent of total health expenditures. National schemes have also defined and limited the benefits available. Possibly because of the misperception that benefits are unlimited, populations have enthusiastically endorsed such schemes and, in particular, the egalitarian basis for the allocation of resources. If such collectivist values continue then there is a pressing need for the development of a method for evaluating the benefits of equity.

However, two factors place the collectivist approach to health under considerable pressure. First, rising health costs imply greater per capita transfers from the healthy wealthy to the unhealthy poor. At present few (outside government itself) appear to question the cross subsidy. As its magnitude grows, social generosity will be increasingly strained. Secondly, and as judged by the (modest) decline in the size of the government sector in most OECD countries, there has been a slow but steady decline in social generosity. This is particularly evident in Australia where (despite mythology to the contrary) the redistributive role of government is small by Western standards and where there has been constant pressure to scale back the government sector and the redistribution of income.

As noted earlier, tax as a percent of the GDP in Australia is the fifth lowest in the OECD.[534] Survey data from the Luxembourg study found that fewer Australians had their relative income changed more then one decile as a result of taxation and cash benefits than in any of the nine countries studied. (The range was from 8.3 per cent of Australians to 47 per cent of Swedes and Dutch for the general population and 2.3 per cent of Australians to 25 per cent of Swedes, for the economically active, [cited from Saunders, 1994]). Reinforcing this impression that Australians are rather less concerned with redistributing income than many, Saunders[565] reports that in 1994 the bottom quintile in Australia received a smaller share of gross family income than in any of the eight countries studied (including the USA): a similar result is reported in the World Development Report for 1996 with respect to the distribution of GDP.[566] In Saunders' study the Australian gini index (of overall inequality) at 0.4 was higher than any other country except the USA (0.41).

This discussion implies that at least two criteria are needed to determine the value of health interventions and the overall level of health expenditures. First, and to the extent to which decisions are still made collectively, it must be decided how individuals evaluate benefits to others (subject to the important caveat that the individual knows that he or she is a potential recipient of benefits). If a major part of the benefit arises from the satisfaction of having a collectivist approach and an equitable health system then this calculation may not be reducible to the evaluation of individual health outcomes. It is for these benefits that economists have not developed a satisfactory evaluation methodology. Yet, paradoxically, it is precisely this situation which is usually used to justify the use of CBA; that is to say, where social values are not simply the summation of the value of individual benefits (or where for technical reasons individual benefits cannot be expressed). This does not imply that CBA is of no potential use. Social values will heavily reflect individual benefits.

The twofold shortcoming of simple CBA as it is usually employed are, first that it does not include the benefits of collectivisation *per se* and that it employs a purely personal notion of value (i.e., what the individual would pay for their own benefits) to measure the value of benefits received by anonymous recipients. Secondly, and to the extent to which decisions are made individually and for the primary benefit of the individual, market principles should govern the evaluation of benefits and the level of expenditures. This does not imply that there should be a simple deregulated market (as the evidence suggests that such markets are very inefficient). It does imply that the value of health services and health outcomes will vary with individuals' incomes and their demand for health. The optimal level of health expenditure in a country will therefore depend on the extent to which it is decided to collectivise the health service, the extent to which there is a (large or small) 'window' for purely individual decision-making and the extent to which health outcome is valued differently under these two systems. Finally, if private markets remain technically inefficient then the optimal level of expenditure will reflect the amount that people are prepared to pay to achieve the personal benefits of a free market component in the system; viz, the reduced subsidy to the poor and unhealthy and the greater flexibility in the purchase of health services.

The way forward

At present we cannot determine the ideal level of health service expenditure or even whether this is above or below the present level. In part this is a result of the methodological problems discussed above and, in part, because of the poor information that is a prerequisite to sensible decision making. Data concerning direct health care costs are now relatively satisfactory. The issue of indirect costs remains problematical. However, as noted earlier the chief problems arise in the measurement of benefits: both tangible systemic benefits but, far more urgently, the benefits of direct interventions measured in medical terms (life years gained, pain alleviation, etc). It is difficult for a health service to determine optimal expenditure when the benefits of many expenditures are not even approximately known and best practice guidelines based upon current knowledge have not been developed or are not used. It is somewhat anomalous that there is such a large budget for medical research and yet so little is known about the most appropriate use of the research findings. This may reflect the common prejudice that evaluative research, and especially the evaluation of service delivery is, in some sense a 'softer'—less rigorous—and less worthy activity than research into the 'harder' sciences.

Information is a prerequisite to the determination of appropriate spending, but equally it is necessary to have incentives to generate and employ the information. This obvious fact suggests that the highest priority in the short run should be health system reform. There is ample evidence of both technical and allocative inefficiency in most health systems and it is a futile exercise to conduct even sophisticated CBA on services which are unnecessarily costly or which would not be provided in an allocatively efficient system. That is, the final decision concerning the inevitable trade-off between the value of life and the value of other benefits can be postponed while health benefits can be obtained at no cost by improved system efficiency.

The difficulty in assessing the various options in the health sector is so great that systemic reform cannot be based upon a model in which the individual consumer/patient is required to judge the options even when he or she is supported by the judgment of a self interested and narrowly focussed provider. To date, this approach has failed to achieve maximum health benefits from the resources made available. This implies an increased reliance upon some form of agency arrangement in which agents are required to inform, advise and/or negotiate and purchase on behalf of patients. The power imbalance between providers and even moderately large agents further suggests that reform will not rely on relatively deregulated and simple markets.

In broad terms there appear to be two chief options for reform. First, it is possible for a government service to attempt to introduce decentralised managed care through the introduction of a purchaser provider separation; i.e., by the creation of an internal market within the government service in which there is a heavy reliance upon contracts to achieve desired objectives.[567] Secondly, and the more radical option, it is possible to introduce competition between purchasing agents in a heavily regulated market; that is 'managed competition'. Efficiency is envisaged as being achieved by competition; equity through regulation and the provision of a risk related subsidy for individual members of competing schemes.[568] With the second option, managed care would be again likely to emerge as the most effective means of achieving allocative efficiency. With either option the era of professional dominance and passive government/private insurance would come to an end.

Conclusions

It is undoubtedly true that health expenditures should not expand until all possible benefits are exhausted. This conclusion must follow from the fact that our resources are scarce and that health expenditures have an opportunity cost. Greater health outlays imply fewer benefits somewhere else. The most fundamental principle of economics is that these competing benefits should be compared before committing resources to any task.

Beyond this self evident statement there is comparatively little we can say with any confidence about the optimal level of spending. It is not true that ageing or even the introduction of new and expensive technologies will inevitably precipitate a crisis. The impact of ageing will be comparatively modest and has already been accommodated in many developed countries. The overall level of health spending is very largely a matter of social choice. If it is believed that greater benefits are obtained through increased health, and specifically for the elderly, than are obtained from alternative uses of our resources, and if these benefits are obtained more efficiently inside than outside the health sector, then there is no reason why the health sector should not expand significantly. Similarly, it is untrue that governments cannot afford to finance these services through taxation. This is, once again, a matter of social and political choice. The reluctance to devote ever increasing sums of money to the health sector is at least in part a result of the limited evidence that substantial benefits will be obtained by further indiscriminate spending.

In principle, the optimal size of the health sector could be determined by the economic evaluation of the cost and benefits of each of the services provided. In practice, this exercise has encountered not only formidable practical problems, but serious conceptual difficulties in the measurement of benefits. The size of the optimal health sector depends largely upon the value placed upon these benefits, and the relationship between health expenditure and benefits is very poorly understood. In CUA the quality and quantity of life are combined into a single unit, the QALY or, more descriptively, the healthy year equivalent. The techniques for doing this are still evolving and CUA has, to date, had little impact upon the allocation of resources.

More intractable problems arise when an attempt is made to convert the value of QALYs into an equivalent number of dollars as is necessary if cost and benefits are to be compared. Current techniques are flawed. Underlying ethical issues are unresolved. Whose values should be used to make this decision? Which values or what mix of values are relevant? How should issues of equity and the distribution of health services affect total expenditures? Satisfactory answers to these questions have not been suggested; indeed, the importance of these issues is often not even recognised.

Fortuitously, there is no urgency in producing answers to these questions. It is not necessary to decide the final marginal trade-off between health and non-health expenditures while the health sector is as inefficient as suggested by the evidence. System reform has the potential for increasing both the quality and quantity of life without additional cost—without the loss of benefits elsewhere. However, as health system efficiency is improved it will become increasingly difficult to postpone the question of the dollar value of life and, following from this, the optimal level of health expenditure. In the meantime, it is appropriate that the greatest attention be devoted to the achievement of efficiency and the improvement of health at given cost.

REFERENCES

518.   Australian Institute of Health and Welfare. *Australia's health 1996*. Canberra: AGPS, 1996, p123.
519.   Australian Institute of Health and Welfare. *Health expenditure bulletin*. Canberra: AIHW, 1996, vol 12.
520.   Richardson J, Wallace R. *Health economics*. In: Gruen F (ed). *Surveys of Australian economics*. Sydney: George Allen & Unwin, vol 3, p125.
521.   OECD Data File, Nov. 1996. Paris: OECD.
522.   Oxley H, McFarlan M. *Health care reform: controlling spending and increasing efficiency*. Paris: OECD, 1994.
522a. Australian Institute of Health and Welfare, *Australia's Health 1996*, Canberra, AGPS.
523.   Newhouse JP. An iconoclast's view of health cost containment. *Health Affairs* Supplement 1993; pp152–171.
524.   Weisbrod RA. The health care quadrilemma: an essay on technological change, insurance, quality of care and cost. *J Economic Literature*, June 1991; 523–52.
525.   Fuchs V. The health sector's share of the GDP. *Science* 1990; 247: 534–8.
526.   Abel Smith B. The escalation of health care costs: how did we get there? In: *OECD health care reform: the will to change*. Paris: OECD, 1996.
527.   Manning W, Newhouse J, Duon N, Keeler E, Leibowitz A, Marquis M. Health insurance and the demand for medical care: evidence from a randomised experiment. *The American Economic Review* 1987; 77: 212–38.
528.   Richardson B, Richardson J. Health outcome with increasing doctor supply. In: Tatchell M (ed). *Economics and health*. Health research project, 1992, Canberra: ANU.
529.   Richardson J. The effects of consumer co-payments in medical care. National Health Strategy, background paper 5, Canberra, 1991.

530. Johnson P. Grey horizons: who pays for old age in the 21st century? *Australian Economic Review* 1996; 3rd quarter, pp261–71.
531. Newhouse, JP. An iconoclast's view of health cost containment, ibid.
532. Evans RB. Health care and the inevitability of resource allocation and rationing decisions. *J Amer Med Ass* 1983; 249: 16.
533. Ashby JL, Craig KL. Why do hospital costs continue to increase? *Health Affairs* 1992, Summer.
534. OECD Data File, 1995. Paris: OECD.
535. Saunders P. Unpackaging equity: wage incomes, disposable income and living standards. In: *The industry commission reference on equity, efficiency and welfare.* Commonwealth of Australia, 1996.
536. Evans RG, Stoddart GL. Producing health, consuming health care. In: Evans RG, Barer ML, Marmor TG (eds). *Why are some people healthy and not others, the determinants of health of populations?* New York: Aldine de Gruyter, 1994.
537. van der Ven PM. Market-oriented health are: reforms, trends and future options. *Social Science and Medicine* 1996; 5: 655–66.
538. Wilson R, Runciman W, Gibberd R, Harrison B, Newby L, Hamilton J. The quality in Australian health care study. *Med J Aust* 1995; 478: 458–71.
539. Bunker JP, Frazier HS, Mosteller F. Improving health: measuring effects of medical care. *Millbank Quarterly* 1989; 72: 225–58.
540. McKinley JB, McKinley SM, Beaglehole R. A review of the evidence concerning the impact of medical measures on recent mortality and morbidity in the USA. *Int J Health Sci* 1989; 19: 181–208.
541. Cochrance AL, Ledger AS, Moore F. Health service input and mortality output in developed countries. *J Epidemiology and Community Health* 1978; 32: 200–5.
542. Richardson B, Richardson J. Health outcome with increasing doctor supply. In: Tatchell M (ed). *Economics and health 1981.* Health Research Project, Australian National University.
543. Kim K, Moody PM. More resources, better health: a cross national perspective. *Social Sci and Medicine* 1992; 34: 837–42.
544. Drummond M, Stoddart G, Torrance G. *Methods for economic evaluation of health care programs.* Oxford: Oxford Medical Publications, 1987.
545. Richardson J. Economic assessment of health care: theory and practice. *The Aust Economic Review* 1991; 1st quarter, pp3–21.
546. Eddy DM. Oregon's methods: did cost-effectiveness analysis fail? *J Amer Med Assn* 1991; 266: 2135–41.
547. Haddorn DC. Setting health care priorities in Oregon: cost-effectiveness meets the rule of rescue. *J Amer Med Assn* 1991; 265: 2218–25.
548. Kaplan RM. Value judgement in the Oregon Medicaid experiment. *Medical Care* 1994; 32: 975–88.
549. Segal L, Richardson J. *Economic framework for allocative efficiency in the health sector. Australian Economic Review* 1994; 2nd quarter, pp89–98.
550. Segal L, Richardson J. *The disease-based allocative efficiency framework: lessons from its implementation.* Research report, Centre for Health Program Evaluation, Monash University, 1997.
551. Robinson JC. Philosophical origins of the economic evaluation of life. *Millbank Mem Fund Q* 1986; 64: 133–55.
552. Mushkin SJ. Health as in investment. *J Pol Economy* 1962; 70: 129–57.
553. Rice DP. *Estimating the cost of illness.* Washington, DC: US DHEW Public Health Service Publications, 1966, pp947–6.
554. Cooper BS, Rice DP. The economic cost of illness revisited. *Social Security Bulletin* 1976; 39: 21–36.
555. Mishan EJ. Evaluation of life and limb. *J Pol Economy* 1971; 79: 687–705.
556. Viscousi K. The value of risk to life and health. *J Economic Literature* 1993; 31: 1912–46.

557. Richardson J. Cost utility analysis: what should we measure? *Social Science and Medicine* 1994; 39: 7–22.
558. Schoemaker P. The expected utility model: its variants, purposes, evidence and limitations. *J Economic Literature* 1982; 20: 529–63.
559. NOAA (National Oceanic and Atmospheric Administration). Report of the NOAA Panel on contingent valuation. *Federal Register* 1993, 58: 4601–14.
560. Nord E, Richardson J, Street A, Kuhse H, Singer P. Who cares about cost: does economic analysis impose or reflect social values? *Health Policy* 1995; 34: 79–94.
561. Nord E, Richardson J, Kuhse H, Singer P. Maximising health benefits versus egalitarianism: an Australian survey of health issues. *Social Science and Medicine* 1995; 41: 1429–38.
562. Nord E, Street A, Kuhse H, Singer P. The significance of age and duration of effect in social evaluation of health care. *Health Care Analysis* 1996; 4: 103–11.
563. Williams A. Intergenerational equity: an exploration of the 'Fair Innings' argument. *Health Economics* 1997; 6, 2: 117–132.
564. Richardson J, Nord E. Perspective in the measurement of quality adjusted life years. *Medical Decision Making,* 1997, in press.
565. Saunders P. *Welfare and inequality. National and international perspectives on the Australian welfare state.* Cambridge: Cambridge University Press, 1994.
566. World Bank. *World Development Report 1996: from plan to market the international bank for reconstruction and development.* Washington, DC: The World Bank, 1996.
567. Jonnson B. Making sense of health care reform. In: OEC. *Health care reform: the will to change.* Paris: OECD, 1996.
568. Scotton R. Managed competition: issues for Australia. *Australian Health Review* 1995; 18: 82–104.

CHAPTER EIGHTEEN

Problems at the Beginning of Life

JOHN YU

'The Child is Father of the Man'[569]

To those who observe babies grow into children and then mature into young women and men, there is little doubt that a well nurtured and cherished baby provides the best chance of a healthy adult outcome, where self image and self esteem will contribute significantly to the achievement of an optimal potential for life.[570] The weight of evidence provides growing support for this, be it the availability of certain fatty acids in breast milk and later brain development, or longitudinal studies in child abuse with its emotional deprivation and calorie deprivation.[571]

The importance of the first years of life to the future health and wellbeing of all people inevitably focuses attention on the major issues of this time. It starts with the intervention of medical technology when conception fails to occur, it involves abortion in other circumstances involving unwanted pregnancy, and the costs of newborn care when things go wrong. In all these situations, emotions and religious dogma speak louder than facts and reasoned logic.

The same divisiveness is met in child abuse and neglect when we are unwilling to make judgments about allegations and accusations of unpalatable actions by people who look and behave, uncomfortably, like ourselves. The best interests of the child invariably suffer when we choose to look the other way.

Lastly, we might look at our own community's record on immunisation and the prevention of killer diseases in children dependent on our protection. We condone inaction and neglect, liking instead to talk about individual freedoms, at the same time assuaging our communal conscience by donating to the cost of vaccination programs in the developing world.

In-vitro fertilisation and abortion

Most governments, either in developing countries or the established industrialised world, are expressing concern about the cost of health care and especially the cost of hospital care. Advances in medical science and technology have allowed miraculous things to happen as everyday events in our referral tertiary care hospitals, but at a considerable cost premium to the health care system. Attempts to reduce management expenditure have seen the integration of many hospitals into networks or multi-unit conglomerates. Often this has placed women's and children's services together, functionally if not geographically, in an uncomfortable but best-fit compromise. It has resulted in in-vitro fertilisation (IVF) programs, abortion services and tertiary neonatal intensive care nurseries being part of the same organisation, sometimes physically juxtaposed, each consuming resources and contributing to a burgeoning expenditure bottom line in the annual financial statements of the organisation that espouses a common vision and mission.

As funds become harder to win from government or insurance companies, where is the common good best met, if indeed there is any agreement on what is the common good? Does the state have any obligation to provide services or subsidise costs of in-vitro fertilisation for married couples, same sex couples or single women who want to have a baby? IVF programs still result in higher than normal rates of multiple pregnancies which, in turn, increase the risks of neonatal morbidity and the need for neonatal intensive care (NIC) services. Logic demands that the costs of NIC must be factored into the costs of IVF, whether or not that IVF program cost were paid by the individual, an insurance company or the state. But we need to acknowledge that means testing, or any other assessment of the ability and hence the need to pay, is not a valid approach when considering social equity or the right to health and well-being in a community.

Whatever the circumstances of preceding events, there is little doubt in my mind that once a baby is conceived and born, contemporary society has a firm expectation that that baby will receive every care that the community can readily or even possibly provide.

If hospital resources are currently unable to meet the expectations and need of the community, then I would not give a priority to publicly funded IVF programs. I reach this position because I am unable to determine what criteria would be used in a gatekeeper system to control the entry of those for whom a publicly funded program is the only possible option of access to IVF. I concede considerable discomfort in the realisation that those who can afford a self-funded IVF program will gain the service and the chance of a much wanted child, while those who don't have the money or insurance, won't.

In a rational world, IVF programs and abortion programs taking place in the same building and provided by the same organisation, are an unacceptable anomaly, made worse by a neighbouring NIC unit costing thousands of dollars each day to keep a baby alive, albeit with the very best prospects of survival and later, a normal existence. But this is not a rational world, and the politics of a growing conservative electorate polarised on the one hand, by vociferous civil rights groups and on the other, a Christian lobby that seems to ignore the New Testament's tolerance and compassion, will ensure that a logical and balanced debate on these important social issues will not occur. Theology has never involved common sense.

In the state of New South Wales, the law provides for termination of pregnancy on medical indications which include the mental health of the mother. This, in practice, allows reasonable access to abortion for a multitude of reasons. In 1993–94 there were 17 532 terminations reported in the NSW Inpatient Statistics Collection as compared with 86 738 deliveries. Terminations are not required to be notified and terminations in private hospitals would rarely be included in the figures quoted, so that this figure can be confidently said to be a conservative estimate.

The most commonly recorded reasons for termination were concerns with finances, change in lifestyle, single parenthood and being too young.[572] Termination of pregnancy following the detection of a congenital anomaly is relatively infrequent, numbering only 150 in 1992. But again, notification is not compulsory and so this figure is also likely to be an under-estimate, but as most of these abortions will take place in referral centres, it is more likely to be accurate than total abortion statistics.

A metabolic defect is an infrequent indication for termination, and so the advent of gene therapy with replacement of deficient or missing enzymes in fetuses or newborn infants is unlikely to make much difference to the termination statistics, though this does not say that such an advance will not significantly change the outlook of babies with inborn errors of metabolism. It will represent an important milestone in man's ability to correct a naturally occurring abnormality.

Termination for a major structural congenital anomaly is more likely. Spina bifida is the most common of the neural tube defects with an incidence of 7.5 per 10 000 in 1982 followed by anencephaly at 5.9 per 10 000. After the introduction of ultrasound for *in utero* screening, the incidence fell to 4.7 per 10 000 and 1.8 per 10 000, respectively. This was before the widespread use of folic acid in women wishing to embark upon a pregnancy, and so most of the fall was attributed to therapeutic abortion.

Table 18.1 Cases of spina bifida, Australia[573]

	1982	1992
Incidence of spina bifida	7.5 per 10 000	4.7 per 10 000
Therapeutic abortions reported	0	45
Number of affected babies born	178	125

These figures show the reduction in the numbers of infants born with spina bifida and clearly demonstrate that the offering of a therapeutic abortion will not alone see the elimination of a major childhood disability. The promise of folate prophylaxis is much more hopeful in reducing this chronic disability.

In countries like Australia where people are allowed to make their own health decisions and where strongly held views are expressed by the Christian Churches and other religious leaders on the sanctity of life, therapeutic abortion will only marginally affect the incidence of congenital anomalies able to be detected early in pregnancy.

A similar story can be told about Down Syndrome or Trisomy 21. It is clear that a great many people in our society are not prepared to make judgments, or allow others to make judgments, on what is a worthwhile quality of life. This, in turn, means that many fetuses with diagnosed Trisomy 21 will proceed to term.

This is a decision for the community and for individual family units to make. Health professionals must provide the facts and as much information as the family can handle. Should a decision to abort be taken, then support must be provided both at the time of the termination and afterwards. Health professionals whose beliefs put them at odds with a family decision must be allowed to withdraw from care of the families without any sense of letting their patient or the team down. They, in turn, must respect the views of others which may differ from their own. Health care professionals must face the fact that they are not missionaries charged with promoting a particular view of life.

Our failure to date has been in providing ongoing support to the family, especially the mother who is at considerable risk of experiencing depression following the abortion. Post-natal depression is estimated to occur in 10–15 per cent of mothers and may persist for many months. The risks following abortion are greater and, as the abortion is often not widely known among the normal community support network of the mother, there is even greater risk of poor recognition, treatment and help.

In some cultures, the death of a baby poses problems of unreasoned blame, and in a multi-cultural society like Australia, these additional burdens for the woman should be appropriately explored and the necessary help initiated. Multiculturalism does not mean that we are all the same, but we are all equally vulnerable to hurt.

There will never be community consensus about abortion, and any society will depend heavily on their political leaders to provide humane and non-prescriptive options to people, without the fear of themselves being targeted during election times by extremists who espouse one cause or another. Unfortunately, contemporary politics is not rich with leaders.

Problems of the newborn

In 1994, Australia's Perinatal Mortality Rate was 8.0 per 1000 births, a middle ranking position among the developed nations.[574] This relatively poor performance becomes more alarming when one looks at a simple analysis of ethnic background, comparing indigenous Aboriginals and Torres Strait Islanders with other Australians.

The state of New South Wales showed in 1994 a low birth weight (2500 gms and less) incidence of 11.7 per cent with maternal Aboriginality, compared with 5.7 per cent in others.[575] A similar finding occurs with prematurity (37 weeks gestation and less) of 11.7 per cent and 6.3 per cent, respectively.[576] The perinatal mortality in Aboriginal babies is double that of non-Aboriginal babies.[577]

Prematurity and low birth weight both result in higher rates of perinatal death, ill health and subsequent disability.[578] It is likely that in a proportion of these small babies, an abnormal baby is the cause of the premature delivery or small size, but in the remaining pregnancies, some maternal factor, some medical condition or obstetrical complication, is important. Many are able to be diagnosed and treated.

In 1994, the NSW Health Department reported that 61 per cent of all New South Wales mothers and 64 per cent of Aboriginal mothers had no major medical condition or obstetrical complication during pregnancy.[579] This is surprising, and suggests that chronic medical problems may be unrecognised in these women, and that diminished wellness and poor health due to poor nutrition, poor hygiene, nonlife-threatening recurrent and chronic infection and infestation, together make a poor basis on which to embark upon a pregnancy.

The challenges of these conditions, and the problem of substance abuse, are very much greater than that of codifiable medical diseases, and less readily recognised. The response must cross many ministerial responsibilities and any solution will involve extraordinary complexity, and risk failure, unless there is government resolve to address the problem.

There has been a Council for Aboriginal Reconciliation established and a well publicised pair of decisions of the High Court of Australia (the Mabo and the Wik decisions) bearing upon Aboriginal rights to land in Australia. The Council has led Australia's debate on Aboriginal reconciliation. With the emergence of a politician (the Independent Member for Oxley) who has highlighted Aboriginal issues, the community is more aware of the problems and possibilities facing Aboriginal Australia than for many years.

Government leadership in finding a way through the multiple difficulties of giving Aboriginal Australians a fair share of the desirable lifestyle that the rest of Australia enjoys seems remote, unless there is a clear commitment by the community generally to fairness and equity for all Australians.

But I think it more likely that true consensus can be reached here than on the previously discussed issue of abortion. The argument will be between rural Australia facing growing financial hardship and big city Australia; between those paying taxes and those receiving social benefit support; between the retirees on fixed incomes and those more able to determine their own destinies. At least there can be some common ground for debate and some prospect of final consensus.

Neonatal intensive care

For most people, however, problems of neonates revolve around neonatal intensive care, the costs that it involves, and knowing when to stop taking extraordinary measures to keep a baby alive.

Health economists alone have no prospect of influencing expenditure in neonatal intensive care, so great is the emotional blackmail that can be exerted on governments when the life of a premature baby is threatened by lack of adequate resources. The only prospect of distributing neonatal services appropriately in logical networks lies in a coalition of clinicians, health bureaucrats and government who reach an agreement based on adequate but realistic funding. Sadly, local advocates will rarely place the public good ahead of parochial ambitions for a local hospital and area budget allocations.

The baby, and hence the community, is best served by the creation of a linked network of neonatal intensive care units of a size large enough to justify a group of expert neonatologists and nurses to sustain a reasonable roster, who can contribute to reasoned discussion, reach out and develop their unit and themselves, supported by a skilled and responsive transport system to retrieve babies from smaller units and to transfer babies needing specialised treatment not available locally.

For most NIC units, this means about six to eight ventilator beds and three neonatologists are required. It also means a consolidation and redistribution of existing resources, and in a democracy, this is easier said than done. Most parliamentary seats that can be won from opposing parties represent growing electorates in new population centres. These are the very areas where community resources, like schools and hospitals, are most valued and where birth rates are highest. Yet if it is politically expedient to establish two neonatal intensive care units in two different areas, each with fewer ventilator beds than optimal, then sadly the political need will invariably win out.

The argument for bigger units relates to their ability to develop and implement treatment guidelines that are not unreasonably influenced by individual idiosyncrasies or local medico-political imperatives. Local peer behaviour and peer evaluation are the best safeguards that health professionals can offer a community, but there have to be enough peers! The larger unit can offer a wider range of services and options for both the health professional and the family. The competence of the health team will engender confidence in the family and contribute to the best decision-making process and best outcome.

For most paediatric health workers, euthanasia is not an option, and euthanasia needs to be very clearly distinguished from treatment that is clearly designed to relieve pain and distress, irrespective of side effects, even those that may also shorten life or compromise life. It needs to be distinguished from withdrawing treatment that is reasonably seen as an extraordinary means of sustaining life. I speak of 'health workers' because this is not a decision taken by the doctor alone. The NICU nurse is a very knowledgeable and skilled professional who is very much concerned with carrying out the treatment, who spends shifts, if not days, with the baby and the family. Doctors come and go but the nurse is always there.

The consultant must include these nurses and junior medical colleagues in the discussion about treatment and likely outcomes. The support and involvement of social workers and spiritual or religious advisers are also essential in the decision-making process. Parents need to be involved as early as possible and their wishes, including their moral views, respected. But the best interests of the infant must be the paramount consideration.

It is often much easier not to embark on a course of treatment than to stop the treatment at some later date. A clear understanding by all parties about likely outcomes and the risks involved in any treatment should be established early when options in treatment remain theoretical considerations and more easily handled than during the emotions of an acute crisis. The question must always be how far to go. I can conceive of no situation where doing nothing is a serious option.

In situations of hopelessness, caring may involve just warmth and fluids or oxygen to minimise discomfort. The basic need to nurture an infant must be provided; it is not intellectually dishonest, it is a positive attempt to help the parents and family to have an experience and, later, memories of care and concern for the baby. It is a positive contribution to the later healing and grieving process for both the family and staff. Professional detachment was never meant to include ignoring discomfort or distress, whether that is physical or emotional. There can be healing without curing and when curing is not possible, healing and caring become even more important.

The cost of neonatal intensive care is high but its results in a variety of measures, such as quality adjusted life years (QALYs), are good and the reality of life is that the community, through its elected government, will demand that the services continue to be provided.

At-risk mothers

In many ways, the greatest challenge to the newborn infant is the 'at-risk' mother. The risk to the baby is not only physical abuse but involves the entire spectrum of child deprivation.

Of the eight Australian states and territories, six have mandatory notification of all suspected cases of child abuse. The Australian Capital Territory will introduce mandatory reporting in mid-1997, leaving Tasmania as the sole state not requiring this basic first step in protecting children and, as such, stands condemned by child advocacy lobbies, if not by all thinking Australians.

During the twelve months 1994–1995, 76 954 reports were made and with 88 per cent of reports finalised, 49 per cent of those found substantiated problems, representing 33 411 children in Australia.[580]

An analysis of this showed:

physical abuse	29 per cent
emotional abuse	28 per cent
sexual abuse	16 per cent
neglect	26 per cent

The gender distribution was marginally higher in boys for each of these types of abuse and neglect, except for sexual abuse where girls outnumbered boys 3:1.

In children with substantiated abuse or neglect, there was an over-representation of children from single female parent families (39 per cent) and from other than natural two-parent families, such as step-parent families (21 per cent). A more detailed study of the type of abuse and relationship of maltreating person showed that physical abuse represented the highest proportion of cases for foster parents, step parents and de facto parents.

The question is, of course, what can society do about an epidemic of child abuse in a cultural environment that is growing less support-ive of the socially disadvantaged who need welfare payments to sur-vive and a society that is blaming the unemployed for their inability to get jobs? Smaller government today means less welfare payments, fewer community workers and the promise of lower taxes.

Most of these challenges fall outside our ability to influence a gov-ernment intoxicated by a sense of fiscal responsibility, but this should not be a reason to stop advocacy for the needs of children and their role in our own society's future. A start must be made to change the pattern that has developed in recent times. In 1994–1995, abused chil-dren represented 8.5 per 1000 children or young people.[581]

Sir Michael Rutter (1996) talks of making children more resilient by promoting self esteem and self efficacy. This comes through secure, supportive personal relationships starting with a good mothering rela-tionship and a sense of being wanted, but also capable of being helped by relationships outside of the family.[582]

One way of achieving this is to identify at-risk mothers, preferably dur-ing pregnancy but certainly in the immediate post-partum period and providing advice and support for them during the first 6–12 months. We need to re-discover the Baby Health Nurse whose misguided demise two decades ago coincided with the social isolation of young mothers from their own family support when they were re-housed in distant housing estates as the cost of inner city property escalated.

It is not hard to recognise the at-risk factors of single parenthood, teen-age pregnancy, substance abuse, chronic illness and handicap, ethnic minority and poverty. A visit to these new mothers in hospital and regu-lar follow-up by a phone call or a home visit could provide the support and confidence that these mothers need to nurture their babies and if a significant number are supported in this way, could break the cycle of neglect by allowing the babies an experience of mothering and care.

In the state of New South Wales, this program could be initiated with $1.0M, or less than 0.1 per cent of the health budget. This would easily be repaid by subsequent savings in the health, community services, justice and corrective services budgets. The consequences to society would be even more worthwhile. Lobby groups for cancer, coronary care, women's and men's health programs gain political preferment, but who will speak up for the next generation of abused children? They don't vote!

Vaccine preventable diseases: parents' rights versus children's interests

Results from the Australian Bureau of Statistics (ABS) survey conducted in April 1995 show that the proportion of children fully immunised was relatively high in younger age groups but worryingly low in older age groups.[583]

At one year of age, 88 per cent were fully immunised against diphtheria and tetanus, but this dropped to 63 per cent for children aged two years and to 45 per cent for six-year-old children. The fall in coverage among older children was not evident for diseases like measles and mumps, for which there is an effective single dose vaccine. The comparative proportions fully immunised at two years of age for the following diseases were:

diphtheria/tetanus	63 per cent
pertussis	58 per cent
poliomyelitis	87 per cent
measles	92 per cent
mumps	90 per cent
rubella	81 per cent

The figure for haemophilus influenzae group B was 51 per cent, but this was omitted from consolidated figures because of its relatively recent introduction. It is anticipated that pertussis immunisation rates will improve with the introduction of the new acellular vaccines with their significantly lower complications.

In 1993–1994, there were 348 admissions to New South Wales hospitals where pertussis was the primary diagnosis. The highest hospitalisation rates were among the under-one-year-old age group (255.9 per 100 000 population) accounting for 64 per cent of all whooping cough admissions. This was followed by the one-year age group (26.9 per 100 000 population) and the 2–4 year age group at 13.7 per 100 000 population.[584] The youngest are the most vulnerable.

These immunisation rate figures show how poorly Australia is performing compared with other parts of the world. In 1992 the immunisation rates for triple antigen (diphtheria, tetanus and whooping cough) were:

China	94 per cent
India	97 per cent
Indonesia	90 per cent
Bangladesh	98 per cent
Vietnam	88 per cent

Only countries like Nigeria (45 per cent), Ethiopia (13 per cent), Zaire (32 per cent) and Myanmar (52 per cent) perform less well than developed Australia.[585]

These abysmal figures have led to the establishment of an Australian Childhood Immunisation Register from 1 January 1996 that will facilitate the follow-up of unimmunised children and the establishment of the Australian Centre for Immunisation Research at the New Children's Hospital at Westmead in Sydney. The National Register will be important, as the ABS survey in 1995 showed that where health cards or records were consulted, much better levels of immunisation were achieved.[586]

	Health card consulted	Health card not consulted
Fully immunised	72.3%	27.8%
Partly immunised	43.3%	56.7%
Not immunised	23.6%	76.4%

The pattern of where immunisations were obtained has gradually changed with more families using their general practitioner (63.3 per cent) rather than local council clinics (22.5 per cent) and baby health clinics (17.3 per cent). Hospitals and other health services provided for a further 4.6 per cent. The source of immunisation is important as some states of Australia are reducing specialised baby services in favour of more generic community health centres, where regular baby check-ups are less likely to take place.[587] Many local government authorities are also abandoning their immunisation services as they face rising costs and try to shift areas of expenditure to some alternative provider.

In the face of these trends, general practitioners need to be encouraged to take up the slack and to be given incentives to promote immunisation. One way would be to increase the reimbursement for immunisation services and provide a bonus at certain key milestones in the immunisation schedules. It seems a vain hope that area health services or local government authorities will allocate greater resources to the prevention of vaccine preventable diseases.

Before looking at how to encourage parents to immunise their children, we need to look at the characteristics of those families who do not immunise their children and the reasons they give for their negligence.

A higher proportion of children from two parent families was considered fully immunised against all diseases recommended on the current NH&MRC schedule than single parent families.[588] This difference between children of two parent and single parent families remained consistent when other variables, such as parental country of origin, work status and family income, were considered.

Language and comprehension seemed more important with new vaccine products. For example, immunisation rates against haemophilus influenzae B was 51.5 per cent in children from six months to six years where English was spoken at home, compared with 33.6 per cent in children from non-English speaking homes. This difference was less with established vaccines, for instance, diphtheria/tetanus was 69.3 per cent and 59.5 per cent, respectively, and rubella was 75.9 per cent and 70.7 per cent.[589]

Children from families with higher weekly incomes were also more likely to be fully immunised than those from lower weekly incomes.

The families of children from three months to six years who had not been immunised were asked the main reasons why immunisation had not been given. The answers for triple antigen were:

Advised against it	8.3 per cent
Concern about side effects	6.6 per cent
Hadn't heard of it	10.1 per cent
Hadn't got around to it	14.5 per cent
Opposed to vaccination	18.4 per cent
Sick when immunisation due	7.4 per cent
Too young	25.4 per cent

This study[590] showed that 31.3 per cent didn't want vaccination for some reason, while another 57.4 per cent were not opposed but for a variety of reasons did not have vaccination done.

The 57.4 per cent of families who did not have vaccination done but were not opposed to vaccination form the easier segment to win over, either by better information or better services. These families need to be provided with better information about immunisation and how to have it done at the time of birth, and followed up at the appropriate times by health staff specifically employed to do what might seem superficially an easy task. But a high proportion of these families is in need of other support and help. Many are the same target group that need support to ensure better baby nurturing and parenting and to prevent the threat of later child deprivation and abuse.

Much of the anti-vaccination lobby comprises misinformed health professionals who may see one or two complications, yet fail to appreciate the alternative greater dangers of the diseases that are being prevented. Perhaps it requires a situation where an affected child who has been denied vaccination is helped to sue the health professionals who gave the original advice.

Another financial incentive may be needed to help convince these families that they not only expose their children to these preventible diseases, but also expose their community to a level of susceptibility that makes others more vulnerable as 'herd' immunity falls and preventible diseases again appear.

If the community finds this unacceptable, then the question arises whether such families should benefit from payments like child endowment or a free school system. Perhaps the need to protect children should extend to withdrawing benefits from those who do not make their own contributions to the protection of the greater child population.

How much personal freedom can a family be allowed when that freedom risks the interests of other children, and old people in the community that the family lives within and whose benefits and community services that family enjoys.

There is a time when the interests of the individual child and the interests of a community must take precedence over the wishes of parents who take a decision that risks others, no matter how well meant the decision may be.

Advocacy for children

Our society is one that shows the most generous response to the needs of the children we know or about whom we are told. Individually they are loved and nurtured. Yet when the needs, interests and protection of children in general are discussed, there is an immediate defensiveness to ensure that those needs and interests do not encroach upon or challenge the individual rights and freedom of parents, guardians or other carers. It is assumed that the needs of children can be best met within the family, yet child abuse and neglect show us every day that the interests of the child and those of the family may not be the same. Not infrequently we find that children may need society to protect them from their family and when society fails the child, then the child's death or chronic incapacity are the result.

The disregard for the child's interest may assume many guises. Over ten years ago, regulations were introduced in New South Wales that forced adult passengers in taxi cabs to protect themselves by the compulsory wearing of seat restraints. After years of agitation, this regulation was extended by requiring taxi cabs to provide suitable safety restraints for small children and infants. Some taxi companies responded by refusing to carry small children as passengers. To me the scandal was not so much the delay in affording small children the same protection as adults, but that in the very beginning when safety restraints were first considered, children were forgotten and no provision for their safety was considered.

Time and again, governments have ignored the needs of children. When pharmaceutical companies apply to have their new drugs included in the Australian Pharmaceutical Benefits Scheme, they are required to provide exhaustive pharmacological data and therapeutic trial data. It is an expensive procedure. But there is no requirement to provide data about children and, as a result, many new drugs are not available for use in children. It does not seem unreasonable to require that children's data to be submitted for appropriate drugs within a reasonable time frame. There are few drugs used in medicine that do not have some role to play in treating children, no matter how infrequent that use may be.

In social security, a Commonwealth allowance is provided for the carers of the chronically ill and handicapped at home, but one needs to be sixteen years or older to be eligible for the allowance. Yet there are over 10 000 children and young people under the age of sixteen years who are the primary carers of parents and guardians, they are not eligible for the allowance but need it just as much if not more than those for whom the rules provide. These young carers are robbed of their childhood and youth as they provide for their families in need. Their burden is doubled by laws that ignore the child carer.

If these children and young people had a vote then there would be many reasons why their interest would be met by our elected representatives in Australia's parliaments and local government councils. There needs to be a coalition of concerned people who say, 'I care for kids and I vote.'

This, of course, will not solve all the problems faced by modern Australian society, but it is an affordable beginning for a new deal for children, starting when they are most vulnerable, in the first years of life.

REFERENCES

569. Wordsworth, William. Ode on the intimations of immortality from recollections of early childhood. In: Aldington R. (ed). *Poetry of the English speaking world*. London: William Heinemann, 1947, p510.
570. Martin HP, Beezley P. Behavioural observations and abused children. *Dev Med and Child Neurology* 1977; 19: 373–8.
571. Oates RK. *The spectrum of child abuse.* New York: Brunner/Mazel, 1996, p123.
572. Adelson PL. In: Frommer MS, Weisberg EA (eds). A survey of women seeking termination of pregnancy in NSW. *Med J Aust* 1995; 163: 419–22.
573. Neonatal Perinatal Statistics Unit, Australian Institute of Health, 1995.
574. Australian Bureau of Statistics. *1996 year book Australia no 78.* ABS catalogue no 131 010. Canberra: Australian Bureau of Statistics, 1996.

575. Rubin G. Mothers and babies. Chapter 3 in: *Health of the people of NSW— report of the Chief Health Officer*, NSW Health, Sydney, 1996.
576. Rubin G. Mothers and babies, ibid.
577. Rubin G. Mothers and babies, ibid.
578. Rubin G. Mothers and babies, ibid.
579. Rubin G. Mothers and babies, ibid.
580. Angus G, Hall G. *Child abuse and neglect in Australia 1994–95*, Australian Institute of Health and Welfare, Canberra, 1996.
581. Angus G, Hall G. *Child abuse and neglect in Australia 1994–95*, ibid.
582. Rutter M. *Protected children, protective families—a global task*. Proc of International Conference on Child Abuse and Neglect, Dublin, 1996.
583. Australian Bureau of Statistics. *Children's immunisation Australia*. ABS catalogue no 43 520. Canberra: Australian Bureau of Statistics, 1995.
584. Rubin G. Mothers and babies, ibid.
585. Australian Bureau of Statistics. *Children's immunisation Australia*, ibid.
586. Australian Bureau of Statistics. *Children's immunisation Australia*, ibid.
587. Australian Bureau of Statistics. *Children's immunisation Australia*, ibid.
588. Australian Bureau of Statistics. *Children's immunisation Australia*, ibid.
589. Australian Bureau of Statistics. *Children's immunisation Australia*, ibid.
590. Australian Bureau of Statistics. *Children's immunisation Australia*, ibid.

CHAPTER NINETEEN

Medicine at the End of Life

MALCOLM FISHER

The nature of death

'Death', said Herman Fiefel, 'is the ultimate thread that binds mankind'.[591] It is the one event that we can consistently predict will happen to everybody.

In the past, death was a natural event. It occurred as a result of accident, disease, or ageing, or, rarely, as punishment at the hands of the rulers. In most societies, death was not the end, but a part of the person continued in either a place of reward or of punishment, or the person was recycled; perhaps into a different species. There is only circumstantial evidence to support the existence of such a hereafter. Anecdotal tales of near death experiences and the work of mediums and spiritualists give support to, but do not validate, the concept which remains an issue of faith rather than fact. The cynic would argue that the promise of rewards for faith and goodness evolved as a means of social control. For many in the past, life had little in rewards or purpose. In a life of drudgery with little chance of acquiring tangible reward for toil, the prospect of equality and comfort in an afterlife was one that made one think twice about resistance or revolution. 'For God and England' was the patriotic cry before the poor gave their bodies to preserve a society, a fair share of whose goods they had no chance of receiving. The home was the desirable place of death.

In Western societies today, science's invasion into death culture has meant that death has become 'worthless and scary like something you flush from your house'.[592] Half of us no longer die at home but in hospitals with all their sterility of habit and emotion. We die of a disease. Old age is not recognised in disease classification systems as a cause of death.

This is not true of all societies, particularly the less affluent. In Western Samoa, for example, the loved one is taken from hospital to die, and buried on the family land as opposed to the institutionalised cemeteries of Western society.

At the other end of the spectrum are the cryogenecists who resuscitate the dead body and then freeze either the body or the brain in the belief that future technology will allow the individual to live again.[593] This group is regarded as lunatic by some, but by others no more lunatic than Magellan setting forth into unchartered seas.

Fifty-three million residents of Planet Earth die each year. A third die of infectious diseases. Four million children die of lung infections and 3 million people die of gastroenteritis and tuberculosis.[594] There are now millions infected by the HIV virus and AIDS related disease is the commonest cause of death in some African countries.[595] In Western societies the causes of death are different. In the USA the main reasons people fail to reach the age of 80 are accidents, homicide, suicide and cirrhosis.[596] In Australia the main reasons are cardiovascular disease, cancer, and accidents.[597] The closest correlation to life expectancy amongst countries is gross domestic product. In the least developed countries life expectancy is 52 years, in developing countries it is 64 years and in the most developed countries it is 77 years.[594]

Across individual countries, even the most seemingly egalitarian, life expectancy is a function of social status and affluence. The manual worker is four times more likely to die in a motor vehicle accident than the business executive.[598] Health, like all of societies attributes, is not fairly distributed. But it is fairer today than it has ever been in the past.

Disease is one of Nature's ways of endeavouring to see that there are not too many people for the environment to support. Crowding leads to animals, including man, becoming short of food and malnourished, which predisposes them to disease, and to death from infection and to turning on one another.[599] The converse also applies: damage to the environment is an inevitable consequence of disease control.

Disease control increases longevity in the populace but has important social consequences as the number of unproductive people increases and they develop new diseases which impose a cost for society to manage. Further, as people live longer more people require assistance. Medicine, housing, water management, peace and road safety all change the main causes of death in a society. But mortality remains at 100 per cent. The Earth could not survive if it were otherwise.

In past times the medical and nursing professions had a major role in easing the passage of their patients from life to death. Indeed, it was one of the few things they could do effectively in the era before antibiotics, vaccination, and anaesthesia. James Robertson notes that not until the decade between 1910 and 1920 was an encounter between doctor and patient more likely to benefit than harm the patient.[600] And he further notes that as doctors' ability to treat effectively has risen, public esteem has fallen.

Progress in the twentieth century led to an unprecedented number of people having a more reasonable life. As they valued their existence more, the rules which allowed the state control over their lives changed. Justice evolved to where the state could use death as a punishment only for serious crimes such as murder or treason, and a 'fair trial' was mandatory prior to execution. Many countries banned the death penalty altogether leaving the state with waging war as its sole means of killing its citizens. The people began to resist war, from the savagely treated conscientious objectors of the First World War to the protesters against the Vietnam War. It is doubtful that a Western society will ever allow the sending of conscripts to war again. Life has become more valuable.

The impact of technology

After the Second World War, technology produced major changes in the ability of the medical profession to cure illness and prolong life. And changes in society meant that fair access for all to this technology was preached as a basic right. Health insurance, particularly employers insuring their workers in the USA, meant that many people in low income groups, gained the ability to pay for the level of health care only traditionally available to the rich, and as more people gained access to health care doctors' incomes and government costs increased.[601]

In the polio epidemic of the 1950s a major advance occurred. Doctors learned that if the patient's breathing was supported, nature would heal some of the patients. The breathing was supported by armies of medical students giving round the clock artificial ventilation on some cases, the iron lung which the patient lived inside in others. But the most successful technology was the ventilator to which the patient was connected by a tube, and was driven by gas or electricity.[602] Its application in polio was followed by its use in barbiturate self poisoning and then tetanus where the mortality went from 90 per cent to almost zero in Western Countries. The mortality from chest injuries fell by 50 per cent.[603]

The biggest impact of the ventilator was what it made possible. For when a patient's breathing could be supported during and after prolonged anaesthesia and surgery, surgical options increased. The addition of drugs to support the failing heart, and then cardiopulmonary bypass so the heart could be temporarily stopped altogether further extended the range of things which medicine could treat. And the wisdom with which the technology was applied did not keep pace with the technology. Medicine averted its eyes from the biological fact of mortality and focussed its attention on the causes of death, fostering the illusions that conquering disease would eliminate rather than change mortality and that death from disease is intolerable.[604]

In other words, Medicine lost the plot.

The departure of medicine from the compassionate care of the dying was fuelled by methods of remuneration for doctors. Doctors were paid for doing things to people. Procedures were more rewarding financially than compassion. Prolonging a patient's life was a continuing source of revenue. Time spent in dealing with families was non-remunerated time.

Three important things became apparent. The first was that the new technology gave doctors the power and skills to prolong life when there was little chance of meaningful recovery. The second was that much of the high technology medicine changed the cause of death but did not improve the overall mortality rate in societies. This remained, not surprisingly, at 100 per cent. The options for an individual to survive to old age still depended more on hygiene and wealth than anything medicine could offer, but medicine did offer more chance of an individual surviving, either well or impaired, than in the past.

The third thing was that there were diminishing returns in using the new options available in medicine. Each new advance produced a lesser improvement in outcome than its predecessor and usually cost more. Right across society, manufacturing and industry deserted the concept of doing it better for less, finding that an affluent society was prepared to pay more for a better television or drug. Medicine, embracing technology that was costing more, improving outcomes less, and available to all members of a society who were increasingly demanding that the state provide the things that traditionally were provided by the family or the insurer, had created a monster.

It was not that doctors were bad or cruel. They were seduced by technology, prospects of cure, and autonomy. Death became a medicalised process rather than a social event. As Ivan Illich said in 1975, 'Death is the ultimate rejection of medical consumerism.'[605] The changing manner of death seemed to increase the problems people experienced in coping with death of their loved ones and led to new specialties such as thanatology and support workers such as bereavement counsellors. Whether the changing ways of dying predicated the need for such support services or whether this was an unrecognised need in times when self sufficiency was more highly regarded is unknown.

Where the new technologies, drugs, and surgical procedures fitted in medicine could only be established by trying them on people. Complex mechanisms were set up to study them in a scientific, ethical, and fair manner. A patient who died was now a failure and could be the subject of litigation. The concept of a person whose time had come dying peacefully at home surrounded by loved ones was no longer acceptable. Death was no longer an event. Death became a process, and often a slow and painful process.

Just how much doctors lost the plot in caring for the dying was shown in the Support study in the USA which was published in 1995. In this study a series of hospitals was provided with a support team to point out the chances of patients dying to the doctors caring for them and to write in the notes if patients had unanswered questions or wished to discuss the appropriateness of their care. It made no difference to the doctors' behaviour.[606]

In 1996 Elisabeth Hansoi wrote a letter to Annals of Internal Medicine[607] about the care of her mother who had a dense stroke which left her right side irreversibly paralysed. A tracheal tube connected her to a ventilator which enabled her to breathe but took away her ability to speak. She had clearly expressed a wish to her personal doctor and daughter that she did not wish to have this sort of treatment and spent five days endeavouring to remove herself from the lines and ventilator until she had to be tied up. She was 87. Her daughter battled with doctors for five days before she was allowed to die. Some of the doctors actively fought her. And she wrote of the feelings of powerlessness when challenging the discipline that she felt the doctors, trained to cure, could not accept. It should be noted that the medical evidence in such cases is that the treatment given would not improve the patient's chances of survival.

The intrusion of lawyers into this process added to its inhumanity. A hospital's legally driven refusal to consider withdrawing care, led the father of 15 month old Samuel Linares, who was in a persistent vegetative state, to hold medical staff at bay with a gun to prevent them from resuscitating his son after Mr Linnares had personally disconnected the ventilator. The doctors agreed that continuing care was inappropriate.[608] In 1996 Asch published a study suggesting that nurses in intensive care units were killing patients covertly.[609]

Such studies are all evidence of the atrocities that may occur when doctors are not realistic about the appropriate care of the dying, and show the reactions of people frustrated by medical ignorance and power, and not involved or empowered to be involved in end of life decisions.

But there are good stories as well.

Jennifer, a 16 year old healthy girl, developed viral encephalitis that made her ventilator-dependent and comatose. She was seen by a number of specialists from a number of hospitals and all agreed that it could not be said accurately whether she would ever improve. All agreed, however, that they had never seen anyone who had not made a major improvement within six months return to useful function. A plan was instituted with Jennifer's parents that she would be kept ventilated for six months then go to an ordinary ward without the ventilator. A few days before the discharge was due she was weaned from the ventilator and at 6 months she was discharged with an agreement that she was not to return to intensive care. Over the subsequent three months she returned to close to normal. The cost of her illness was approximately $A250 000. Few would begrudge this to a 16 year old girl in an affluent society. But if she had been significantly impaired or had died, which the odds favoured, it would have been regarded as money wasted. And a similar amount could have prevented 12 000 African children from dying of malnutrition.

How much society is prepared to pay for the life of a sick individual is a serious and important issue distinguished by its lack of easy answers.

The provision of expensive care with little chance of a favourable outcome has important implications for society, as such care must be paid for and may preclude us being able to fund more cost effective programs in health care, or even things apparently more valued by our political masters (such as ensuring we had sufficient politicians and staff in Atlanta to receive the Olympic flag, or that our Prime Minister spent money refurbishing Kirribilli House as his home). It is, however, perceived by politicians as political suicide to say publicly that we want to spend less on health and that we do not want to spend money on high risk expensive treatment. So politicians employ covert rationing by speaking of inappropriate use of resources and have recently adopted the slash and burn managerialism of industry and applied it to health care.

The doctor, who has traditionally dealt with individual rather than societal problems, believes the government should be honest, say what it does not wish to fund, and take the consequences. The government wishes to manoeuvre the doctor into the position of gatekeeper. So far no Western societies have shown a way to get the two groups to combine to produce a medical system that is appropriate, affordable, universal, moral and accountable to the taxpayers who fund it.[610]

Medicine and dying

Medicine has valid options available to it today to use in caring for the family unit of the dying patient. These options can be pursued without fear of prosecution, or discipline by medical boards.

Western societies emphasise the right of patients to participate in decisions regarding their treatment and their right to refuse treatment. There must be proper informed consent before any treatment can be started.

When patients are not able to give informed consent our society may permit either a legally appointed representative or ask a guardian to decide in the patient's interest what is appropriate, or, more commonly, it uses an informal process. This involves doctors and relatives or loved ones who attempt together to ascertain what the patient would want if the patient could participate in the decision. Rarely, patients will be referred to an ethics committee to decide what is appropriate, but many ethicists believe the decision about care for individual patients is inappropriate material for ethics committees' discussion.[611]

The living will or advance directive is becoming more common and is given legal validity in some countries. In practice, it is little help to the decision makers as it depends on the words 'no hope of meaningful survival'. The patient's wishes in situations where there may be a five per cent chance of survival or a 5 per cent disability remains. Where the wording is 'no reasonable chance' the interpretation of the patient's wishes becomes even more difficult. What is 'reasonable' is an emotive judgment.

The withholding of treatment from a patient who competently demonstrates no wish to receive the treatment is regarded as the patient's right, even when death is an inevitable consequence. Intervention by authorities has only occurred when the refusal of treatment may affect the life of another, such as the unborn child.

The right to refuse treatment by proxy or to have others decide that you would not wish treatment is more complex. Society accepts the wishes of a Jehovah's Witness to refuse blood, and the assumption that if a patient not capable of being involved in a discussion is a Jehovah's Witness that the patient would not wish to receive blood. But the right of the Jehovah's Witness to make a decision that blood be withheld in a child, or even that child to make such a decision is not granted in some societies. And yet parental decision about withholding treatment in children is usually honoured by the medical profession. But the rights of surrogates and parents in reality are often dependent on how many other people share their view. As beliefs diverge from the mainstream they are more likely to be overridden by doctors or the law.

Our society also condones the use of 'double effect' drugs. This means that a suffering patient who has no chance of survival or refuses treatment may be given whatever amount of drug it takes to control their pain and suffering even if such treatment shortens life. The patient is deemed to have died of their disease and if pain control is achieved it is regarded as good medicine.

Society also appears to accept the concept that withdrawing ventilators or drugs which are maintaining life in the absence of any chance of an outcome acceptable to the patient is allowable. Often this type of treatment involves moving into grey areas which cloud the difference between killing and letting die. For example, a quadriplegic patient who is unable to move or breathe and will never be able to function independently or feed or clean herself may not wish to continue such an existence. It is usual to sedate such patients so they will not be aware of the disturbing effects of lack of oxygen and remove the ventilator so the patient dies peacefully in 15 to 20 minutes. This action is justified on the basis of the patient refusing treatment and the treatment having no chance of an acceptable outcome. But there is no doubt that the act of removing the ventilator will lead to death. Whether the death is due to the disease or the act becomes an important distinction, emphasising the difficulty in determining the difference between killing and letting die. Society and the law accept the latter but not the former. There is disagreement on this dilemma between ethicists,[612] but the acceptance by society carries greater weight than these, often academic, opinions.

The hypothetical scenario may be taken further. The quadriplegic with a head injury has an illness from which rehabilitation is not possible. That the treatment will not influence the outcome is not in question, but it is now no longer possible for the patient to refuse the treatment. The discussion between health care worker and family is fraught with ethical hazard. Everyone in the discussion may be disadvantaged by allowing the patient to continue to survive. The doctor needs the bed for another patient, the family cannot be unbiased if it has clearly been explained to them the devastating consequences that will occur to their lives if it is decided to send the patient home in their care. If the patient is compensable because the injury occurred at work or while as a passenger in a car, or if the patient has health insurance, financial resources are available to help the family keep the patient clean, comfortable and alive. If the patient has no such backup the persistence of futile care will provide an enormous emotional and financial burden to the family.

A new set of dilemmas occurs if a patient who is quadriplegic decides that he or she wishes to continue to live. In New South Wales there are very limited resources for such ventilator dependent patients. The patient will require a bed in intensive care and then the spinal injuries unit indefinitely, a bed which may have been used to save the life of a patient with potentially reversible disease. The patient will have a devastating effect on the lives of those who love and care for him or her, and one could legitimately ask what right has the patient to put self interest before the lives of others. And the economic demands the patient makes diverts money from more cost effective pursuits. A similar economic dilemma is posed by the Jehovah's Witness. Skilled physicians and nurses may nurture the Jehovah's Witness through a major illness without using blood or blood products, but this may be at a cost 10 to 15 times greater than treating the same illness with blood products. Does an individual's religious belief entitle that person to use a greater slice of the health dollar?

Then there is the dilemma faced by the decision makers with respect to the validity of outcome prediction. While a range of tools is used to predict outcome, they are only reliable for groups and not individuals.[613]

Mr JD was a 65 year old retired diplomat and an ex-president of a voluntary euthanasia society. He entered hospital with a severe 'mystery illness' and required artificial ventilation, dialysis and massive doses of drugs to support his heart. On the first day his living will was delivered to the doctors which clearly stated he did not wish to be treated if there was no hope of survival. Over the ensuing seven days he deteriorated. The drugs needed to support his heart caused gangrene of his toes and were producing a lack of oxygen to his bowel which looked as though it was dying at laparotomy. His wife delivered a letter asking the doctors to cease treating him and stating that he wished his body to be left to medical science. Of four scientific tools used to predict outcome one gave him a 3 per cent chance of survival and three others no chance.

The doctors caring for him all believed his request was reasonable except one who argued that we could not say there was no hope unless we knew what was wrong and that his living will clearly stated 'no hope'. The dissenting doctor spoke to the patient's wife and said he was uncomfortable with withdrawing care, although his colleagues believed him incorrect. He guaranteed that the patient would feel no physical or mental discomfort, and asked for another 48 hours after which he would be comfortable to withdraw life support if there was no improvement. If there was any deterioration there would be no escalation of treatment and the patient would be allowed to die.

The wife acquiesced. In 48 hours there were minor improvements and it was agreed to persist another 48 hours. Over this period there were marked improvements and now three doctors felt the patient had a chance. He is alive and well six years later.

The problems encountered by doctors facing a patient who cannot say what he wants or is suffering to such a degree that the doctors cannot be sure his requests are rational, are immense. If there was a 10 per cent chance of full recovery what would be his wish? Or what would be his wish if there was a 10 per cent chance of a recovery with blindness or paraplegia? Or both? Many who have either condition live meaningful and happy lives. The burden of such decision-making lies in its uncertainty. Acting on a decision to withdraw care leads to death. The need to feel confident about the validity of the decision is great. The decision to persist is easier as there is a preserved option to change one's mind later.

The relatives, without experience of similar patients or knowledge of medicine, medical decision making, or the science of prediction, face an even greater dilemma if the doctors cannot honestly say there is absolutely no chance. They read in the press and see on the TV a number of miracles. Surely their loved one may be the one and how can we abandon her. If there is only a 5 per cent chance how do we know that Aunty Belle will not be in the 5 per cent group?

In the absence of information as to the patient's wishes, the fallback position is even more fraught with ethical compromise. In practice the decisions are based on what the stakeholders believe a reasonable person would wish.

In seriously ill patients most tools used to predict outcome are only right 80 per cent of the time on day one. The only redeeming way of dealing with these inaccuracies is collective medical wisdom. The opinions of all doctors involved must be that there is no reasonable chance of an acceptable outcome before treatment is withdrawn. One important practical objection to the solo euthanasia practitioners is that the soloist deprives the patient of access to the benefits of collective wisdom.

The move by health professions to improve care of the dying began after the technological invasion of the process. Specialised hospitals, called hospices, are provided in many societies with varying degrees of success. Out of these places a new medical speciality called palliative care, which deals with the needs of the dying, has arisen. And the medical literature is full of debate on how to restore appropriate care of the dying.

We are relearning the processes addressed by GK Dunstan in 1985.

> An intensive care unit should not be judged by the statistics of survival as though each death was a failure. We should judge it rather by the quality of survival of those who survive, the quality of the dying

of those in whose best interests it is to die, and the quality of the relationships involved in each death.[614]

That the process of change is slow is more an index of how today even powerful people cannot act independently in a society with diverse ethical, moral and religious culture, than a desire to perform better.

Killing and letting die

The societal licence to withdraw treatment given to the medical profession is dependent on a perceived difference between killing and letting die. Some ethicists argue that this distinction is invalid and cruel. Allowing death by withdrawing care is a slower and sometimes more painful process than a speedy injection for euthanasia and asserted by some to be therefore less humane. The consequentialist ethicists maintain the end is the same and whether the person involved achieves the end by withdrawing something or being active is of no consequence. Others argue that there are major differences between doing harmful things and not performing beneficial things.

There is no question that the distinction between the actual acts of killing and letting die may blur on occasions and be vastly different on others. The quadriplegic patient who will be continually unable to move and attached to a breathing machine may not wish to live in this manner and ask that the treatment be withdrawn. To continue the treatment would be regarded by most as an infringement of the patient's autonomy and right to refuse treatment. The doctor who removes the ventilator has the intent of fulfilling the patient's wishes, but death is an inevitable consequence.

In contrast, the patient racked with pain from disseminated cancer who has a cardiac arrest and is not resuscitated is a more clearcut difference: indeed this patient has died and although it may be possible to bring the patient back to a wretched existence, accepting death is obviously different from applying extraordinary treatment to allow the patient a few more days of suffering.

In the end, the important thing is that our society seems to accept a difference, and thus gives the medical profession a solution to the problem of caring appropriately for most fellow humans in whose best interests it is to die. Passive euthanasia has not attracted the interests of either the courts or special interest groups. But there are still those who wish to die in whom there is nothing that can be stopped that will lead to death. To help these people die peacefully in accordance with their wishes would require active euthanasia.

Active euthanasia

Active voluntary euthanasia is an act upon a patient at the patient's request which will lead to the death of the patient. The intent to end life is greater than the intent to relieve suffering. It is illegal in every Western society and has been found unacceptable by government consensus in the USA, England, and Canada.[615,616] It is ethically different from instituting therapy which relieves suffering even if such therapy shortens life.

Euthanasia is probably being practised more now than in the past, and it is generally believed in the United States that partner euthanasia (not involving doctors) is more common because of the medical profession being legally restricted from helping. If euthanasia is being practised and is acceptable to society there is a reasonable argument that it should be controlled by legislation, in spite of arguments (see below) that the law is a poor tool for dealing with abstract concepts like suffering or dignity, and laws that permit taking of another's life have potential for abuse. That potential may be greater than if there are no laws regulating dying at all.

Antagonists argue that good care of the dying will almost eliminate the need for euthanasia and quote data that most people who wish to die have clinical depression, the treatment of which will lead to a change of mind. But even if the care of the dying were done well there is a small group of patients whom medicine cannot fix and whose suffering or potential for future suffering, when they cannot control the situation, makes death the most acceptable alternative to them. Some believe it is illogical to consider that painful suffering can be treated but suffering which is not interpreted as pain cannot. Thus the treatment of this group of patients appropriately and legally cannot be done without allowing euthanasia. This group includes patients with diseases like AIDS and muscular dystrophies whose absence of physical pain makes the provision of assisted death, that is legally acceptable, difficult. These people are unable to take their own lives. The dilemma of individual versus society reemerges.

Cassell believes that pain and suffering are different and that it is purposeless suffering that is unacceptable.[617] When suffering occurs there is a threat to the integrity of the person that continues if the person cannot be made whole. In our practice in Australia it is apparent most people fear suffering and pain and how they will react to them more than they fear death. Callahan emphasises that fear of dying alone is a greater fear than death itself.[618]

Where the combatants in the euthanasia debate disagree, their differences lie in simple questions. Will the introduction of laws which allow the taking of life on request do more harm than good, or will those advantaged by the laws be of greater numbers than those disadvantaged? And the second question is that if one person is disadvantaged are the laws acceptable?

The arguments become emotive and are usually based on 'hard case' scenarios. The protagonists of euthanasia paint pictures of patients for whom it is difficult for a fair minded and compassionate person to say euthanasia would not be a good thing. The antagonists' hard case scenarios involve patients whose relatives coerce them into seeking death, and the patient whose depression was not treated. They may invoke the spectre of Nazi Germany, pointing out that the holocaust began with the mentally ill, was condoned by doctors and worked on the basis of devaluing the lives of other human beings, starting with little things. The advocates argue that the excesses of Germany are very unlikely to occur in Australia in the 1990s. The protagonists of euthanasia point out that Dutch society has not crumbled because of euthanasia and the antagonists point out publications emanating from Holland (some emotive and some not) suggesting voluntary euthanasia leads to involuntary and financial euthanasia, the latter being where people are killed because of the cost of their treatment, or are coerced into seeking euthanasia. Such events probably occur and return us to the more good or harm arguments. The advocates of euthanasia suggest that its misuse emphasises the need for laws and regulations and does not support a no euthanasia argument.

In reality the covert practice of euthanasia is unlikely to be influenced by legislation. Doctors and patients make decisions in private and act in private. As Callahan says:

> Short of putting a policeman in every doctor's office, there is no possible way of knowing what doctors and patients decide to do except insofar as they are willing to make that known. It is a mistake to believe otherwise.[618]

The question the antagonists have no answer for is what our society should do about those in whom there are legal and cultural barriers to assisting death by the only effective means: voluntary euthanasia or assisted suicide. Such people must often die alone and clandestinely when they should die with those they love around them and be cared for up to the moment of death.

The weakest argument of the pro euthanasia group is that euthanasia will have no downside for other members of society, but the reality of the downside is difficult to forsee in an individual society.

Assisted suicide

As an alternative to euthanasia, the decriminalising of assisted suicide is favoured by some. In assisted suicide the patient commits suicide and friends and loved ones or doctors may help in ways such as advising as to the means, providing the means, or even placing the tablets on the disabled patient's tongue so they can be swallowed. Suicide *per se* is not an illegal act. Thus to assist in suicide seems logically an inappropriate act to be labelled a crime. At present a disabled patient who wishes to end their life must dismiss the loved ones and die alone which is not in keeping with any concept of an appropriate and peaceful death. Assisted suicide removes from the scenario the perceived but very questionable right to ask another to kill you. The responsibility for the act of ending life returns to the patient and is a better example of autonomy than euthanasia. Many objectors to euthanasia have no such objection to assisted suicide.

Assisted suicide seems more acceptable than euthanasia legally. Dr Jack Kevorkian, the celebrated USA doctor who has been tried unsuccessfully on a number of occasions is a provider of the means to commit suicide rather than a provider of euthanasia. In 1996, in NSW, a lay person was convicted of assisting a close friend with AIDS to die and given a suspended sentence. Bob Dent, the first person to use the Rights of the Terminally Ill Act in the Northern Territory of Australia, actually used assisted suicide.

The main objections to assisted suicide are the uncertainty, incidence of treatable depression in people who wish to die, possibility of coercion and the consequences of society relaxing standards of the way human life is valued.

Requests for inappropriate treatment

At the other end of the scale the doctor has the dilemma of dealing with the requests of patients or families for treatment which has little or no chance of being successful. In most countries in the world it is accepted that there is no ethical or legal obligation for a doctor to institute or continue treatment which is in accord with the relatives wishes but not the patient's, or unlikely to influence the ultimate outcome. In the United States, this situation is different as individual court cases have led to doctors being legally forced to continue inappropriate care at the families' request. In Australia a case has been made for doctors over-riding the wishes of patients and families when such requests are made and the situation cannot be resolved by negotiation.[613]

Brain death

The introduction of organ transplantation led to the concept of brain death. Previously, death was defined by cessation of breathing or heartbeat. Initially organ removal teams waited until the heart stopped after a ventilator was discontinued, but convenience and the demonstration that better organs were procured if the heart was beating led to the institution of legal and medical guidelines for brain death. This may be clinical or radiological. Radiologically, an absence of cerebral blood flow is the diagnostic criterion for death. Clinically, the absence of reacting pupils, cessation of breathing, absence of blink and cough reflexes lead to a declaration made by one or more doctors at one or more times (depending on local rules) that the patient is legally dead, although the heart remains beating.[619]

The time of death is recorded. The family is informed and consent for organ donation requested. If the correct procedure is followed it is certain that no-one has ever recovered from the state in which death has been diagnosed, in spite of 'The Doctors Said I was Dead' headlines. Recent work has shown that the clinical diagnosis of brain death may not be associated with 'irreversible cessation of all brain function' and some minor functions may persist. This has led to conflict among philosophers and between ethicist and doctor. The procedures in Australia have not been changed in response to this conflict. The transplant program has led to other dilemmas in dying. In the beginning, the needs of consenting families were ill-defined and inevitably not well managed. The family may have great difficulty in accepting that a loved one whose heart is beating and whose skin is pink and warm is now dead when they looked exactly the same and were alive minutes before. The process of decay which begins within minutes of the cessation of heartbeat in a 'conventional' death does not begin in the brain dead patient until the heart beat ceases.

The continuing shortage of organs for transplantation has led to other assaults upon the cultural processes occurring after death, including the removal of organs immediately upon death from patients in hospital and prisoners immediately after execution.

In the United Kingdom, patients who have died have been resuscitated until organ transplants can be arranged, then had their organs harvested and been allowed to die again. It has been suggested that the wishes of a patient to be an organ donor, when documented, should over-ride family wishes. While this is ethically sound, appropriate care of the dying patient involves care of the family unit and most doctors would honour the family's wishes at the expense of the patient's in the interests of harmony and conflict prevention. It has also been suggested that unless a patient had specifically stated they did not wish to be a donor then organs should be available, an extension of the 'reasonable person' test.

The role of the law

Our society is a regulated one. We value freedom but only up to a point. We regulate actions that may hurt others or their property, physically or financially.

Our laws are made by government and interpreted by judges. Access to the law is expensive and only for the very rich, the very poor, or the citizen bold enough to risk all for justice. In an adversarial legal system the courts are about winning and losing under rules designed to see fair play for both sides. However, the outcomes may not reflect truth and justice but that the rules of the game are more important than a just outcome. 'Justice?' said William Gaddis. 'You get justice in the next world; in this world you have the law.'[620]

In the USA there is an increasing tendency to attempt to resolve the dilemmas about dying using a judicial approach. The extraordinarily foolish outcomes that arise in many of these cases illustrate the impropriety of attempting to apply adversarial legal principles to complex medical decisions. The law is not good at dealing with abstract processes such as dignity, suffering, and love. Even in the USA few would regard recourse to the courts as desirable and would acknowledge such recourse as a breakdown of common sense and bedside medicine.

In New South Wales, Australia, in the early nineties the legal advisers to the Health Department were asked if a doctor who withdrew life support could be prosecuted for murder. The answer was 'Yes'. This led to the drafting of legislation on withdrawing and withholding treatment, which was discussed at a public meeting. Such legislation was rejected by the public. At the meeting it was pointed out that the wrong question had been addressed. If the question had been, 'Is it likely that a doctor would be prosecuted for withdrawing life support?', or, 'Is it likely that a doctor prosecuted for withdrawing life support would be convicted or if convicted receive other than a derisory or token sentence?', the answer would have been, 'No'.

There were a number of reasons for this. Firstly, there is a legal principle known as the 'mischief' principle. Applying laws about murder or manslaughter to withdrawing care was not considered when such laws were written and therefore they should not be applied. A second principle, the 'nonsense' principle suggests that if a law punished an act of compassion the law would be producing a nonsense result. The third major reason that prosecution was unlikely was that the public prosecutors in NSW had no wish to become involved in the area.

Instead of legislation, the NSW Health Department produced guidelines describing what was appropriate.[621] There was ethical concern at these guidelines, especially from the legal profession who felt doctors were writing the laws. In August 1996 a State Coroner examined a case where treatment was withdrawn, and publicly endorsed the guidelines and commented favourably on how they had been followed.[622] Other states have passed laws regarding enduring power of attorney, empowered surrogates, and giving legal status to the living will. Keeping the adversarial legal system at bay in the decisions surrounding peaceful death is the mark of an extraordinarily mature society.

Many of those who are not opposed to voluntary euthanasia *per se* are opposed to its legalisation, believing that it should be left to doctor and patient. In favour of this argument is the extreme difficulty in writing laws that are workable. Those in favour of legislation believe it may reduce inappropriate clandestine euthanasia and permit doctors prepared to practise euthanasia to do so openly and without fear.

As a general principle the law is a poor and expensive tool for dealing with social and ethical problems. There is a tendency for modern societies to believe that outlawing a practice legally will control it and mean that the more difficult task of understanding the practice is not necessary. We have laws against sale of cigarettes and tobacco to minors and against paedophilia; the former is a growth industry and perhaps the second is also.

Autonomy

To many, the management of the end of life is a simple matter of autonomy, the right of an individual to make decisions about him or herself. But autonomy is one ethical value only. To the doctor faced with end-of-life decisions the concept is often unhelpful. Is the patient's advance directive valid under the new circumstance? Is the patient's wish to die prompted by treatable suffering or reversible depression? Has the patient been coerced into the request by relatives? If the living will says 'no chance' what would the patient think of a 2 per cent or 10 per cent chance? And the even more difficult question is, what right does this patient have to receive a huge share of society's money that could be spent on other things?

Who should decide?

Under most circumstances these situations are dealt with by health workers and family in a manner acceptable to both. Conflict arises when agreement on appropriateness cannot be reached. In these circumstances there is no societal consensus on whose view should prevail. Continuing treatment, being the option that allows attempts to resolve the conflict, is usual under these circumstances.

When conflict occurs it is between families and doctors. Families of moribund patients have difficulty making critical decisions regarding life support systems based on the complex information necessary to assimilate and comprehend. Logically, rational patients and their families should not be willing to continue life support and prolong suffering after a reasonable trial has demonstrated that a satisfactory outcome is not possible. However, placed in the position of decision-maker, a family member, who may have neither the benefit of medical knowledge and experience, nor confidence in the validity of medical prediction, is also placed in a situation where it is legitimate to err on the side of prolonging life and where the family member sees responsibility to the individual totally outweighing the responsibility to the collective i.e., to see society's money is spent wisely.

While the rights of patients to regulate their medical treatment, particularly their right to refuse treatment, is accepted by doctors, there is less certainty of the patient's or family's right to demand treatment, especially expensive treatment, with a high risk of a poor outcome.

Often the burden of such decision-making about people they love in complex unfamiliar situations means that most families are happy for the decisions to be made for them, and is the reason that in many societies acquiescence is sought with medical decisions rather than seeking from the family a decision *per se*.[610]

The strong argument for entrusting the care of complex life support systems to physicians is that they have the knowledge and experience to manage these resources in an objective manner. The physician has two major problems. The first is the uncertainty of prediction of outcome in some patients. We have no societal consensus on how much expense individual societies are prepared to spend on a small chance of survival. The only tool we have to protect the patient from incorrect decision-making is that prior to discussions with families regarding withdrawal of life support, the physicians involved in care must all agree that further treatment is futile.

All the benefits of physician expertise involve some kind of external assessment of the patient's quality of life. Ethically, the only person who can validly assess the quality of an individual's life is that person. In practice, much of the discussion between doctor and family is based on the best possible, albeit flawed, assessment of what the wishes and values of the patient would be if we could ask the patient.

Conclusion

The complexities of the decisions that face patients, relatives and health care workers at the end of life are enormous. The interests of our society are best served by these decisions being dealt with by doctors and nurses trained in dealing with such decisions who must provide accurate information of potential outcomes, preferably before the patient is in a state where the information cannot be processed accurately because of coma, drugs, or pain and suffering. The health care workers must work as a team with empowered patients and families, who are given the odds and outcomes and play a major part in deciding what is appropriate. There is no ethical or legal compulsion for health care workers to provide continuing treatment that will not provide an acceptable outcome. Requests for such treatment should be met with firmness, but negotiation rather than conflict, wherever possible. And we must acknowledge that to take the process away from the carers to committees, courts, or statutory bodies is a failure of the correct, the ethical, and the humane processes.

A peaceful death, preferably in the home surrounded by loved ones, has been valued by civilised societies from the beginning of civilisation. 'A good death,' said Petrach, 'is a tribute to a good life.'[623] To recapture this lost concept should be an important goal for all members of society. There is a further need for society to craft effective processes for the use of high technology medicine. The community that has to pay for the resources has a right to be involved in their use, and this right extends not only to how the health care dollar is used but in how much of society's wealth is appropriately spent on health and disease.

Ultimately, to deal with death appropriately and fairly in terms of the cost of health care and our environment, our society will require us to acknowledge the concept of acceptable death. Further efforts to defer dying are likely to increase suffering, and there is a good fit between biological inevitability of death and the circumstances of that death in the life of the individual.[624] Whether legislation and discussion can resolve the dilemma between the needs of the individual and the individual as a member of society is unknown.

REFERENCES

591. Civetta JM. Beyond technology: intensive care in the 1980s. *Crit Care Med* 1981; 9: 763–7.
592. Itami J. A director boasts of his scars. *New York Times*, 30 August 1996, E7.
593. Fisher M. Retractor column, Hoping to come in from the cold. *Australian Doctor Weekly*, 31 May 1996; 104.
594. McGregor A. 'Fatal complacency' over health says WHO. *Lancet* 1996; 347: 1478.
595. Pindborg JJ. Global aspects of the AIDS epidemic. *Oral Surgery, Oral Medicine, Oral Pathology* 1992; 73: 138–41.
596. Maloney JV. Presidential Address: the limitations of medicine. *Ann Surg* 1981; 247–55.
597. National Heart Foundation of Australia. *Heart and stroke facts 1996 report.* Canberra: National Heart Foundation of Australia, 1996, pp7–8.
598. Hetzel BS, McMichael T, *The LS factor: lifestyle and health.* Ringwood, Vic: Penguin Books, 1987.
599. Watson L. *Dark nature; natural history of evil.* London: Hodder & Stoughton, 1995.
600. Robertson JC. Seed corn; the impact of managed care on medical research. *Ann Sur* 1996; 223: 453–63.
601. Thompson WL. Critical care tomorrow: economies and challenges. In: Shoemaker WS, Thompson WL, Holbrook PR (eds). *Textbook of critical care,* 1st edition. Philadelphia: WB Saunders, 1984, pp1028–35.
602. See Colice GL. Historical perspective on the development of mechanical ventilation. In: Tobin M (ed). *Principles and practice of mechanical ventilation.* New York: McGraw Hill, 1994, pp28–9.
603. Rogers RM, Weiler C, Ruppenthal B. Impact of the respiratory intensive care unit on survival of patients with acute respiratory failure. *Chest* 1972; 62: 94–7.
604. Callahan D. *The troubled dream of life. In search of a peaceful death.* New York: Simon & Schuster, 1993, pp59–67.
605. Illich I. *Medical nemesis: the expropriation of health.* London: Calder & Boyars, 1975.
606. Support Principal Investigators. A controlled trial to improve care for seriously ill patients. *J Amer Med Ass* 1995; 224: 1591–1636.
607. Hansoi E. A letter from a patient's daughter. *Ann Int Med* 1996; 125: 149–51.
608. Truog RD. Allowing to die. *Crit Care Med* 1990; 18: 700–91.
609. Asch DA. The role of critical care nurses in euthanasia and assisted suicide. *New Engl J Med* 1996; 334: 1734–39.
610. Fisher MM, Raper RF. Withdrawing and withholding treatment in intensive care. Part 1: Social and ethical dimensions. *Med J Aust* 1990; 153: 217–20.
611. Annas GJ. Do ethics committees work? No. *Hospitals & Health Networks* 1994; 68: 6.
612. Johnson K. A moral dilemma: killing and letting die. *Brit Nursing J* 1993, 2:635–40.
613. Fisher MM, Raper RF. Withdrawing and withholding treatment in intensive care. Part 2: Patient assessment. *Med J Aust* 1990a; 153: 220–2.
614. Dunstan GR. Hard questions in intensive care. *Anaesthesia* 1985; 40: 479–82.
615. Emmanuel EJ. The history of euthanasia debates in the United States and Britain. *Ann Int Med* 1994; 121: 793–802.
616. Griffith G, Swain M. *Euthanasia Volume II*, NSW Parliamentary Library Research Service, background paper 1995/3, 41–53.
617. Cassell EJ. *The nature of suffering and the goals of medicine.* Oxford: Oxford University Press, 1991.
618. Callahan D. *The troubled dream of life. In search of a peaceful death*, ibid, p115.

619. Halevy A, Baruch B. Brain death: reconciling definitions, criteria, and tests. *Ann Int Med* 1993; 119: 519–25.
620. Gaddis W. *A frolic of his own.* New York: Poseidon Press, 1994.
621. NSW Health. *Dying with dignity. Interim guidelines on management.* State Health Publication no (HPA) 93–93, 1993.
622. Sydney Morning Herald, 14 August 1996.
623. Petrach FP. *De Vita Solitaria,* 1346.
624. Callahan D. *The troubled dream of life,* ibid, pp180–1.

CHAPTER TWENTY

Nurses and the End of Life: Dying in the Margins or a Good Death?

Dorothy Angell

The current debate on active voluntary euthanasia so far has failed to recognise the central role that nurses play in the care of the dying. Because of this neglect, active, voluntary euthanasia has now become a complex and worrying issue for the nursing profession.

In their position statement on assisted suicide, the American Nurses Association acknowledges that:

> Nurses witness firsthand the devastating effects of debilitating and life-threatening disease and are often confronted with the despair and exhaustion of patients and families. At times, it may be difficult to find a balance between the preservation of life and the facilitation of a dignified death. These agonising tensions may cause a nurse to consider intentionally hastening a patient's death as a humane and compassionate response.[625]

Such a consideration is despite the traditional goals and values of the profession which mitigate against it.

Recently, the Royal College of Nursing, Australia, released a professional development document, the *Politics of Euthanasia*.[626] In this document, Dr. Megan-Jane Johnstone draws attention of nurses to the fact that in March, 1995, the Court at Groningen in the Netherlands gave a two months suspended prison sentence to a 38-year-old registered nurse for performing active, voluntary euthanasia on a patient suffering from end-stage AIDS. The sentence was passed despite the fact that:

(1) the patient (who was a friend and colleague of the nurse) had specifically requested that the nurse perform the final deed, and
(2) the procedure fully complied with legal regulations governing euthanatic practices in the Netherlands.

Although Dutch law permits nurses to perform certain 'medical procedures' under the direction of a qualified medical practitioner, the court in this instance totally rejected the position that doctors could delegate the task of performing active voluntary euthanasia to a nurse. The court determined that the deed of 'ultimate care', that is, the act of euthanasia itself, could only be performed by a doctor and could not be delegated to anyone else. It now seems highly likely that unless policies and procedures are carefully formulated for nurses in Australia this situation may well be repeated in this country.

In her book *Illness as Metaphor*[627] Susan Sontag states that everyone who is born holds dual citizenship—in the kingdom of the well and in the kingdom of the sick—and although we all prefer to use only the good passport (to wellness), sooner or later each of us is obliged, at least for a spell, to identify ourselves as citizens of that other place, the darker side of life—illness. We are all border-crossers and as such, we cannot overlook the way in which the industrial revolution of the last century, with its technological consequences, has actually transformed the experiences of illness and of death in people's lives.

All of us should voice a concern for the gradual disappearance of the representation of death from our modern society. For the nature of death is now repressed by the dazzling achievements of modern science and by our current systems of communication such as television, computer and the news media, which publicly revere the world of medical technique. Death has become almost a taboo now.

Hans-Georg Gadamer,[628] one of this century's leading philosophers, sees the real depersonalisation of death becoming more deeply entrenched in our modern day hospitals. Dying patients and their relatives are now removed from the domestic environment of the family to an environment where the artificial prolongation of life, through modern technological advances, becomes a prolongation of death, with a fading away of the experiences of the self.

Whilst modern anaesthetic and analgesic drugs can completely sedate the suffering person, the artificial maintenance of vegetative functions makes the person into a mere link in the chain of causal processes.[628] Death itself becomes like an arbitral reward dependent on the decision of the doctor treating the case and, throughout all this, except for palliative care, the living are excluded from attendance and participation in what is irrevocably taking place. Even care of the soul, offered by the church, for example, often fails to gain admittance, and is received neither by the dying person nor by those others who are involved.

Gadamer (1996) writes that:

... For every living person in our modern society there is now something incomprehensible in the fact that a human consciousness, capable of anticipating the future, will one day come to an end. Likewise, for those who witness it, this final coming to an end has something uncanny about it.[629]

In our enlightened modern day world, it is not now inappropriate to speak of an almost systematic repression of death. Such a repression of death reflects the will of life, an elementary human reaction to death each of us takes up with respect to our own lives in order to strengthen, in every possible way, the will to survive when threatened by death. The force of illusion, with which the gravely ill or dying keep a hold on their will to live, is to be marvelled at, but as Gadamer states 'it speaks a language which cannot be understood'.[629] He then concludes that it can now rightly be claimed that the world of modern civilisation has eagerly and enthusiastically brought this tendency to repression (which is rooted in life itself) to institutional perfection,[630] and has pushed the experiences of death wholly into the margins of public life. In support of this claim, Elias believes that:

Never before in the history of humanity have the dying been so hygienically behind the scenes of social life; never before have human corpses been expedited so odourlessly and with such technical perfection from the deathbed to the grave.[631]

Our society has constructed a lack of meaning of death or dying and we now do not know how to respond when a person is dying or has died. Even some health workers reflect this societal construct by regarding dying as a medical event and death as a failure of their medical expertise.

In the care of people living with a terminal illness, nurses have always played a vital role. They are well used to accompanying the person and those closest to them on the journey through the difficult choices that need to be made at the end-stage of life.[632] Because of their close proximity to the bedside, nurses are often in the foreground as the first professional confidante to whom the patient expresses their wishes and fears, and it is difficult to deny a doctor's reliance on the nurse for information about the patient as well as assistance in many medical procedures, including acts of euthanasia. However, in the end, it will be the nurse who will lay out the body and, inevitably, it will be the nurse who will provide grief support for the loved ones left behind. Yet nurses' voices are silenced in the euthanasia debate and it is this silence which negates the skills that nurses have in being able to relieve much of the suffering at the end of life. It is also this silence which has failed to give expression to the difficulties that nurses experience in their involvement in planning and implementing care for the terminally ill person.

The basic dictum of nursing (to be compassionate, humane and caring toward those for whom we provide care) is to be concerned with the 'whole person', and to practise with compassion, consideration and sensitivity. The integrity of the human self is basically our ethical injunction. Caring, as a professional and personal value, is of central importance for nurses as it provides a normative standard by which to govern our actions and attitudes toward those for whom we care.[633]

In care of the person in the final stages of life, the central concerns of nursing pertain to suffering and the role of the nurse in patient decision-making, whereas an understanding of the individual and the subjective experience of suffering will always be problematic for a scientific discipline like medicine.[634]

It would now appear that the current health care system increasingly seems to have little time or no room for people who have chronic and debilitating illnesses; who do not necessarily respond to the increased possibilities of cure from our modern technologies.[635] Further to this, the exercise of authority by some health professionals, conferred on them by the power of clinical science and technology, would seem to carry with it the frightening potential for tyranny, overshadowing individuals who do not belong in the mainstream, reducing them to objects or abstractions. Such individuals become and will remain marginalised in the mainstream healthcare system.

The story of Min

Let me now relate to you the story of Min.

> Min was a person with severe dementia, 'person' being the key word. Unfortunately Min was diagnosed in the days before there was the opportunity for her to prepare an Advance Directive or Living Will on how she wished her health state to be managed and whom she wished to be made the decision maker when she became mentally incompetent.
>
> Min was a person who enjoyed the theatre and concerts. She collected fine porcelain and appreciated antique furniture. She was an expert dress designer and dress maker, and was considered by her husband to be the business head of the family. Yet she was never given the opportunity to determine the nature of her own journey into dementia.
>
> For seven years Min was taken every month to her local GP by her husband, who loved her very much. Religiously, her GP would order the same heart medication without examination and carry on small talk with her husband, never acknowledging Min as a person, but only

as an elderly dementia. The process continued, and even when her weight had fallen from 13 stone to 7 stone, she remained on the same medication and sedation year in and year out.

Finally Min's physical condition deteriorated and her daughter was summoned from interstate. She went to see the local doctor whose opening words were 'You know she's BND' (meaning 'bloody near death!'). The daughter requested that no active 'rescue' measures be taken, as her mother had suffered enough. 'Your mother has not suffered!' yelled the doctor, to which the daughter replied, 'I'm not talking about physical suffering, I'm talking about mental anguish. She and my father have had enough.' Although difficult for him, the doctor finally agreed to let nature take its course and Min died. Not peacefully, however, and certainly without dignity.

How do I know so much about Min? You see, Min was my mother.

Suffering at the end of life

O'Connor[636] states that:

> Physical pain is not necessarily the same as suffering, but those who suffer are pained in some way. A difficulty inherent in much medical treatment is the amount of suffering that must be endured by the person receiving the treatment.

Both my mother and my father suffered throughout her illness, and although I don't know whether they would have availed themselves of an opportunity to end her suffering, I do believe that it would have eased their burden to just know that the opportunity was there should they have needed it.

Wisdom and compassion are required from those who accompany the sufferer on their end of life journey, for each person's journey will naturally be different. Respect must be shown for the different cultural, philosophical and religious traditions, which may have different interpretations and understandings of suffering and dying.[637]

Kanitsaki[638] points out that:

> Marginalised groups of people from non-English speaking backgrounds genuinely fear that the powerful members of society (including doctors and nurses) may, under the provisions of the euthanasia legislation, continue to perceive and treat them in dismissive ways. These groups fear that their 'best interests' may be neglected if not by deliberate acts, . . . (then by) . . . deliberate ommisions, such as: failure to inform them of all available treatment options; not using available life saving technologies and treatments; and withholding or withdrawing treatments deemed 'extraordinary' by standards with which they do not agree.

However, suffering is a complex and multi-faceted part of individual human experience which may not always be amenable to relief by another person or intervention. In speaking about palliative care, Roger Hunt[639] suspects that many psychological and existential problems of patients cannot be solved and believes that the hospice ideal of a pain-free, comfortable death is a myth which should not be promised.

As early as 1964, Virginia Henderson[640] believed that the unique function of the nurse was to assist the individual, sick or well, in the performance of those activities they would ordinarily carry out for themselves if they had the necessary strength, will or knowledge. In the end-of-life situation, the nurse's role should be to support the person as they weigh up the options available to them; it should not be to influence the person one way or the other. The nurse's role is strictly a facilitatory role, as these patients negotiate the myriad of decisions that need to be made. The nurse's role is also a protective one, as nurses seek to protect the patient's right to:

- make informed choices about care;
- receive expert care;
- withdraw from or continue treatment;
- have one's symptoms controlled;
- consider the family and significant others;
- die in the place of one's choice.[641]

We can now add to this list the need to protect a patient's right to *request assistance in ending their suffering*.

The central concern of nurses is to enhance the total circumstances of the dying process—we have a duty of care to the patient. Therefore to negate the right to end one's life could now be seen as the abandonment of that duty of care.

Current debate in nursing ethics involves conflict between those nurses who follow an ethic of care and those nurses who practise by the general rule, principle and justice notions of traditional biomedical ethics. In recent years, there has been a growing debate surrounding the sufficiency of any rule-and-principle, duty-based ethical tradition for nursing ethics, in the belief that the moral point of view for the theory of nursing ethics itself should not be defined by reference to any external system of justification.[642] There is now a strong incentive for the nursing profession to look beyond the current dominant models of biomedical ethics to a more inclusive framework which addresses the professional concerns of caring and other relationships that have traditionally characterised nursing.

In an attempt to find a relationship between the two ethical stances of justice and care, Bartlett[643] explores Albert Camus' ethic of 'rebellion'.

She puts forward that through this approach justice and care can, and indeed do become fruitfully interrelated. She points out that Locke, Kant, and others claimed to have arrived at their universal principles of justice through the application of a disinterested and impartial reason; that Rawls[643a] set up his 'veil of ignorance' to ensure that our interests and our caring did not interfere with our ability to clearly perceive and derive principles of fairness. However, this is not so for Camus, as Camus believes that we demand justice, and clearly perceive its incumbent rights and claims precisely because we do care.

In examining Camus' ethic of 'rebellion', Bartlett states that, 'Justice and rights originate from a passionate and compassionate concern for oneself and for others'.[644] Therefore, as with the right to life and our duty of care, then so too with the right to die and our duty of care. For Camus would argue that it is the element of caring which defines the boundary between those actions which are just, and those actions which are unjust; that if justice becomes a devotion to the ideal of justice in and of itself, rather than caring for particular persons, then it becomes a tool of oppression; that once justice has 'abandoned care', it ceases to be justice and results instead in acts of oppression. Justice, losing touch with humanity, becomes unjust.[643]

If this be the case, then those persons wanting to end their suffering must be listened to, for to deny these patients their right places a serious limitation on their autonomy and one becomes guilty of patriarchy and oppression. The availability of voluntary euthanasia in the Northern Territory now extends that autonomy and it may now be more compassionate and appropriate to accede to these patients' wishes.*

Nurses and voluntary euthanasia

For those persons previously marginalised because of the dominance of the 'sanctity of life' discourse, the changes to the legislation in the Northern Territory offers them new hope, for it now centres their end-of-life journey toward a good death. It would appear to make health care services more just and more equitable for all clients and for all health professionals. However, under the existing Northern Territory Government's Rights of the Terminally Ill Act (1995)[645] there is no specific provision for ensuring that the role of nurses (and other health professionals) is not compromised. Whilst the Act confers immunity

---

* In February 1997 the Federal Parliament overturned the Northern Territory Right of the Terminally Ill Act (which permitted the practice of voluntary euthanasia under closely specified conditions). This Chapter was written before that event occurred.

from any form of penalty for assistance with euthanasia, nurses will be judged according to professional standards of competence. Therefore, the obligation of nurses taking part in euthanasia is to be competent to do so, otherwise nurses could still be subjected to claims of negligence or of unprofessional conduct.[646]

The role of nurses participating in voluntary euthanasia needs to be clearly established at law. Once such a law is passed, then nurses will need guidance on how to respond to the law. Position statements on the nurse's role in active euthanasia will need to be compiled by the major nursing organisations and these documents will need to provide standards of nursing practice related to:

- the nurse's legal and clinical responsibilities in relation to the practice of euthanasia,
- what nurses are required to do in the event of a patient/client requesting assistance to die, and
- what mechanisms should be in place for appropriate protection of employment for the conscientious objector.[647]

Employers will need also to provide a set of policies and protocols that are consistent with the legal framework on active voluntary euthanasia and that will guide nursing practice in respect to this procedure.

Currently, voluntary active euthanasia does not fit into nursing practice, but a request for assistance to die does not mean the abandonment of the patient to make the final journey alone. Each nurse's response will depend very much on the context in which the request is made.

O'Connor[648] points out that it is difficult for nurses to respond either one way or the other without isolating the patient and states that

> perhaps then this is not a situation calling for a conscientious objection action of 'opting out' ... (but) ... rather it calls for a 'hanging in there' to support, in a holistic way, patients as they explore their options ... If nurses will not maintain their presence at the bedside of those who are dying—then who will?

It is the professional responsibility of all nurses (regardless of their ethical stance on euthanasia) to be fully informed about all aspects of care of the client seeking euthanasia. Therefore, educational opportunities will need to be made available for nurses in order to maintain professional standards.

In the multidisciplinary team, the nurse has a unique role as confidante, carer and advocate, and her or his involvement with the patient contributes vital knowledge to the careful consideration of, and decision on the request to die. It is highly desirable, therefore, that he or she be involved in the decision-making process.

Finally, at the end of the day, the unique function of the nurse will be as advocate on behalf of the vulnerable, against carrying a disproportionate burden of suffering because of the enforcement of inadequate or ill devised public policies (whether for or against voluntary euthanasia). Finally, the unique function of the nurse will be to assist those currently dying in the margins toward a more dignified death and in the future, to be more actively involved in the decision-making process about voluntary euthanasia.

REFERENCES

625. American Nurses Association position statement on assisted suicide. In: Johnstone MJ (ed). *The politics of euthanasia: a nursing response*. Deakin, ACT: Royal College of Nursing, Australia, 1996.
626. Johnstone, MJ. The political and ethical dimensions of euthanasia. In: Johnstone MJ (ed). *The politics of euthanasia: a nursing response*, ibid, p21.
627. Sontag Susan. *Illness as metaphor*. London: Penguin Books, 1991, p3.
628. Gadamer HG. *The enigma of health*. Cambridge: Polity Press, 1996, p62.
629. Gadamer HG. *The enigma of health*, ibid, p63.
630. Gadamer HG. *The enigma of health*, ibid, p65.
631. Elias N. *The loneliness of dying*. Oxford: Blackwell, 1985, p23.
632. O'Connor M. Euthanasia and its implications for the bedside nurse. In: Johnstone MJ (ed). *The politics of euthanasia: a nursing response*, ibid, p97.
633. Carpenter, BA., *The Ethics of Caring*. Advances in Nursing Science, 1979, 1:11–20.
634. O'Connor M. Euthanasia and its implications for the bedside nurse, ibid, p98.
635. O'Connor M. Euthanasia and its implications for the bedside nurse, ibid, p102.
636. O'Connor M. Euthanasia and its implications for the bedside nurse, ibid, p98.
637. O'Connor M. Euthanasia and its implications for the bedside nurse, ibid, pp98–9.
638. Kanitsaki O. Euthanasia in a multicultural society: some important considerations for nurses. In: Johnstone MJ (ed). *The politics of euthanasia: a nursing response*. ibid, p87.
639. Hunt Roger. Palliative care—the rhetoric-reality gap. In: Kuhse H (ed). *Willing to listen, wanting to die*. Melbourne: Penguin Books, 1994, p121.
640. Henderson, Virginia. The nature of nursing. *American Journal of Nursing* 1964 (August): 62–65.
641. O'Connor M. Euthanasia and its implications for the bedside nurse, ibid, p105.
642. Cooper MC. Reconceptualizing nursing ethics. *International Journal of Scholarly Inquiry for Nursing Practice* 1990; 4: 209–18.
643. Bartlett EA. Beyond either/or: justice and care. In: Browning Cole EC, Coultrap-McQuin S (eds). *Explorations in feminist ethics: theory and practice*. Bloomington: Indiana University Press, 1992, pp82–88.
643a. Rawls J. *A theory of justice*. Oxford: Oxford University Press, 1972.
644. Bartlett EA. Beyond either/or: justice and care, ibid, p84.
645. Northern Territory Government. *Rights of the Terminally Act*. Darwin: NTGP, Northern Territory Government Publications, 1995.
646. Johnstone MJ (ed). *The politics of euthanasia: a nursing response*, ibid.
647. Johnstone MJ (ed). *The politics of euthanasia: a nursing response*, ibid.
648. O'Connor M. Euthanasia and its implications for the bedside nurse, ibid, p113.

INDEX